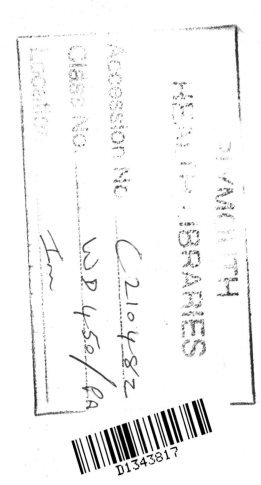

OXFORD MEDICAL PUBLICATIONS

Emergencies in Clinical Medicine

Published and forthcoming titles in the Emergencies series:

Emergencies in Anaesthesia
Edited by Keith Allman, Andrew McIndoe, and Iain H. Wilson

Emergencies in Cardiology
Edited by Saul G. Myerson, Robin P. Choudhury, and Andrew Mitchell

Emergencies in Clinical Surgery
Edited by Chris Callaghan, Chris Watson and Andrew Bradley

Emergencies in Critical Care
Edited by Martin Beed, Richard Sherman, and Ravi Mahajan

Emergencies in Nursing
Edited by Philip Downing

Emergencies in Obstetrics and Gynaecology
Edited by S. Arulkumaran

Emergencies in Oncology
Edited by Martin Scott-Brown, Roy A.J. Spence, and Patrick G. Johnston

Emergencies in Paediatrics and Neonatology
Edited by Stuart Crisp and Jo Rainbow

Emergencies in Palliative and Supportive Care
Edited by David Currow and Katherine Clark

Emergencies in Primary Care
Chantal Simon, Karen O'Reilly, John Buckmaster, and Robin Proctor

Emergencies in Psychiatry
Basant Puri and Ian Treasaden

Emergencies in Radiology
Edited by Richard Graham and Ferdia Gallagher

Emergencies in Respiratory Medicine
Edited by Robert Parker, Catherine Thomas, and Lesley Bennett

Head, Neck and Dental Emergencies
Edited by Mike Perry

Medical Emergencies in Dentistry
Nigel Robb and Jason Leitch

Emergencies in Clinical Medicine

Edited by

Piers Page
SHO Intensive Care Medicine,
James Cook University Hospital
Middlesbrough, UK

Greg Skinner
SHO Neonatology,
Derriford Hospital
Plymouth, UK

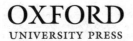

OXFORD
UNIVERSITY PRESS

OXFORD

UNIVERSITY PRESS

Great Clarendon Street, Oxford OX2 6DP

Oxford University Press is a department of the University of Oxford.
It furthers the University's objective of excellence in research, scholarship,
and education by publishing worldwide in

Oxford New York

Auckland Cape Town Dar es Salaam Hong Kong Karachi
Kuala Lumpur Madrid Melbourne Mexico City Nairobi
New Delhi Shanghai Taipei Toronto

With offices in

Argentina Austria Brazil Chile Czech Republic France Greece
Guatemala Hungary Italy Japan Poland Portugal Singapore
South Korea Switzerland Thailand Turkey Ukraine Vietnam

Oxford is a registered trade mark of Oxford University Press
in the UK and in certain other countries

Published in the United States
by Oxford University Press Inc., New York

British Library Cataloguing in Publication Data

Data available

Library of Congress Cataloging in Publication Data

Data available

Typeset by Newgen Imaging Systems (P) Ltd., Chennai, India
Printed in Italy
on acid-free paper by
Legoprint S.p.A.

ISBN 978-0-19-920252-2

10 9 8 7 6 5 4 3 2 1

Foreword

Napoleon always asked supporters of potential generals 'Yes—but is he *lucky?*' *Emergencies in Clinical Medicine* might just make you lucky, because luck often turns out to consist in well prepared minds seizing half-apprehended opportunities. To the outsider, it looks like luck and, some-times even to ourselves our successes look like luck—because we do not understand just how important our intuitions have been. Intuitions are particularly important in emergency care. This is a problem for newcom-ers to the world of emergencies. How do you get to the state where your intuitions can guide you? But as with luck, so with intuitions: they are not the dark products of unknowable processes. Intuition is under-pinned by as thorough and detailed a history and examination as time allows—coupled with common sense and pattern recognition. For exam-ple, you may be about to arrange intubation of an unconscious man with stridor when, percolating through your dreary early morning mind, comes a sentence from *Emergencies in Clinical Medicine*—'don't forget to distinguish between peaceful snoring and respiratory obstruction'. A quick jab in the ribs, and suddenly you are a hero to the nursing staff. Unfortunately it often takes a bit more than a jab in the ribs to impress our colleagues, so where better place to start than *Emergencies in Clinical Medicine*?

We all need more luck at emergency bedsides, and in facing (and help-ing) bereft relatives and damaged patients come to terms with their ordeals. During one such encounter I was expecting difficulties for I had committed a senseless error, diverting a boisterously delirious patient to the psychiatrists rather than to the medics (his haemoglobin turned out to be less than 6 g/dl). So I was surprised to be greeted by smiles: 'Thank goodness for your help, doctor. At least you *did* something…*you took command*'. This 'taking command' is all very well, and there *is* a vital role for leadership at emergency bedsides. But nobody wants to be led into the jaws of death if a well timed offer of blood transfusion is a valid alternative. My mistake was not to have ordered my thoughts before acting (first of all be in command of your facts—then you can command events). My mistake, in other words, was not to have read *Emergencies in Clinical Medicine*. Now that this book is in your hands, should I, one day, become boisterously delirious, I am confident that you will do me proud. Good luck!

Murray Longmore
Author, Oxford Handbook of Clinical Medicine
Ferring
2007

Preface

Why another handbook, and what's so different to the *Oxford Handbook of Clinical Medicine (OHCM)?* Both pertinent questions, asked of us by others and of ourselves during the title's development. Over its 21 years in print, the *OHCM* has evolved from a condensed set of aides-mémoire to the colourful, information-rich seventh edition found on wards everywhere today.

Emergencies in Clinical Medicine is a text to get you out of trouble, featuring basic detail on core topics. Its focus is on being useful at the bedside, in that lonely time between your realisation that this patient is unwell and the arrival or phone call of someone senior enough to help further. This is not to say it is solely a title for the most junior of doctors—we hope that the structured list approach will be invaluable to those more senior who would perhaps benefit from a checklist in going about their reviews.

As such, this is an unapologetically basic text, with every topic featuring references to more detailed coverage elsewhere. As with the other *Emergencies* handbooks, it is intended as a companion, in this case to the *OHCM*. Murray Longmore has spent many years collating this mine of information; we suggest with all the topics that you do follow up the suggested further reading to give a background to the treatment plan from which you have been working.

This approach has been new to all involved in the project and we would be very interested to hear how the book works (or doesn't work) for you. A reader card is included, or feedback may be submitted via *www.oup.com*. The topic spectrum was initially chosen after discussion with many colleagues—we have chosen also to follow the *OHCM's* chapter structure as far as possible for ease of reference. As with any first edition title, we are sure there will be topics the reader would like to see included—we urge you to get in touch and tell us!

Enormous thanks are due to the team at OUP; Chris 'CK' Reid (who has worked tirelessly as the interface between junior doctors and the world of medical publishing), Fiona Goodgame, Sara Chare and Catherine Barnes.

Our writers, have all worked around the constraints of busy house or senior house officer jobs to produce well researched, evidence-based management plans from the outlines provided. Special thanks to WGPE, who organized the entire surgical section, including senior review, practically single-handedly. As the original *OHCM*, this is also a text by junior doctors for junior doctors. We sincerely thank them all for their hard work, especially in this stressful climate of uncertainty.

Thanks are also due to our expert team of senior advisors—Murray Longmore, Jane Metcalf, Malcolm Louden, Andy Port, Neil Ineson, Jennifer Logue and Tim Reynolds, whose generous contributions of 'spare' time and clinical wisdom made the title possible. Equal thanks, of course, go to the anonymous but thorough peer reviewers engaged by OUP!

The list of other people who have helped us in these past 2 years is long and diverse (including Andrew Hall, who has offered many a sensible word and comfortable working environment), but must be ended with our fiancées and families, whose tolerance of late nights, exasperation, seemingly endless emails, many trips to Oxford and yet-to-be-planned weddings has been limitless. Thank you.

PRJP
GJS
Oxford, Spring 2007

Contents

Contributors

Adam Stannard
Research Registrar
Heartlands Hospital,
Birmingham

Alan Weir
PRHO General Surgery
James Cook University Hospital
Middlesbrough, Cleveland

Asif Shah
SHO Emergency Medicine
Sunderland Royal Hospital
Sunderland

Ben Skinner
SpR Anaesthetics
Wessex Rotation

Brendan Wooler
SHO General Surgery
University Hospital of
North Durham
Durham

Giles Moseley
SHO Intensive Care Medicine
James Cook University Hospital
Middlesbrough, Cleveland

Hilde Andersen
SHO Psychiatry
County Durham and Darlington

Jeanette Lahai-Taylor
SHO Plastic Surgery
James Cook University Hospital
Middlesbrough, Cleveland

John Page
Team Rector
Parish of Hale with Badshot Lea

Kate MacDougall
SHO Pathology
Royal Victoria Infirmary,
Newcastle upon Tyne

Mark Garside
SHO Medicine
Sunderland Royal Hospital
Sunderland

Mark Harrison
SHO Paediatrics
James Cook University Hospital
Middlesbrough, Cleveland

Martin Taylor
SpR Orthopaedics and Trauma
Yorkshire Rotation

Matthew Mudford
SHO General Practice
James Cook University Hospital
Middlesbrough, Cleveland

Simon Hutchinson
SHO GP VTS
James Cook University Hospital
Middlesbrough, Cleveland

Steven Land
SHO Medicine
James Cook University Hospital
Middlesbrough, Cleveland

Suzanne Elcombe
SHO Medicine
Freeman Road Hospital,
Newcastle upon Tyne

Will Eardley
SpR Orthopaedics and Trauma
Northern Rotation

Senior Reviewers

Mr Andy Port
Consultant Orthopaedic Surgeon, James Cook University Hospital,
Middlesbrough, Cleveland
Visiting Lecturer, University of Teesside
Middlesbrough, Tees Valley
Deputy Programme Director, Northern Deanery Orthopaedic rotation

Dr Jane Metcalfe
Consultant, General Medicine, University Hospital of North Tees
Senior Lecturer, University of Newcastle upon Tyne,
Newcastle upon Tyne

Dr Jennifer Logue
Specialist Registrar, Chemical Pathology
Western Infirmary, Glasgow

Mr Malcolm Louden
Consultant Colorectal and General Surgeon
Aberdeen Royal Infirmary, Aberdeen

Dr Neil Ineson
Consultant Cardiologist, Frimley Park Hospital, Camberley

Professor Tim Reynolds
Consultant, Chemical Pathology
Queens Hospital, Burton-on-Trent

Symbols and abbreviations

AAA	Abdominal aortic aneurysm
ABC	Airway, breathing, circulation
ABG	Arterial blood gas
ABx	Antibiotics
ACE	Angiotensin-converting enzyme
ACS	Acute coronary syndrome
ACTH	Adrenocorticotrophic hormone
AF	Atrial fibrillation
AFB	Acid-Fast bacilli
AG	Anion gap
ALP	Alkaline phosphatase
ALS	Advanced life support
ALT	Alanine transaminase
ANA	Anti-nuclear antibody
ANP	Atrial natriuretic peptide
APTT	Activated partial thromboplastin time
ARF	Acute renal failure
ASDH	Acute subdural haematoma
ASMA	Anti-smooth muscle antibody
ASOT	Antistreptolysin O titre
AST	Aspartate transaminase
ATN	Acute tubular necrosis
AV	Arteriovenous or atrioventricular
AVNRT	Atrioventricular nodal re-entrant tachycardia
AVRT	Atrioventricular re-entrant tachycardia
AVPU	Conscious scale: alert, response to voice, responds to pain, unresponsive
AXR	Abdominal X-ray
BD	Twice daily
BE	Base excess
βhCG	Beta human chorionic gonadotrophin
BIPAP	Bilevel positive pressure support
BM	Bedside finger-prick blood glucose test
BMI	Body mass index
BNF	*British National Formulary*
BNP	B-type natriuretic peptide
BP	Blood pressure

Ca^{2+}	Calcium
CKMB	Myocardial-bound creatine kinase
Cl^-	Chloride
CMV	Cytomegalovirus
CNS	Central nervous system
CO_2	Carbon dioxide
COPD	Chronic obstructive pulmonary disease
CRF	Chronic renal failure
CRP	C-reactive peptide
CRT	Capillary refill time
C&S	Culture and sensitivity
CSF	Cerebrospinal fluid
CSM	Committee on safety of medicines
CT	Computer tomography
CTPA	Computed tomography pulmonary angiogram
CVP	Central venous pressure
CVS	Cardiovascular system
CVST	Central venous sinus thrombosis
CXR	Chest X-ray
DC	Direct current
DHx	Drug history
DIC	Disseminated intravascular coagulation
DKA	Diabetic ketoacidosis
DM	Diabetes mellitus
DNAR	Do not attempt resuscitation
DT	Delirium tremens
DVT	Deep vein thrombosis
EBV	Epstein–Barr virus
ECF	Extracellular fluid
ECG	Electrocardiogram
EDH	Extradural haematoma
EEG	Electroencephalogram
eGFR	Estimated glomerulofiltration rate
ERCP	Endoscopic retrograde cholangiopancreatography
ESR	Erythrocyte sedimentation rate
FBC	Full blood count
FFP	Fresh frozen plasma
FiO_2	Fraction of inspired oxygen
GCS	Glasgow coma score
GFR	Glomerulofiltration rate
GGT	Gamma glutamyl transferase
GI	Gastrointestinal

G&S	Group and save serum
GTN	Glyceryl trinitrate
Hb	Haemoglobin
HCO_3^-	Bicarbonate
Hct	Haematocrit
HDU	High dependency unit
HELLP	Haemolysis elevated liver enzymes and low platelets
HIV	Human immunodeficiency virus
HONK	Hyperosmotic non-ketotic hyperglycaemia
HR	Heart rate
HSV	Herpes simplex virus
HUS	Haemolytic uraemic syndrome
IBD	Inflammatory bowel disease
ICF	Intracellular fluid
ICH	Intracranial or intracerebral haemorrhage
ICP	Intracranial pressure
Ig	Immunoglobulin
IHD	Ischaemic heart disease
INR	International normalized ratio
ITP	Idiopathic thrombocytopenic purpura
ITU	Intensive therapy (care) unit
IV	Intravenous
IVT	Intravenous (fluid) therapy
IVU	Intravenous urogram
Ix	Investigations
JVP	Jugular venous pressure
K^+	Potassium
KUB	Kidneys, ureters and bladder
L	Left
LBBB	Left bundle branch block
LDH	Lactate dehydrogenase
LFTs	Liver function tests
LMP	Last menstrual period
LMWH	Low molecular weight heparin
LP	Lumbar puncture
LUQ	Left upper quadrant
LV	Left ventricle
MAOIs	Monoamine oxidase inhibitors
MCV	Mean cell volume
Mg^{2+}	Magnesium
MHRA	Medicines and Healthcare Products Regulatory Agency
MI	Myocardial infarction

MMSE	Mini mental state examination
MRCP	Magnetic resonance cholangiopancreatography
MRI	Magnetic resonance imaging
MRSA	Methicillin-resistant Staphylococcus aureus
MS	Multiple sclerosis
MSU	Midstream urine
Na^+	Sodium
NBM	Nil by mouth
NCEPOD	National confidential enquiry into peri-operative deaths
NG	Nasogastric
NHL	Non-Hodgkins lymphoma
NIV	Non-invasive ventilation
NSAID	Non-steroidal anti-inflammatory drug
NSTEMI	Non-ST elevation myocardial infarction
O_2	Oxygen
OCP	Oral contraceptive pill
OD	Once daily *or* Overdose
OGD	Oesophagogastroduodenoscopy
OHCM	*Oxford Handbook of Clinical Medicine*
$PaCO_2$	Arterial blood partial pressure of carbon dioxide
PaO_2	Arterial blood partial pressure of oxygen
PCI	Primary coronary intervention
PCP	*Pneumocystis carinii* pneumonia
PCR	Polymerase chain reaction
PE	Pulmonary embolism
PEF	Peak expiratory flow
PEFR	Peak expiratory flow rate
PICH	Primary intracerebral haemorrhage
Plt	Platelets
PMHx	Past medical history
PO	Per oral
PO_4^{2-}	Phosphate
PPI	Proton pump inhibitor
PR	Per rectum
PRN	As required
PSA	Prostate specific antigen
PT	Prothrombin time
PTC	Percutaneous transhepatic cholangiogram
PTH	Parathyroid hormone
PV	Per vagina
QDS	Four times daily
R	Right

RAPD	Relative afferent pupillary deficit
RR	Respiratory rate
RS	Respiratory system
RTA	Road traffic accident
rTPA	Recombinant tissue plasminogen activator
RUQ	Right upper quadrant
SAH	Subarachnoid haemorrhage
SaO_2	Arterial blood oxygen saturation
SDH	Subdural haematoma
SHx	Social history
SIADH	Syndrome of inappropriate antidiuretic hormone secretion
SIRS	Severe inflammatory response syndrome
SLE	Systemic lupus erythematosis
SOB	Shortness of breath
SpO_2	Peripheral blood oxygen saturation
STEMI	ST elevation myocardial infarction
SVT	Supraventricular tachycardia
TB	Tuberculosis
TCA	Tricyclic antidepressants
TDS	Three times daily
TFT	Thyroid function tests
TH	Thyroid hormone
TIA	Transient ischaemic attack
TIPSS	Transjugular intrahepatic portosystemic shunt
TLS	Tumour lysis syndrome
TOE	Transoesophageal echocardiography
TPN	Total parenteral nutrition
TRALI	Transfusion-related acute lung injury
U&Es	Urea and electrolytes
UO	Urine output
USS	Ultrasound scan
UTI	Urinary tract infection
VBG	Venous blood gas
VF	Ventricular fibrillation
V/Q	Ventilation/perfusion
VSD	Ventricular septal defect
VT	Ventricular tachycardia
VTE	Venous thromboelism
WCC	White cell count
ZN	Ziehl–Nielson stain

No minute gone comes ever back again—take heed and see ye nothing do in vain

Inscription on the clock bridge,
Liberty of Regent Street
Anon

For Caroline—PRJP

For Hilde—GJS

The basics

ABC assessment

Introduction

The bread and butter of clinical assessment, the ABC approach gives a rapid analysis of the patient's vital physiological parameters. The panic induced by being faced with the unfamiliar is a remarkable way of losing one's train of thought—this checklist ensures all necessary first-line assessments are made and should not be dismissed as one purely for managing trauma.

This guide is no substitute for hands-on training; there is now a wealth of courses such as Advanced Life Support or Care of the Critically Ill Surgical Patient. These will give much greater confidence in handling medical emergencies and should be viewed as essential for the first few years of clinical practice.

A simple premise...

- **Airway**—oxygen (either as a constituent of room air or as medical gas) must be able to get to the bronchial tree for ventilation to occur
- **Breathing**—gas exchange will not occur without some kind of ventilatory movement and the right gases being supplied
- **Circulation**—the overall goal of oxygenating blood is to perfuse the body's organs
- **Disability**—central nervous system problems cause multiple sequelae: unprotected airways, Cushing's response and status epilepticus are but a few
- **Everything else**—once the above have been covered, it's time to begin thorough secondary assessment

Airway

- Start talking to the patient now—one doctor's obstructed airway is another doctor's snoring, sleepy patient!
- Is the patient talking without any other abnormal noises?
  - If yes, the airway is patent—proceed to breathing assessment
- Head tilt, chin lift and jaw thrust to open the airway
  - Simple and effective manoeuvres which will give a surprisingly high degree of control
- Is there obstruction evident?
  - Suction any vomit or excess secretions (and file it in the back of your mind that the patient has likely aspirated)
  - Magill forceps carry greater 5-year survival for doctors' fingers in removal of solid objects! (Think of status epilepticus)

- Airway adjuncts can help you now
  - In the absence of basal skull trauma, nasopharyngeal airways can be tolerated by patients with a relatively high GCS. Size by using the patient's little finger as a diameter guide, lubricate, pass directly posterior via right nostril, ensuring that safety pin is in place at flared end of tube to avoid misplacement
  - A Guedel airway will likely only be tolerated by a patient with lowered consciousness, and carries its own risk of causing airway obstruction by posterior displacement of the tongue. Size from the distance between the angle of the mouth and the earlobe, and insert flat over the tongue with the curve upwards. On reaching the back of the tongue, rotate through 180° so the curve is downwards (minimizing chances of taking the tongue back with the airway). It has a useful secondary function as a bite block for an intubated patient
  - Remember that adjuncts primarily aid oxygenation by holding airways open—this also renders them highly susceptible to aspiration. Manual control is always desirable until the airway is either self-managed or secured by intubation.

Breathing

Oxygenation

- 15 l/min oxygen via a non-rebreathing face mask (giving around 85% FiO_2)
  - In a medical emergency, this is almost always indicated in the initial management
  - Use caution in patients in type 2 respiratory failure (i.e. with a hypoxic respiratory drive) owing to the risk of CO_2 retention. In this situation, it is advisable to use a Venturi mask and to titrate FiO_2 to the patient's condition
  - △ Remember that hypoxia kills before hypercapnia—ensure that oxygenation is adequate. Non-invasive ventilation (e.g. BIPAP) may be required if a balance between oxygenation and CO_2 retention cannot be found.

Assess breathing

- How effective is the breathing?
  - Respiratory rate, in the context of clinical condition. For example, the severely asthmatic patient with a normal respiratory rate but poor chest movements after 20 minutes is not improving but tiring.
  - Monitor SpO_2, again in the context of clinical condition. If peripherally poorly perfused, the oximetry probe will not give useful information and an ABG is far more appropriate.
  - Work of breathing (accessory muscle use, subcostal/intercostal recessions, tracheal tug)
  - Auscultate chest (assess air entry, any added sounds?)
- Have a very low threshold for taking ABG sample
- Augment breathing if required, by use of bag and mask.

Circulation

Assessment of circulatory state

- Does the patient have a pulse? If no, initiate basic life support. If yes, what is its character?
- Blood pressure
- What does the combination of blood pressure and pulse tell you? (think about high vs. low output cardiac failure, etc.)
- Is there evidence of overfilling?—chest creps, pedal and sacral oedema, raised JVP
- Is there evidence of underfilling?—dry mucous membranes, skin turgor, sunken eyes, thirst
- Does the patient have a fluid balance chart to help with your assessment?
- Better still, do they have a urinary catheter? If so, what is urine volume and colour?
- Further guidance on fluid balance and what to do about it is in the next section.

Haemorrhage

- Is there any history of trauma or bleeding conditions?
- Abdominal examination should always be performed as part of circulatory assessment—in the absence of trauma, this is the most likely site of concealed blood loss.

Points of access

- Now is the time to take stock of the situation. What access does the patient have, and do they need more?
- If regular fluid and drug administration is required, more than one IV cannula is desirable as it enables intercurrent administration (and offers a small degree of redundancy)
- Is invasive monitoring going to be required?
  - Arterial lines offer beat-on-beat blood pressure monitoring and mean arterial pressure, as well as a portal for repeated ABG sampling
  - Central venous lines normally have four lumens, allowing rapid fluid administration, greater electrolyte replacement rates and monitoring CVP (a more direct means of ascertaining the patient's intravascular filling)
  - As well as the individual competence required for line insertion, nursing and management must be considered. A patient with this much access will normally be in a higher dependency environment than the ward, and so should be discussed at an early stage with the critical care team.

Cardiac monitoring and ECGs

- As a first line, cardiac monitoring offers continual visualization (normally of lead II) pending a formal ECG
- Although monitors are often in short supply, modern defibrillators normally offer monitoring either through separate leads or via the main electrodes if adhesive.

Disability

Assess GCS

Although only strictly validated for head injury, the GCS is now almost universally used as a means of expressing level of consciousness across three domains:

- Eyes (also take this opportunity to note pupillary size and reflexes)
  - 1—not opening
  - 2—opens in response to pain
  - 3—opens on command
  - 4—spontaneously opening
- Voice
  - 1—no vocalization
  - 2—noises
  - 3—incoherent speech
  - 4—confused speech
  - 5—talking and oriented
- Movement
  - 1—no movement
  - 2—extension
  - 3—abnormal flexion
  - 4—withdrawal from pain
  - 5—localizes to pain
  - 6—movement on command

If there is no neurological history and a normal GCS, there is little to justify further neurological examination. Weakness, headache, back pain, new retention of urine or altered sensation should all prompt full neurological assessment.

Everything else

If corrective management has been instituted throughout this process, you should now be in a position to find out more information from nursing staff and clinical notes. Will imaging help your management? If not sought already, is senior review required? Continuous reassessment is also a key principle here—check your measures are still working frequently.

❶ Don't struggle out of your depth with this approach. Almost all encounters with the seriously sick are frightening—if you can't manage, seek help. Most crucially, don't be afraid to put out an arrest call—a patient in 3rd degree AV block, for example, hasn't arrested but you will not be faulted for calling the team. Early escalation of care for seriously ill patients is associated with better outcome, and there is little more frustrating than for a critical care team to see a potentially salvageable patient through the retrospectoscope 3 hours later.

Fluid management

An adult has total body water accounting for around 60% of body weight—roughly 42 litres for a 70-kg man. By convention, this water is considered as being divided between fluid compartments.

Fluid Compartments

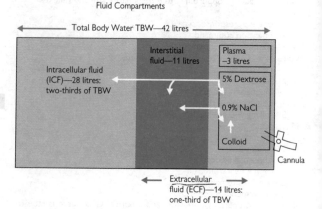

Fig. 1.1 Body fluid composition, and distribution of IV fluids.

Ionic substances distribute freely within the ECF, whereas the ICF composition varies between tissue and cell types, and is controlled by cellular homoeostasis.

Basal requirements

Average minimum daily requirements (totals in parentheses) for an adult weighing 70 kg are:

Water	25–35 ml/kg/day	(1.75–2.5 litres/day)
Sodium	1–1.4 mmol/kg/day	(70–100 mmol/day)
Potassium	0.7–0.9 mmol/kg/day	(50–70 mmol/day)
Calcium	0.1 mmol/kg/day	(7 mmol/day)
Magnesium	0.1 mmol/kg/day	(7 mmol/day)

In health, renal and endocrine mechanisms ensure maintenance of water and electrolyte homoeostasis, and daily intakes generally exceed the above minima considerably.

Intravenous fluid therapy

Intravenous fluids may be classified as:
- Crystalloids
  - True solutions which may pass though semi-permeable membranes (e.g. dextrose solutions, saline solutions, Hartmann's)
- Colloids
  - Homogeneous non-crystalline particles of one substance dispersed through another (e.g. Gelofusine®, Haemaccel®, human albumin solutions (HAS), starch solutions).

Crystalloids will tend to distribute more rapidly throughout the ECF, and hence, volume for volume, will have a smaller plasma expansion effect. However, there is no evidence demonstrating better outcomes following fluid resuscitation with colloid in preference to crystalloid. Crystalloid preparations are considerably cheaper. The electrolyte composition of various intravenous fluids is shown in the table below (ions in mmol/l; osmolality in mosmol/l):

Table 1.1 Composition of IV fluids

Solution	Na$^+$	K$^+$	Ca^{2+}	HCO$_3$	Cl$^-$	Osmolality
5% Dextrose	—	—	—	—	—	280
4% Dextrose/ 0.18% NaCl	30	—	—	—	30	255
0.9% NaCl (normal saline)	150	—	—	—	150	300
Hartmann's Solution	131	5	2	29	111	278
Gelofusine®	154	0.4	0.4	—	125	279
Haemaccel®	145	5.1	6.25	—	145	301
HAS 4.5%	100–160	<2	—	—	100–160	270–300
HAS 20%	50–120	<10	—	—	<40	135–138

Potassium is often added to fluids in specified quantities—usually 20 or 40 mmol/l. Concentrations larger than this can cause phlebitis if infused into a peripheral vein.

Choice of intravenous fluid

Maintenance intravenous fluid should provide adequate water and electrolytes. Baseline requirements as described above, in combination with knowledge of the composition of the various available solutions, may guide initial prescription. Bear in mind that fluid losses due to, for example, burns, pyrexia, post-surgical drains, enteral output, renal pathology, etc., may necessitate far greater volumes of maintenance fluid than these minima.

Certain disease states will also require larger amounts of electrolytes than those mentioned above. For example, sodium is lost in large amounts when vomiting or in patients with polyuric renal recovery. Potassium is lost in large amounts in diarrhoea, and in patients with paralytic ileus.

Pathological processes, complicated by the stress response in a sick patient—promoting sodium and water retention—mandate that ongoing therapy must be guided by repeated clinical assessment, alongside serial serum electrolyte measurements, with prescriptions adjusted accordingly.

Assessment of hydration

First, ask the patient if they are feeling thirsty and dehydrated! HR, BP, distal perfusion/CRT, JVP, GCS, skin turgor, examination of mucous membranes and UO will afford further information. Invasive monitoring of CVP may also help, although absolute values are of less value than trends and response to fluid challenges.

Fluid resuscitation

This refers to the administration of fluid to a patient who has inadequate circulation to their peripheries due to hypovolaemia. The aim is to increase the plasma volume to increase cardiac preload, and hence cardiac output. Fluid used should therefore expand plasma volume.

Colloids contain large molecules, which do not permeate the endothelial membrane, so therefore hold water within the plasma compartment. Fluids containing large amounts of charged ions (e.g. normal saline, Hartmann's) will distribute throughout the ECF, though will not enter cells so easily. Fluid containing uncharged (e.g. dextrose solutions) particles will distribute throughout the entire body, and will thus not give rapid increases in plasma volume. For this reason, resuscitation is usually undertaken with normal saline, Hartmann's or colloid solutions. 5% dextrose should not be used as a resuscitation fluid.

Repeated fluid challenges (e.g. 250–500 ml) with frequent evaluation of changes in HR, BP, JVP, CRT, GCS and UO, alongside surrogate markers of tissue perfusion (e.g. serum lactate), will guide further therapy; a urine output of >0.5 ml/kg/h should be maintained.

If the patient does not improve clinically, consider sources of ongoing fluid loss (e.g. drains, third space losses) or cardiogenic shock, and call for senior help. Further investigations, alongside invasive monitoring and circulatory support may be required, and critical care involvement at an early stage should be sought.

Further reading

- *OHCM*, 7th edn. Oxford: Oxford University Press, p. 778.

Pain control

Possibly one of our most frequently requested tasks as junior doctors, this is too often approached with no system or thought towards progressive management. There is a wealth of analgesia available in hospital; timely prescription with a next step already planned ensures maximum patient comfort and fewest calls back to the ward.

The simplest model to work from is that of the World Health Organization (WHO), who have developed a 3-step ladder.

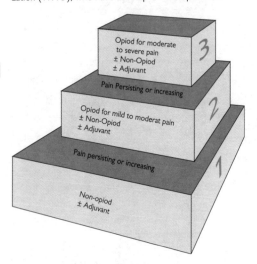

Fig. 1.2 WHO Pain Ladder. Reproduced with kind permission of the WHO.

Care should be taken in the choice of agent at each level on the ladder. Particular issues to consider include:

- Renal function and NSAID use
  - There is significant risk using NSAIDs in patients with established renal failure, so non-opioid medication is far better confined to paracetamol
  - Diclofenac is around eight times more nephrotoxic than ibuprofen—they should not, therefore, be used interchangeably
- Tramadol
  - Although a potent analgesic offering alternative options to morphine, it can make patients very unwell, causing disorientation, nausea and vomiting
  - Frail, elderly or slight patients are at particular risk from this
- Codeine
  - Codeine is good analgesia for headaches
  - Chronic administration should always be accompanied by a laxative. Elderly patients have died from perforations secondary to as little as 1 week on codeine.

Make use of specialist pain services where available if failing to control the pain with the ladder approach. Other options that may be available this way include patient-controlled analgesia, capsaicin creams and nerve blocks.

Death and dying—a hospital chaplain's perspective

None of us views death impartially. Our attitude towards it will depend heavily on our beliefs about it, which in turn will form part of the more general and wideranging spiritual (often a distinct concept from religion) perspective we hold. Whether we view it as total extinction, or a welcome release from a condition of pain and suffering, or as a transition from one form of existence to another—all of this will have a bearing on how we cope with it emotionally.

It is inevitable that you will be affected by the death of a patient, especially if you have been closely involved with them during their treatment. In my work as a hospital chaplain, I have frequently come across medical professionals profoundly upset by the death of a patient, yet also struggling with the feeling that they shouldn't be letting their emotions 'get the better of them', that somehow such a response was unprofessional. So, in addition to coping with the patient's death, they also had to cope with their own sense of inadequacy and failure regarding how they handled it.

You are human beings first and foremost, before you are 'professionals'. What is more, I would suggest that what patients value in you, at least as much as your professional expertise, is precisely your humanity, and your ability to respond to them empathically as one person to another. If that is so, then your vulnerability to an emotional response at a patient's death will be the inevitable 'flip side' to those qualities in you which made you a good doctor for them when they were alive.

So, be prepared to be upset by death; however, rather than seeing this as a weakness on your part, or a failing of professionalism, rejoice in it as evidence of that human gift of empathy which will enable you to be, not a medical professional, but a true healer.

In situations like this, remember that you too are a person with needs. Give yourself time and space to work through your feelings; make use of others who can accompany you in this—if your hospital has a chaplain, then you may well find him or her a valuable resource at such times, irrespective of whether or not you subscribe to his or her particular creed.

Consider the patient facing his or her own death, the family of that patient, the loved ones of a patient who has died, maybe suddenly or unexpectedly—all these have in common the fact that they need to grieve. Patients who have lost limbs, or important physical functions, will experience grief; even the loss of independence and control which a stay in hospital can entail, especially if it is a long one, will produce some of the symptoms of grief. Second, as far as death is concerned, grief is not experienced only by others; the patient himself, facing the prospect of the loss of his life, with all that that means, will experience grief too.

It is important for the physician, who is used to working with a model of illness and cure, to appreciate that grief does not fit this model. It is not there to be cured, but endured; and those who deal with grieving people are not striving to solve a problem, but to support a person who is experiencing a quite natural, and indeed necessary, process. This can induce a feeling of helplessness in those who have to deal with a grieving patient or relative, and that in turn might tempt one to offer quick fixes or facile responses.

Above all, grief is a process; it takes time. A bereaved spouse, for instance, might spend up to 2 years working through this process, before achieving some sort of resolution whereby, though life will never be the same again, he or she feels able to 'pick up the pieces' and move on. Though it is important to note that this process is different for everyone, both in its duration and its shape, it does tend to follow a common pattern. In 1970, Dr Elisabeth Kubler-Ross published a seminal work entitled *On Death and Dying*, in which she outlined the main 'stages' of the grief process, namely denial, anger, bargaining, depression and acceptance.

From this, it follows that you will often see and deal with people—especially relatives—who are in the early stages of the process, particularly denial and anger. Thus it is that a member of the medical professions will get the feeling that the patient or relative has not heard, or cannot have been listening to, what they have been saying. You feel that you have made the situation clear, but it is as if you have not said anything. You may find this puzzling and frustrating, but be aware that this is simply a manifestation of denial by those in the early stage of the grief process. Also potentially difficult is the anger, which may often be directed at you personally, maybe even in the form of accusations of negligence or error. Understandably, this can be distressing for the doctor on the receiving end; nevertheless, bear in mind where it is really coming from, and this will enable you to keep a sense of perspective about such accusations and continue to work with a 'difficult' family.

Finally, remember that working with the dying and their families, though it is undoubtedly at times difficult, is also a great privilege, and your approach and attitude to them before and after death can make a significant difference to their experience of the death, whether it be their own or that of their loved one.

Capacity and consent

'It is for the patient, not the doctor, to determine what is in the patient's own best interest'. Seeking patients' consent: the ethical considerations (GMC)

Practical and legal aspects of capacity and consent vary between countries. This section will focus on the law and guidelines in England and Wales and, although many principles are the same elsewhere, it is important that you familiarise yourself with the relevant legislation where you work. Note that the situation is different when working with children; this will not be discussed here.

Consent

Consent is needed for all examinations and treatments. It is the responsibility of the treating clinician to make sure valid consent has been obtained. For the consent to be valid, the patient must:

- Have capacity
- Be informed
- Give consent freely, without being pressured.

In most cases it is important to seek explicit consent (verbal or written). Consent can also be implied; when the way someone acts communicates clearly that they consent, for example, to having their BP checked. At other times it may not be appropriate to spend time obtaining consent, such as when immediate treatment is necessary.

Giving information

Do what you can to make it easier to understand, such as using leaflets, asking if the person would like someone else present and allowing plenty of time for questions. Individuals differ in how much and what they need to know but, to come to a decision, it is important to know:

- Broadly what the condition is
- The purpose and nature of the proposed treatment
- What options there are
- What is likely to happen if the treatment is not given
- Likely benefits and risks of options
- That the person can withdraw consent at any time.

If you have been asked to take consent for a treatment suggested by a more senior doctor, make sure you understand the treatment and that you are able to answer any questions the patient may have. If you do not feel confident doing this alone, don't!

Assessing capacity

Capacity is the ability to make a decision for one's self, and is a requirement for consent to be valid. It is specific to the decision and may change with time. If you find that a person has capacity to make the decision, you must respect it, even if the decision is likely to cause serious outcomes (e.g. death).

The Mental Capacity Act 2005

The Mental Capacity Act (MCA) for England and Wales is currently being implemented (April 2007). It replaces common law principles when treating patients who may lack capacity to make some decisions. Professionals caring for people who may lack capacity will have a duty to comply with the Act, and need to be familiar with it.

Principles of the Mental Capacity Act

- A person must be assumed to have capacity unless it is established that he lacks capacity
- A person is not to be treated as unable to make a decision unless all practicable steps to help him to do so have been taken without success
- A person is not to be treated as unable to make a decision merely because he makes an unwise decision
- An act done, or decision made, under this Act for or on behalf of a person who lacks capacity must be done, or made, in his best interests
- Before the act is done, or the decision is made, regard must be had to whether the purpose for which it is needed can be as effectively achieved in a way that is less restrictive of the person's rights and freedom of action.

According to the MCA, a person is unable to make a decision for himself if he is unable:

- To understand the information relevant to the decision
- To retain that information
- To use or weigh that information as part of the process of making the decision
- To communicate his decision (whether by talking, using sign language or any other means).

Take care of yourself!

Use these criteria systematically when assessing capacity, and document them clearly in the case notes. Treatment of a person with capacity against their will is assault, and not giving treatment that is in the best interest of a person who lacks capacity is negligence. In real life, you may also find that there are degrees of capacity, or that you are uncertain about what to do. Ask someone more senior for advice, as a wrong decision may violate the patient's human rights as well as causing you serious problems with the law, the GMC or the press.

When a patient lacks capacity to make a decision

Assess whether anything is likely to improve the patient's capacity to make a decision (e.g. different communication style). If the patient still does not have capacity to make the decision, it is your responsibility to act in the patient's best interest.

It has been a principle that no-one can give consent on behalf of another person, but be aware that the MCA introduces 'designated decision-makers' who can act on behalf of a person who lacks capacity (Lasting Powers of Attorneys and Deputies). Advance decisions must also be respected if they are valid and applicable.

What is in the person's best interest?

This can be a difficult question to answer. Take into account:

- Risks and benefits of options. Which option is the least restrictive?
- The person's background, beliefs and values
- The person's wishes
  - Present feelings
  - Previously expressed wishes or advance directives
- The views of others
  - Family, carers or others close to the patient
  - Any Lasting Power of Attorney or Deputy.

Further reading

- *The Mental Capacity Act 2005* (subject to Crown Copyright protection). http://www.opsi.gov.uk/acts/acts2005/20050009.htm
- *Seeking patients' consent: the ethical considerations.* GMC, 1998. http://www.gmc-uk.org/guidance/current/library/consent.asp
- *Consent. A complete guide for consultants.* The Medical Protection Society http://www.medicalprotection.org/Default.aspx?DN=ea688602-e427-49d7-8b64-7ec720905bac
- *Reference guide to consent for examination or treatment.* Department of Health. http://www.dh.gov.uk/assetRoot/04/01/90/79/04019079.pdf
- *Mental Capacity Act Code of Practice* 2007. http://www.dca.gov.uk

Help! I need somebody...

The junior doctor who can deal with the emergencies in this book without feeling the strain is rare; maybe they are in fact non-existent. For all the educational reform and career management taking place, medicine has not become less stressful. It is inevitable that some days will be better than others—if the bad days start outnumbering the good, take action.

The frightening feeling of not coping is not one you should keep to yourself. Your educational team will be able to offer you support locally, and without judgement. If, however, you prefer to discuss it outside work in the first instance, there are several ports of call. Your medical school (or postgraduate deanery if you have moved out of area) should have contacts with a university counselling service. There is also the Doctors' Support Network or the Samaritans—sometimes the adages about problems shared ring true.

If, however, you feel your performance at work is being affected, informing your clinical tutor or supervisor is wise. If you feel out of your depth, both your patients and you should be protected from potential adverse outcome. Also, with the advent of near continuous formal assessment, a sudden drop in performance without explanation has potential to create difficulties in later years.

Simple steps to help avoid this situation arising can be taken. The concept of 'protected time' can be applied to personal life equally as to education—ensure that you set aside time to see your friends and to do the things you enjoy. It inevitably takes far more effort to do this around a busy clinical rota, but brings great benefits.

If you are lucky and enjoying stress-free jobs, look around you. Do any of your colleagues need you?

Where to turn

The Samaritans

Samaritans is available 24 hours a day to provide confidential emotional support for people who are experiencing feelings of distress or despair, including those which may lead to suicide.

☎ 08457 90 90 90

🖳 www.samaritans.org

Doctors' Support Network

The Doctors' Support Network (DSN) is a warm, friendly self-help group for doctors with mental health concerns. These concerns include stress, burnout, anxiety, depression, manic depression, psychoses and eating disorders.

☎ 0870 321 0642

🖳 www.dsn.org.uk

BMA Counselling Service

The BMA Counselling Service is staffed by professional telephone counsellors, 24 hours a day, 7 days a week. All counsellors are members of the British Association for Counselling and Psychotherapy and are bound by strict codes of confidentiality and ethical practice.

The service is confidential, and when making contact you can choose to remain anonymous. It is available to you and members of your family who normally live with you, including children up to the age of 21 even if they are at university.

The counsellors are there to help you deal with a wide variety of issues, including the pressures and stresses of work (and the impact of this on family life), relationship problems, concerns about children and other family members, and issues relating to mental health. The service can also help address alcohol or drug misuse, and provides information about other specialist resources available to you.

☎ 08459 200 169

🖳 www.bma.org.uk

Section 1

Presentations

:۞: **Chest pain**

Chest pain can be a frightening symptom for both patient and doctor alike. Given the incidence of ischaemic heart disease, this is often top of the list of differential diagnoses, though consideration must be given to other causes.

Immediate management

- ABC
  - Remember the association between conditions causing chest pain and cardiovascular collapse
- Keep patient on cardiac monitor until cardiovascular cause is ruled out
- Observations must be checked frequently (i.e. every 15 minutes) until patient is stable
- Gain IV access and take bloods for investigation as detailed below
- Consider IV fluid boluses if the patient is haemodynamically unstable (see p. 6–8)
  - ⚠ Use caution if any evidence of heart failure (e.g. ↑JVP, hepatomegaly, peripheral/sacral oedema, bibasal fine crepitations)—consider using smaller fluid boluses (e.g. 5 ml/kg)
- Administer adequate analgesia
  - e.g. diamorphine, 2.5–5 mg by slow IV injection
  - *and* metoclopramide, 10 mg by IV
- 12-lead ECG
- ABG if SpO_2 low or any respiratory distress
- Check temperature—pyrexia may indicate pneumonia (see p. 208–211), pericarditis (see p. 148–151) or SIRS/sepsis (see p. 304–306)

History

The key aspect of the history is to determine the system involved, i.e. cardiovascular, respiratory, gastrointestinal or musculoskeletal. Patients rarely have a completely 'classical' picture of pain from a defined cause, but a good impression can often be formed from a well explored history.

- Site
  - Well localized—pleuritic or musculoskeletal cause
  - Diffuse, central chest—characteristically cardiac
  - Retrosternal—classically oesophageal or cardiac (often difficult to differentiate)
- Onset
  - Sudden onset—abrupt vascular ischaemia (e.g. MI, PE, aortic dissection) or pneumothorax
  - Gradual onset—unstable angina or pleuritic pain
- Character
  - 'Heavy, crushing, tight' pain—cardiac
  - 'Stabbing' pain—pleuritic
  - 'Tearing' pain—consider aortic dissection
- Radiation
  - Left arm, neck and jaw—cardiac pain

- Interscapular—aortic dissection
- Abdominal—basal pneumonia or inferior MI
- Subphrenic pathology can cause radiation to the chest and shoulder
- Associated symptoms
  - SOB—respiratory or cardiac causes (see p. 28–31)
  - Nausea, vomiting and sweating—↑sympathetic tone associated with cardiac pathology (also consider sepsis)
  - Palpitations—arrhythmia (especially if fast) or hyperdynamic circulation (see p. 40–43)
  - Cough—respiratory pathology
  - Sputum—purulent (pneumonia), haemoptysis (PE)
  - Syncope/presyncope—cardiac pathology (particularly arrhythmia)
- Timing
  - Duration of pain may have implications for administration of thrombolytics
  - If previous angina, ↑duration or crescendo pain can indicate unstable angina (see p. 140–143)
  - Retrosternal pain worse at night or stooping—gastro-oesophageal reflux
- Exacerbating/relieving factors
  - Worse on deep inspiration/coughing—pleuritic and musculoskeletal pain
  - Worse sitting forward—pericarditis
  - Worse lying down—gastro-oesophageal reflux
  - Relief from GTN—cardiac ischaemia
  - Relieved by eating or taking antacids—gastro-oesophageal reflux
- Severity
  - Severity of pain should guide analgesic use
  - 'Worst ever' pain—acute MI (NB elderly patients and patients with DM can have milder pain, however)
- Past medical history
  - Similar pains previously
  - IHD
  - Hypertension
  - Diabetes
  - COPD
  - Thrombophilia, previous DVT or PE
- Recent OGD (risk of oesophageal rupture)
- Recent chest infection or trauma
- Family history of cardiorespiratory disease
- Smoking and alcohol history

Examination
Cardiovascular
- Heart rate and rhythm
  - Consider arrhythmia if rate >120/min
  - ❶ ☎ 2222 if arrhythmia is causing haemodynamic instability
- JVP and neck veins
  - ⚠ Raised JVP can indicate R ventricular failure, caution should be used when giving IV fluids

- ❶ Distended neck veins + hypoxia + ↓BP may indicate late stage tension pneumothorax (see p. 204–207), cardiac tamponade (see p. 152–155) or large PE (see p. 200–203)—☎ **2222** if in any doubt
- Heart sounds
  - Muffled heart sounds—consider tamponade (difficult to elicit)
  - New murmurs—papillary muscle rupture, acute VSD, endocarditis or aortic regurgitation 2° to aortic dissection
- Blood pressure
  - Monitor BP and treat if hypotensive (see p. 96–100)
  - Check BP in both arms—>20 mmHg difference may suggest aortic dissection (see p. 160–162)

Respiratory
- Tracheal deviation
  - ❶ With hyper-resonance + absent air entry on the opposite side is a late sign of tension pneumothorax—consider immediate needle decompression (see p. 204–207)
  - NB Ensure patient has not had previous pneumonectomy on that side
- Inspect and palpate chest
  - If history of trauma—look for flail segments, bruising and surgical emphysema
  - Localised tenderness reproducing the presenting pain indicates a musculoskeletal cause
- Percussion note
  - Hyper-resonant—pneumothorax
  - Dull—consolidation or pulmonary oedema
  - Stony dull—haemothorax or pleural effusion
- Auscultation
  - Bibasal fine crepitations—pulmonary oedema
  - Coarse focal crepitations + bronchial breathing—pneumonia
  - Reduced air entry—pneumothorax, pleural effusion, haemothorax or lobar collapse

Abdominal
- Abdominal tenderness
  - ?Referred pain from a basal pneumonia or inferior MI
  - ?Atypical presentation of pancreatitis, cholecystitis or peptic ulcer disease
- Hepatomegaly—R heart failure

Investigations
- Serial ECGs
  - Check regularly to detect evolving changes
  - Cardiac ischaemia—see p. 134–143
  - Arrhythmia: see p. 164–186
- FBC & CRP
  - ↓Hb can precipitate or worsen cardiac ischaemia
  - ↑WCC + ↑CRP—inflammatory condition
- U&Es, Ca^{2+}, PO_4^{2-}, Mg^{2+}
  - Electrolyte disturbance (especially ↑K^+) can cause arrhythmia

- Troponins & cardiac enzymes
  - Only rise 12 h after myocardial damage
- Well's score ± D-dimer—see p. 188–190
- CXR
  - Check for consolidation, pulmonary oedema and pneumothorax
  - Globular heart shadow—pericardial effusion or tamponade
  - Pneumopericardium—oesophageal rupture
- Transthoracic echocardiogram
  - Indicated if new murmurs or haemodynamic compromise

Causes

Cardiovascular
- MI/ischaemia (see p. 134–143)
- Aortic dissection (see p. 160–162)
- Pericarditis/pericardial effusion (see p. 148–155)
- Arrhythmia (see p. 164–186)

Respiratory
- Pneumonia/empyema (see p. 208–211)
- Pneumothorax/tension pneumothorax (see p. 204–207)
- Pleural effusion (see p. 216–218)
- PE (see p. 200–203)

Gastrointestinal
- Oesophagitis/gastro-oesophageal reflux
- Oesophageal rupture
- Pancreatitis (see p. 372–375)
- Cholecystitis (see p. 380–382)
- Peptic ulceration
- Subphrenic abscess

Musculoskeletal
- Trauma/rib fracture
- Muscle strain
- Costochondritis
- Bony metastases/myeloma
- Cervical spondylitis

Other
- Psychogenic/panic attacks
- Herpes zoster infection (shingles)

Further reading
- *OHCM*, 7th edn. Oxford: Oxford University Press, p. 80.
- *Oxford Textbook of Medicine*, 4th edn, vol. 2, Oxford: Oxford University Press, p. 829.
- *Oxford Handbook of Emergencies in Cardiology*, 1st edn, Oxford: Oxford University Press, p. 15.
- Erhardt L *et al.* (2002) Task force on the management of chest pain. *European Heart Journal*, **23**:1153–76.

⊙ Shortness of breath

SOB is a common complaint, which has the potential to become life-threatening very quickly. Prompt assessment and action can be life-saving. There is an extensive list of causes for SOB, so it is vital to work systematically to exclude or treat serious problems first, using the ABC approach.

Immediate management

Airway
- Inability to talk, stridor or gesticulating to neck—consider upper airway obstruction
- Compromised airway—☎ **2222** or fast bleep anaesthetist
- ❶ If the patient is in dire straits—needle cricothyroidotomy may buy time

Breathing
- Assess respiratory rate and work of breathing
- Monitor SpO_2 and check ABGs
- Give high flow O_2 via non-rebreathing mask— ⚠ use caution in COPD (see p. 212–215)
- Consider nebulized bronchodilators
  - e.g. Salbutamol 5 mg, nebulized
  - Check response, and repeat as necessary
- ❶ If evidence of tension pneumothorax—perform immediate needle decompression (see p. 204–207)
- ❶ Beware of failing of respiratory effort (e.g. decompensating asthma)
  - Fall in RR can be falsely reassuring
  - Accompanied by ↓SpO_2, ↓GCS and ↑$PaCO_2$—☎ call for senior/ITU help

Circulation
- Establish IV access
- Assess heart rate and rhythm
  - Arrhythmias can manifest as SOB
  - Place patient on a cardiac monitor
- Check BP and CRT
  - Is the tachypnoea a physiological response to shock?
  - Give IV fluid bolus if haemodynamically unstable (see p. 6–8)
- Is there evidence of acute heart failure? (see p. 144–146)

DEFG
- Don't Ever Forget Glucose
- Check BM—DKA can present with Kussmaul's respiration

History
SOB is most commonly due to primary respiratory disease, but don't fall into the trap of not considering other causes (e.g. acute heart failure).

- Speed of onset
  - Sudden (within seconds)—PE, pneumothorax, airway obstruction, arrhythmia
  - Fast (within minutes)—MI, asthma, pulmonary oedema
  - Over hours or days—asthma, pneumonia, exacerbation of COPD, pleural effusion, cardiac failure
  - Weeks or months—fibrosing alveolitis, pneumonitis, cardiomyopathy
  - Intermittent—asthma, arrhythmias, L heart failure
- Chest pain
  - Cardiac or respiratory? (see p. 24–27)
- Associated symptoms
  - Cough—pneumonia (purulent sputum), PE (haemoptysis), pulmonary oedema (pink frothy sputum)
  - Pyrexia—pneumonia, SIRS/sepsis, anaphylaxis
  - Palpitations—arrhythmia, psychogenic
  - Parasthesiae (circumoral/hands and feet)—psychogenic
- Exacerbating and relieving factors
  - Relief with bronchodilators—reversible airway constriction (i.e. asthma, COPD)
  - Relief with GTN—cardiac cause
  - Orthopnoea/paroxysmal nocturnal dyspnoea—heart failure
- Past medical history
  - Cardiac or respiratory illness
  - Asthma—establish number of previous admissions, and severity of these (e.g. ITU admissions, IV treatment required)
  - Medications can give clues as to underlying pathology (e.g. inhalers, cardiac medications, oral hypoglycaemic agents)
  - Allergy history, especially any anaphylactic reactions
- Risk factors for cardiac or pulmonary disease
  - Smoking
  - Diabetes
  - Hypercholesterolaemia
  - Occupation (e.g. mining, asbestos exposure)
  - Family history

Examination

- Look around the patient
  - Inhalers/cigarette packets at the bedside?
- General examination
  - Clubbing (chronic suppurative lung disease, fibrosing alveolitis, carcinoma of the lung), clinical anaemia, body habitus (obesity, cachexia)
  - Signs of CO_2 retention—coarse tremor, bounding pulses, warm peripheries, hyperaemic conjunctivae
  - Cervical lymphadenopathy—infection, malignancy
- Assess work of breathing
  - Respiratory rate
  - Accessory muscle use
  - Pursed lips/nasal flaring
  - Intercostal/subcostal recession

- Inspection of chest wall—trauma, previous surgery/chest drains, deformity
- Percuss chest
  - Hyper-resonant—pneumothorax
  - Dull—consolidation
  - Stony dull—pleural effusion or haemothorax
- Vocal resonance and fremitus
  - Increased—consolidation
  - Decreased—pleural effusion, haemothorax, pneumothorax
- Auscultation
  - Localised crackles + bronchial breathing—pneumonia
  - Bibasal fine crackles—pulmonary oedema
  - Wheeze, reduced air entry + prolonged expiratory phase—asthma (⚠ beware of 'silent chest' in life-threatening asthma)
  - Pleural rub—PE, pleural effusion/inflammation
- Cardiovascular
  - Pulse rate and rhythm—arrhythmia
  - BP + CRT—shock (cardiogenic, hypovolaemic, septic)
  - Murmurs—acute heart failure
  - Peripheral/sacral oedema—R heart failure

Investigations
- ABGs (see p. 422–424)
  - Will usually show $\downarrow PaCO_2$ owing to increased ventilation, often due to $\downarrow PaO_2$
  - Metabolic acidosis may cause tachypnoea (respiratory compensation)
  - ⚠ If patient is retaining CO_2 and requiring O_2 therapy, they may require non-invasive ventilation
- Full blood count & CRP
  - Anaemia can exacerbate SOB of any cause. Raised WCC + CRP can indicate infective cause
- U&Es + bone profile
  - Electrolyte imbalance can precipitate arrhythmia
  - Check anion gap in presence of metabolic acidosis
- Glucose and lactate—could this be DKA or lactic acidosis?
- BNP
  - If <100—cardiac failure unlikely
  - If >500—makes cardiac failure very likely
- Blood culture if pyrexial (prior to starting ABx if possible)
- CXR—can reveal pneumothorax, pleural effusion/haemothorax, consolidation, pulmonary oedema, cardiac dilatation
- ECG—look for ischaemia, hypertrophy, strain, arrhythmia
- Echocardiogram—how good is the cardiac function?

Causes
Respiratory
- Acute exacerbation of asthma (see p. 196–198)
- Exacerbation of COPD (see p. 212–214)
- Pleural effusion (see p. 216–218)

- Pneumonia (see p. 208–211)
- Pneumothorax (see p. 204–207)
- Pulmonary embolism (see p. 200–203)
- Anaphylaxis (see p. 192–194)
- Fibrosing alveolitis
- Aspiration of foreign body
- Pressure on larynx (abscess, haematoma, thyroid mass)
- Acute epiglottitis
- Chest trauma (e.g. flail chest, open pneumothorax)

Cardiac
- MI/angina (see p. 134–143)
- Acute heart failure (see p. 144–146)
- Arrhythmias (see p. 164–186)
- Pericardial effusion/tamponade (see p. 148–155)

Other
- Pain (see p. 10–11)
- Anaemia
- Metabolic acidosis with respiratory compensation, e.g. DKA (see p. 422–424)
- Shock/sepsis (see p. 304–306)
- Central causes, e.g. head injury, malignant hypertension (see p. 102–106)
- Acute respiratory distress syndrome, e.g. following trauma, hypovolaemia, shock, sepsis, etc.
- Guillain–Barré syndrome
- Carbon monoxide poisoning
- Psychogenic

Further reading
- *OCHM*, 7th edn. Oxford: Oxford University Press, p. 58, 770.
- *Oxford Textbook of Medicine*, 4th edn, vol. 2. Oxford: Oxford University Press, p. 1285.

① **Haemoptysis**

This refers to blood being coughed up from the lower respiratory tract, but is easily confused with haematemesis or upper airway bleeding. Large haemorrhages are quite rare, although it is important to deal with them promptly. Small streaks of haemoptysis in association with vigorous coughing are most often found with acute exacerbations of COPD. Often, though, haemoptysis is an indicator of serious underlying disease, and should be investigated thoroughly.

Immediate management

- ABC assessment
    - In heavy haemorrhage, airway maintenance can be very tricky. Place patient on their side (try to place on the side from where the bleeding is thought to come), and perform airway opening manoeuvres (e.g. jaw thrust) whilst waiting for experienced help
    - Give high flow O_2 via non-rebreath mask, as oxygenation is likely to be compromised
    - Gain large bore IV access (preferably ×2) and send blood for crossmatch
    - Assess circulation regularly and give IV fluid/blood boluses to maintain perfusion
    - Check coagulation and correct any coagulopathy
- ☎ Call chest physician or cardiothoracic surgeons for definitive management
    - Patient may require urgent bronchoscopy, pulmonary angiography + embolization or surgery to stop the bleeding
- Is aggressive treatment appropriate if patient has terminal illness?
    - Discuss with patient and family
    - Consider giving IV diamorphine and midazolam to relieve distress
    - e.g. Diamorphine, 2.5–5 mg IV (with antiemetic, e.g. metoclopramide, 10 mg IV)
    - *and* midazolam, 2 mg IV over 1 min, *then* give in 1 mg steps and titrate to response

History

- Take a careful history of the episode, to determine whether it was a true haemoptysis
    - True haemoptysis should come from a cough as opposed to a retch
    - Haemoptysis will usually be frothy to some extent, owing to mixing with air
    - Bleeds from the lower respiratory tract are likely to be arterial, therefore will be bright red
    - Sputum will be alkaline in haemoptysis, and acidic with GI bleeds
    - Ask about nosebleeds or dental problems (possible source for the bleeding)

- How long has the haemoptysis been evident?
  - Short or one-off history may indicate acute event—e.g. bronchial infection, PE
  - Frequent episodes may indicate a more long-term problem, e.g. bronchial carcinoma, pulmonary TB
- PMHx
  - Any history of carcinoma—primary/secondary tumour, ↑risk of PE
  - Is there a history of coagulopathy, or is the patient on warfarin?
  - Chronic fever and weight loss may suggest TB or neoplasia
  - Any history of bronchiectasis—may be the cause
  - Risk factors for DVT/PE (see p. 188–190, 200–203)
  - Risk factors for bronchial carcinoma—smoking, industrial exposure to carcinogens (e.g. asbestos), family history
  - Any cardiac history—acute pulmonary oedema, mitral stenosis
  - Significant diseases—hereditary haemorrhagic telangiectasia (Osler–Weber–Rendu syndrome), Goodpasture's syndrome, polyarteritis nodosa

Examination

- General examination
  - Cachexic appearance should make you suspicious of TB or malignancy
  - Clubbing may suggest chronic suppurative lung disease (e.g. bronchiectasis) or bronchial carcinoma
  - Fever suggests infection
  - A swollen leg should make you suspicious of PE
  - Lymphadenopathy may be present in infection and malignancy
  - Rashes may be present in systemic illnesses (e.g. vasculitic disorders)
- RS
  - Bronchial breathing, coarse crackles and dull percussion indicate infection
  - Bibasal fine crackles suggest pulmonary oedema
  - Stony dull percussion and reduced air entry may reveal a pleural effusion—is there an underlying malignancy?
- Abdominal
  - Hepatomegaly or splenomegaly can be present in systemic diseases or malignancy

Investigations

- ABGs
  - Can give an indication of lung function if the patient is severely unwell—check the A–a O_2 gradient (see p. 422–424)
- FBC, CRP, coagulation screen
  - Raised inflammatory markers will suggest infective cause
  - Coagulopathy may be revealed as cause or exacerbating factor
- U&Es
  - ↑Urea may make you consider whether this is haematemesis (but large bleeds may make patients swallow significant quantities of blood)

- Autoantibody screen
  - May highlight connective tissue/autoimmune disease
- CXR
  - Look for pulmonary tuberculous granulomas or opacities suggestive of neoplasia
  - Wedges of decreased density in the lung fields may indicate PE (although will often not be present)
  - Consolidation will suggest pneumonia, but may obscure an underlying neoplasm
  - Pleural effusion should make you suspicious of underlying malignancy
- ECG
  - May show changes suggestive of PE (see p. 200–203)
- Bronchoscopy
  - Should be considered for most patients, as it will allow visualisation and tissue diagnosis of proximal bronchial lesions. Bronchioalveolar lavage can be sent for cytology as well
- V/Q scan
  - Good for revealing PE
- CT chest
  - CT pulmonary angiography is the gold standard for detecting PEs
  - High resolution CT scan can give detailed images of lesions, and is particularly useful for showing distal lesions inaccessible to bronchoscopy, and showing lymph node involvement

Causes

- Bronchial
  - Carcinoma (primary or secondary)
  - Bronchiectasis
  - Acute bronchitis
  - Acute exacerbation of COPD (see p. 212–214)
  - Foreign body
- Parenchymal lung disease
  - Pneumonia—can cause bleeding, but early pneumococcal infection can produce 'rust coloured' sputum (see p. 208–211)
  - Pulmonary TB
  - Lung abscess
  - Lung trauma
  - Aspergilloma—usually in immunosupressed patients
  - Wegener's granulomatosis
  - Actinomycosis
  - SLE—lupus pneumonitis
  - Pulmonary endometriosis
- Pulmonary vascular disease
  - PE (see p. 200–203)
  - Polyarteritis nodosa
  - Goodpasture's syndrome
  - Arteriovenous malformation—more common in patients with hereditary haemorrhagic telangiectasia

- Idiopathic pulmonary haemosiderosis
- Pulmonary hypertension (e.g. secondary to mitral stenosis)
- Cardiovascular disorders
  - Acute left ventricular failure (see p. 144–146)
- Coagulopathy
  - Leukaemia
  - Haemophilia
  - Anticoagulant use (see p. 112–115)

Further reading

- *OHCM*, 7th edn, Oxford: Oxford University Press, p. 62.
- *Oxford Textbook of Medicine*, 4th edn, vol. 2. Oxford: Oxford University Press, p. 1284, 1480.

☼ Reduced oxygen saturation

This can be a very common call to see a patient owing to the widespread use of pulse oximeters. It is vitally important to differentiate this from hypoxia (failure to deliver adequate oxygen to the body tissues), which requires urgent treatment. Pulse oximeters are a useful screening/monitoring tool for this, but can also be falsely reassuring or worrying. This is where a good grounding in basic physiology will enable treatment of patients correctly and safely.

The pulse oximeter

The pulse oximeter works by measuring the absorbance of known wavelengths of light (660 nm and 940 nm) in arterial blood flow, and from this it can determine what percentage of the haemoglobin is saturated with oxygen in the arteries (SpO_2). It does not tell you concentration of haemoglobin, oxygen (PaO_2) or carbon dioxide ($PaCO_2$) in the arterial blood. These measures are required for an accurate assessment of respiratory function and oxygen delivery, and can only be obtained from an ABG sample. The pulse oximeter requires adequate peripheral perfusion to give an accurate reading.

Immediate management

- Assess ABC
  - Ensure airway obstruction is not the cause
  - Give high flow O_2 via non-rebreath mask initially—hypoxia kills before hypercapnia
  - Take ABGs (see below)
  - ☎ Involve ITU team early if intubation/mechanical ventilation is looking likely (i.e. poor response to treatment)
- If patient has COPD (see p. 212–214)
  - Give minimum FiO_2 required to prevent hypoxia (aim for PaO_2 >8 kPa)—use Venturi mask
  - If this is causing retention of CO_2, then NIV should be considered
- Rapid identification of the underlying cause, and treatment of it, is vital

History

- How long has the patient had a low SaO_2?
  - ↓SaO_2 can be acceptable in certain circumstances—stable COPD, cyanotic congenital heart disease, large pulmonary AV shunts
  - Does this patient need any intervention? (i.e. are they hypoxic?)
- Any symptoms to suggest cause?
  - Cough—pneumonia (purulent sputum), PE (haemoptysis), pulmonary oedema (frothy, pink sputum)
  - SOB (see p. 28–31)
  - Chest pain (see p. 24–27)
  - Pyrexia—sepsis
- Are there any symptoms of end organ hypoxia?
  - Confusion/↓GCS

- Angina
- SOB
- Arrhythmia/palpitations
- Nausea/vomiting
- Hypotension or hypertension
- Is there any PMHx suggestive of chronic respiratory illness?
  - Do you need to be cautious with O_2 therapy?
  - COPD, heavy smoking, restrictive chest pathology (e.g. severe kyphoscoliosis), occupational history (e.g. mining, asbestos exposure)
- Is there any PMHx of likely causative disease
  - e.g. asthma, IHD/heart failure, DVT/PE

Examination

- General
  - Check GCS—hypoxia causes confusion initially, then coma
  - Clubbing (may suggest chronic suppurative lung disease), signs of anaemia, body habitus (obesity, cachexia)
  - Signs of CO_2 retention—coarse tremor, bounding pulses, warm peripheries, hyperaemic conjunctivae
  - Check for cervical lymphadenopathy
- Assess work of breathing
  - Usually increased in most acute situations
  - If decreased, think about hypoventilation (e.g. failure of hypoxic respiratory drive, opiate overdose, decompensating respiratory illness)
- Full respiratory examination

Investigations

- Arterial blood gases (see p. 422–424)
  - Determine if the patient is in respiratory failure ($PaO_2 < 8$ kPa) and, if so, what type?
  - If the patient is chronically hypoxic and clinically well, do they require treatment?

Pattern of changes in ABGs with type 1 and type 2 respiratory failure				
	Type 1		Type 2	
	Acute	Chronic	Acute	Chronic
PaO_2	↓↓	↓	↓	↓
$PaCO_2$	↔/↓	↔	↑	↑
pH	↔/↓	↔	↓	↓/↔
HCO_3^-/BE	↔	↔	↔	↑

- FBC and CRP
  - ↓Hb will exacerbate hypoxia and ↑Hb will occur in chronic hypoxia
  - ↑WCC + ↑CRP should make you seek infection
- CXR
  - Check for any respiratory pathology

Causes

The vast majority of causes for ↓SpO$_2$ are respiratory, either primary (e.g. PE, pneumonia) or secondary (e.g. pulmonary oedema due to acute heart failure). The clinical picture will help to guide your diagnosis.

Acute type 1 respiratory failure

A primary insult will cause hypoxia, and the response will be to increase ventilation. The patient will have increased work of breathing. Acidosis may be caused by tissue hypoxia leading to anaerobic metabolism (lactic acidosis).

- Acute exacerbation of asthma (see p. 196–198)
- Acute exacerbation of COPD—with normal respiratory drive (see p. 212–214)
- Pulmonary oedema—e.g. due to acute heart failure (see p. 144–146)
- PE (see p. 200–203)
- Pneumonia (see p. 208–211)
- Pneumothorax (see p. 204–207)
- Acute respiratory distress syndrome

Acute type 2 respiratory failure

This will be caused by failure of ventilation (owing to ↓respiratory rate ± ↓tidal volume). The patient may have reduced work of breathing, or may be severely compromised despite working hard. Hypercapnia may cause a respiratory acidosis.

- ❶ Life-threatening asthma—decompensating (see p. 196–198)
- ❶ Severe manifestation of causes of type 1 respiratory failure
- Inhaled foreign body
- Drug overdose—e.g. opioids (see p. 420–421)
- Flail chest
- Brainstem lesion
- Respiratory muscle paralysis (e.g. Guillain–Barré syndrome)
- Acute epiglottitis

Chronic type 1 respiratory failure

These patients will have longstanding lung disease, but will still have a normal respiratory drive. They may have a chronically low PaO$_2$, but they can easily develop acute on chronic failure if there are any additional insults (e.g. infection).

- COPD (see p. 212–214)
- Fibrosing alveolitis
- Anaemia
- Carcinoma
- Lymphangitis
- Right to left shunt (intracardiac or extracardiac)

Chronic type 2 respiratory failure

These patients will have chronic obstructive and/or restrictive lung disease, and will have developed a hypoxic drive due to chronic hypercapnia. An acute insult can severely compromise oxygenation. Caution must be used with oxygen therapy, as too much O_2 will reduce respiratory drive and lead to hypercapnia and respiratory acidosis. NIV will be necessary if a balance between hypoxia and hypercapnia cannot be achieved. Prognosis if mechanical ventilation is required is very poor, so failure of NIV should be discussed with the patient and their family.

- COPD (see p. 212–214)
- Severe kyphoscoliosis
- Severe ankylosing spondylitis
- Respiratory muscle failure (e.g. muscular dystrophies)

Further reading

- *OHCM*, 7th edn. Oxford: Oxford University Press, p. 148, 172.
- *Oxford Textbook of Medicine*, 4th edn, vol. 2. Oxford: Oxford University Press, p. 1308.

① **Palpitations**

Palpitations describe the increased awareness of the heartbeat, and can be very worrying for patients. The common usage of the word 'palpitations' can vary, however, so it is important to ask the patient specifically what they mean if they describe this as a symptom. Often they will not cause serious problems, but it is essential to rule out the rarer, more serious causes.

Immediate management

- Assess ABC
  - Start high flow O_2 via non-rebreath mask—tachyarrhythmias may reduce cardiac output leading to reduced tissue oxygen delivery
  - ❶ Check central pulse—if absent or inadequate start ALS (see Inside cover)
  - Attach cardiac monitor—observe rate, rhythm (regular or irregular) and QRS complexes (broad or narrow)
  - Gain large bore IV access into large, proximal vein
  - Any IV drugs given may require large flushes and elevation of the limb as circulation might be sluggish
- ❶ Are there any signs of imminent collapse?
  - Heart rate <40/min or >150/min (broad QRS) or >200/min (narrow QRS)
  - Systolic BP <90 mmHg
  - Low cardiac output (pallor, sweating, SOB, ↑CRT, ↓GCS)
  - Chest pain
  - History of heart failure (can decompensate quickly)
- ►► If YES ☎ Seek help (ideally from a cardiologist)
- Bradycardia
  - Atropine, 0.5 mg boluses IV (repeat up to total 3 mg if required)
  - Transthoracic or percussive pacing
  - For further management, see p. 164–166
- Tachycardia
  - Will require sedation or general anaesthetic (demands experience of giving sedation/anaesthesia)
  - ⚠ Cardioversion whilst conscious is excruciatingly painful and should be avoided
  - **Synchronized** DC cardioversion—100J: 200J: 360J (or biphasic equivalent)
  - ⚠ Ensure that machine is set to synchronized mode. If it is not, R on T can precipitate VF

History

This can be vital in paroxysmal episodes, as definitive ECG diagnosis can often be difficult to attain (patient has to be monitored during episode).

- What is the rhythm? It is helpful to ask the patient to clap out how they feel their heart beating
  - Irregular—AF, frequent ectopics, atrial tachycardia/flutter with variable AV block

- Fast (especially >120/min)—tachyarrhythmia (SVT/AF, VT)
- Normal/slightly fast (i.e. 90–120/min) 'pounding' heart—most likely physiological/psychogenic
- 'One-offs' or 'missing beat'—ectopics
- Slow rate (i.e. <60/min)—bradyarrhythmias (rarely) can present with palpitations, usually with forceful, slow beats felt. Runs of VT can also occur with slow heart rates
- Onset
  - Sudden—SVT/AF, VT
  - Gradual—physiological
  - Associated with anxiety—psychogenic
  - Related to exertion—physiological, SVT/AF
- Frequency of attacks
  - Guides further investigation and management—are they actually troublesome for the patient?
- Duration
  - Seconds—ectopic beats
  - Minutes/hours—SVT/AF
  - Continuous—physiological
- Associated symptoms
  - Angina, syncope/presyncope, SOB—is there underlying cardiac disease
  - Polyuria—SVT (due to ANP release)
- PMHx and SHx
  - History of rhythm disturbance
  - Previous IHD, valvular disease, cardiac surgery—risk factors of arrhythmia
  - Known heart failure—arrhythmia more likely to cause haemodynamic compromise
  - Hyperthyroidism and other endocrine conditions
  - Alcohol, caffeine, drugs and smoking—can all precipitate arrhythmias
- DHx
  - β_2 agonists, digoxin, L-dopa, tricyclic antidepressants, adriamycin, doxorubicin—can trigger arrhythmias

Examination

Apart from the initial survey to check for circulatory sufficiency, examination is mainly to find evidence of underlying heart disease.

- General examination
  - Look for signs of hyperthyroidism
- Assess pulse
  - Rate (apical vs. peripheral), rhythm, volume and character
- JVP
  - Is it raised?—R heart failure, volume overload
  - A waves—absent in AF, enlarged in tricuspid stenosis and pulmonary hypertension
  - Large V waves—tricuspid regurgitation
  - Cannon waves—3rd degree heart block, atrial flutter, ventricular ectopics

- Inspect and palpate precordium—look for underlying cardiac disease
  - Scars from previous surgery?
  - Any heaves or thrills?
  - Assess apical impulse
- Auscultate heart
  - Check rate—not all beats may be palpable as pulses
  - Listen for murmurs—mitral stenosis commonly causes AF
  - Any added heart sounds?
- Auscultate chest—any evidence of pulmonary oedema

Investigations

- ECG
  - This is the most important investigation, and is often diagnostic if captured during an attack. For this reason, telemetry and ambulatory ECGs can be very valuable
  - Remember to record a rhythm strip when doing anything to correct an arrhythmia
  - Bradycardias—rate <60 bpm—see p. 164–166
  - SVT—rate >100 bpm, regular rhythm, QRS <120 ms—see p. 172–176
  - AF—rate >100 bpm, irregularly irregular rhythm, absent P waves—see p. 178–182
  - VT—rate >100 bpm, QRS >120 ms—see p. 184–186
- FBC
  - Anaemia can cause sinus tachycardia
- U&Es and bone profile
  - Electrolyte disturbance can cause arrhythmia (especially $\uparrow K^+$)
- TFT
  - Thyrotoxicosis can cause sinus tachycardia or precipitate other arrhythmias (e.g. AF)
- 24-hour urine catecholamines
  - Small print. Send to exclude phaeochromocytoma in hypertensive patients (very rare)

Causes

Cardiac (further causes listed in related chapters)

- SVT (see p. 172–176)
- AF (see p. 178–182)
- VT (see p. 184–186)
- Ectopic beats (atrial or ventricular)
- Sinus node disease/AV block (see p. 164–166)

Non-cardiac

- Pain (see p. 10–11)
- Exertion
- Psychogenic/abnormal awareness of normal rhythm
- Hypoxia (see p. 36–39)
- Sepsis (see p. 304–306)
- Hypovolaemia (see p. 96–100)
- Anaemia
- GORD

- Thyrotoxicosis (see p. 234–235)
- Phaeochromocytoma (rare)
- Carcinoid syndrome (rare)
- Autonomic instability (rare)

Further reading

- *OHCM*, 7th edn. Oxford: Oxford University Press, p. 66, 80.
- *Oxford Textbook of Medicine*, 4th edn, vol. 2. Oxford: Oxford University Press, p. 845.
- *Oxford Handbook of Emergencies in Cardiology*, 1st edn. Oxford: Oxford University Press, p. 37.

☠ Haematemesis

Haematemesis is the vomiting of blood from an upper GI bleed. Often, it is only small flecks of blood in the vomitus, but it can be very severe and lead to exsanguination within minutes. This can be the terminal illness in chronic liver disease, in which case thought should be given to discussing with the patient and family how far treatment should go.

Immediate management

Airway
- The patient should be positioned on their side to protect against aspiration
- Consider large bore NG tube if patient is struggling to maintain airway
- Airway management can become extremely difficult. ☎ Call anaesthetist if there are any difficulties

Breathing
- Administer high flow O_2 via non-rebreath mask
  - Oxygenation of tissues may be compromised owing to blood loss
  - Remove whilst patient is vomiting, as it may encourage aspiration
- Check ABGs regularly
  - Lactic acidosis may indicate failure to oxygenate tissues—give more O_2 or transfuse blood

Circulation
- Regularly assess for haemodynamic compromise
  - Check HR, BP, CRT, JVP and UO
- Insert at least two large bore cannulae and take bloods as detailed below
  - ⚠ Remember to label G&S correctly to avoid delay in processing
  - Send crossmatch for at least 4 units of red cells
- Measure vomit volume to aid impression of blood loss
- Catheterize and monitor UO—should be >0.5 ml/kg/hr
- Reverse anticoagulation if on warfarin (see p. 112–115)
- Give fluid boluses if haemodynamically compromised (see p. 6–8)
  - Initially, use colloids or normal saline to maintain BP
  - Give blood if there is significant bleeding—if waiting for cross-match, consider using O negative or type-specific
  - If large volumes are being transfused, heat the blood/fluid to avoid hypothermia
  - Consider platelet and FFP transfusions if large volumes of red cells are being transfused. ☎ Discuss with haematologist
- Consider central line insertion to guide fluid management

Stop the bleeding
- ☎ Call surgical, endoscopic and anaesthetic teams to arrange definitive treatment in theatre (e.g. endoscopy or surgery)
- If suspicious of variceal bleeding
  - Give vasopressin analogue to reduce splanchnic blood flow, e.g. terlipressin, 2 mg IV every 4–6 h
  - Insert Sengstaken tube (if you are familiar with the technique) to buy time for endoscopy
  - Consider prophylactic ABx, e.g. ciprofloxacin, 200 mg IV over 30 min
- Start PPI
  - Omeprazole, 40 mg in 100 ml normal saline IV over 30 min

History
- Has the patient had any melaena? (dark, smelly, sticky stool)
  - This indicates a significant bleed
  - Red blood PR can occur in rapid haemorrhage (haemochezia)
- PMHx
  - Any previous significant GI haemorrhage? This increases the risk of severe haemorrhage
  - Is there any history suggestive of liver disease or portal hypertension? Be very suspicious of bleeding varices and consider coagulopathy
  - Does the patient have a history of *Helicobacter pylori* infection or peptic ulcer disease?
  - Has the patient been vomiting recently? Consider Mallory–Weiss tear
  - Are there any symptoms of underlying malignancy (anorexia, weight loss, altered bowel habit, pain)? Could there be liver metastases?
- DHx and SHx
  - Drugs which increase risk of peptic ulcers—NSAIDS, corticosteroids, smoking, alcohol
  - Take a careful alcohol history—don't forget to plan for alcohol withdrawal if patient is going to be admitted (see p. 258–260)

Examination
- General examination
  - Is the patient cachexic?
  - Are there any stigmata of chronic liver disease? For example, encephalopathy, clubbing, palmar erythema, bruising, jaundice, spider naevi, gynaecomastia, oedema
- Chest
  - Has the patient aspirated? Remember to cover anaerobes as well if suspicious (i.e. metronidazole)
  - Is there a pleural effusion? This can be caused by hypoalbuminaemia
- Abdomen
  - Signs of liver disease—hepatomegaly, ascites, caput medusa
  - Epigastric tenderness may suggest peptic ulcer
  - Peritonitis may be due to perforated ulcer
  - Perform PR and check for melaena

Investigations

- FBC
  - Get baseline Hb level, and monitor daily. NB There is often a delay of several hours between a large bleed and a drop in Hb
  - Is the patient thrombocytopenic? If so, consider platelet transfusion
- Coagulation screen
  - Check for and treat any coagulopathy. ☎ Discuss with haematolgist
  - Is also good indicator of liver synthetic function
- U&Es
  - ↑Urea is a good indicator of significant GI bleed (caused by gut absorption of protein from digested blood)
  - Carefully monitor electrolytes if patient is requiring large amounts of IV fluid
- LFTs
  - Derangement may suggest a hepatic cause giving rise to portal hypertension; however, patients with severe liver impairment may have normal liver enzyme levels
- Erect CXR and AXR
  - If patient is peritonitic, check for evidence of perforation
  - Check for aspiration pneumonitis if patient is SOB
- Upper GI endoscopy
  - Often both diagnostic and therapeutic

Causes

- Peptic ulcer disease
- Gastroduodenal erosions
- Oesophagitis
- Varices
- Mallory–Weiss tear
- Swallowed blood from upper respiratory tract (e.g. epistaxis)
- Upper GI malignancy
- Vascular malformations
- Aortoduodenal fistula following aortic graft (rare)

Further reading

- British Society of Gastroenterology Endoscopy Committee. Non-variceal upper gastrointestinal haemorrhage: guidelines. *Gut* 2002; **51**(Suppl. IV):iv1–iv6.
- Jalan R, Hayes PC. UK guidelines on the management of variceal haemorrhage in cirrhotic patients. *BSG Guidelines in Gastroenterology*, June 2000.
- *OHCM*, 7th edn. Oxford: Oxford University Press, p. 244, 804.
- *Oxford Textbook of Medicine*, 4th edn, vol. 2. Oxford: Oxford University Press, p. 511
- Transfusion management of acute blood loss. UK blood transfusion and tissue transplantation services. *Handbook of Transfusion Medicine*, 3rd edn. (www.transfusionguidelines.org.uk)

☼ **Severe acute lower gastrointestinal bleeding**

This is passage of large amounts of maroon diarrhoea or fresh blood from the rectum, accompanied by evidence of hypovolaemic shock. This is a potentially life-threatening presentation, and has a mortality rate of 10–20%. If the patient has melaena (passage of black, tarry stool), treat as for haematemesis (see p. 44–46).

Initial management

- ABC assessment
  - Give high flow O_2 via a non-rebreath mask
- Regularly assess for haemodynamic compromise
  - Check HR, BP, CRT, JVP and UO
- Insert at least two large bore cannulae and take bloods as detailed below
  - △ Remember to label G&S correctly to avoid delay in processing
  - Send sample for crossmatch
- Measure blood losses to aid impression of blood loss
- Catheterize and monitor UO—should be >0.5 ml/kg/h
- Reverse anticoagulation if on warfarin (see p. 112–115)
- Give fluid boluses if haemodynamically compromised (see p. 6–8)
  - Initially, use colloids or normal saline to maintain BP
  - Give blood if there is significant bleeding—if waiting for crossmatch, consider using O negative or type-specific
  - If large volumes are being transfused, heat the blood/fluid to avoid hypothermia
  - Consider platelet and FFP transfusions if large volumes of red cells are being transfused. ☎ Discuss with haematologist
- Consider central line insertion to guide fluid management
- ☎ Call for urgent surgical/gastro team help
- Consider antibiotic treatment
  - If peritonitis/perforation is suspected: cefuroxime, 1.5 g TDS IV *and* metronidazole, 500 mg TDS IV
  - If *Clostridium difficile* infection is suspected: metronidazole, 400 mg TDS PO *and* consider stopping other antibiotic therapy
- Bleeding will most often stop spontaneously, but if it does not
  - More definitive management may involve colonoscopy, selective embolization or surgery

History

- Nature of the bleeding
  - Bright red blood surrounding stool is suggestive of anorectal cause
  - Bleeding mixed with diarrhoea and mucus suggests colitis
- Any previous bleeding?
  - Can give a clue as to underlying diagnosis (e.g. diverticular disease, angiodysplasia)
  - Risk factors for diverticular disease—age, low fibre diet, constipation

- Any risk factors for upper GI bleed?
  - Could this be a large upper GI bleed? (haemochezia)
- Recent colonoscopy/surgery
  - Bleed may be from polypectomy or surgical site
- Past history of inflammatory bowel disease
- Has the patient had any history of weight loss or altered bowel habit?
  - May indicate neoplastic cause (although this rarely causes large haemorrhage)
- DHx
  - Check for anticoagulant use
  - Angiodysplasia most often occurs in patients on long-term anticoagulation, e.g. aortic valve replacement
  - History of antibiotic use predisposes to pseudomembranous colitis (*C. difficile* infection)

Examination

- General examination
  - Are there any signs suggestive of neoplasia? For example, cachexia, signs of chronic anaemia (e.g. nail changes), jaundice (suggests liver metastases)
- Abdomen
  - Check for peritonitis—rigidity, guarding, rebound/percussive tenderness
  - Left iliac fossa tenderness is common with diverticular disease
  - Hepatomegaly may suggest liver metastasis of GI malignancy
- PR examination
  - Check for perianal indications of IBD—skin tags, fistula, inflammation
  - Are there any haemorrhoids?
  - Extreme pain/inability to tolerate examination could suggest anal fissure
  - Feel for any masses suggestive of rectal carcinoma
  - Examine stool—fresh blood suggests rectal pathology, blood mixed with stool suggests bleeding from high up, mucus suggests IBD or colitis

Investigations

- FBC and CRP
  - Monitor Hb and consider transfusion if low. NB Hb may not drop for several hours after a large bleed
  - ↑WCC and ↑CRP occur with diverticulitis, IBD and colitis
  - ↓MCV may indicate chronic iron deficiency owing to GI malignancy
- U&Es
  - Monitor electrolytes if patient is requiring large amounts of IV fluid
  - ↑Urea could indicate bleeding from higher up in the GI tract
- LFTs
  - Deranged LFTs should make you consider liver metastases
- Lactate
  - Markedly raised lactate occurs with bowel infarction/ischaemia (but will also occur in severe hypovolaemic shock)

- Erect CXR/AXR
  - Check for signs of perforation if patient is peritonitic
  - Check for a toxic megacolon if IBD/colitis is suspected
- Colonoscopy
  - Can be diagnostic and therapeutic
  - Extreme caution should be used if colitis is suspected as there is a greatly increased risk of perforation
  - There are differing views on whether bowel preparation is necessary—use local guidelines

Causes

- Diverticular disease—accounts for 60% of patients
- Inflammatory bowel disease (see p. 252–255)
- *C. difficile* infection (pseudomembranous colitis)
- Colonic angiodysplasia
- Inferior mesenteric artery ischaemia/infarction
- Meckel's diverticulum
- GI malignancy (rarely causes severe haemorrhage)
- Coagulopathy
- Arteriovenous malformation
- Anorectal disease, e.g. haemorrhoids, anal fissure (rarely causes severe haemorrhage)
- Intussusception
- Colonic polyps, e.g. idiopathic, familial adenomatous polyposis, Peutz–Jegher's syndrome

Further reading

- *OHCM*, 7th edn. Oxford: Oxford University Press, p. 589.
- *Oxford Textbook of Medicine*, 4th edn, vol. 2. Oxford: Oxford University Press, p. 512.

☼ **Abdominal pain**

Abdominal pain may be the presenting symptom of numerous conditions both within and without the abdominal cavity. Although there is an extensive list of differential diagnoses, common things will always be common. Management may often be more symptomatic; of the group of patients admitted to hospital with abdominal pain, not all will leave with a diagnosis.

Immediate management

- ABC

⚠ If, after ABC assessment, a worrying clinical picture is emerging, call for help immediately. There is little merit in delaying senior assessment of a pulsatile abdominal mass in the presence of hypotension to permit completion of a detailed history
- History and examination
- Request a minimum of hourly observations until patient has been reviewed by senior colleague
- Ask nursing staff to check capillary blood glucose level
- Initiate accurate fluid balance
- Make nil by mouth, communicating this to patient, relatives and staff
- Request an urgent ECG
- Administer analgesia with antiemetic as required
- Urinary catheterization
  - In critically ill patients or those with urological co-morbidities
  - Essential for accurate fluid balance assessment, particularly in pancreatitis
- Nasogastric tube
  - Decompresses upper GI tract, reducing risk of vomiting and subsequent aspiration
  - Use in the critically ill or those with vomiting secondary to obstruction
  - NG tubes should not be used routinely
- Investigations as detailed
- Consider antibiotic administration if infection suspected (see local protocols)
- If by now any operative decisions have been made, do the on-call theatre team leader and anaesthetist know?

History

With the range of conditions that present as abdominal pain, it is vital to take a detailed history and perform a thorough examination. Where the patient is unable to provide a history, family or carers should be questioned. Alternatively, GP surgeries will hold information on medication and chronic diseases.

Nature of the pain

- Timing
  - Sudden or gradual onset. Be very suspicious of 'snap' onset of abdominal pain, given its association with aneurysmal causes
  - Constant or intermittent
- Location (see Figure 2.1)
- Previous episodes—has the patient experienced this pain or other abdominal symptoms previously, if so, establish nature of investigations and presumed diagnosis
- Description
  - Colicky, wavelike, cramping, burning, stabbing, sharp, dull, aching, throbbing?
  - Remember that renal colic is a true colic, whereas biliary colic is in fact a much more constant pain
- Aggravating or precipitating factors
  - Did anything happen before the pain came, such as eating?
  - Does anything make the pain worse or better (eating, drinking, coughing, movement, lying still, urination, defecation)?
- Radiation
  - Does the pain spread or does it stay in one place?
  - Has it moved from where it was first felt? (e.g. the classic migration of appendicitis pain from vague central abdomen to right iliac fossa)
  - Does it radiate to the back, round to the side, to the tip of the shoulder or the groin?

Associated features

- Bowel habit
  - When was last stool and what was its nature?
  - Alteration of bowel habit and stool nature, particularly the presence of mucus, blood (fresh or altered) and tar-like stool
- Genitourinary features
  - Frequency, polyuria, haematuria, dysuria, discharge, pneumaturia and frequent UTIs
  - PV bleeding
  - Sexual history and contraceptive usage (could this be an ectopic pregnancy?)
- Diet and appetite
  - General assessment of nutritional status
  - Nature of appetite, weight loss (intentional or otherwise), fit of clothes
- Nausea and vomiting
  - Timing of nausea and relation to other factors
  - Nature of vomit—foodstuffs, bilious, bloodstained, effortless or retching
- Systemic features
  - Fevers, rigors, sweating, headaches, visual disturbance, rash, allergy

Past medical history

- Previous admissions with abdominal symptoms
- Previous abdominal, pelvic, genitourinary or gynaecological surgery

- Obstetric history
- Cardiovascular and respiratory disease?

Drug and alcohol intake
- Full history of nature and quantity of alcohol and drugs consumed
- Important for diagnosis and also in perioperative management (withdrawal)
- Triangulate information with friends and family if clinical suspicion of dependency

Pharmaceutical history
- Special attention to steroid and NSAID use, hypoglycaemic agents, anticonvulsants, antihypertensives, anticoagulants and antiarrhythmics

Examination
- General appearance
  - In pain, comfortable
  - Well nourished, dehydrated, dishevelled, neglected, unkempt
  - Flushed, jaundiced, pale
  - Walking aids, medic alert bracelets, tattoos
- Cardiovascular
  - Pulse rate, rhythm and character
  - Blood pressure, JVP
  - Auscultation—cardiac and carotid
  - Hands—tobacco use, clubbing and tremors
  - Peripheral pulses, ankle oedema
- Respiratory
  - Rate and pattern of breathing
  - Auscultation—dullness, hyper-resonance, wheeze
  - Cyanosis (peripheral and central)
  - Gynaecomastia and spider naevi
- Abdomen
  - Scarring, stoma and drainage systems
  - Bruising, erythema, visible masses, distension, dilated veins or peristalsis
  - Rigidity, guarding and rebound tenderness
  - Area of maximal tenderness and its relationship to the area of pain
  - Auscultation—bowel sounds and bruits
  - Palpable masses—pulsatile or expansile?
  - Urinary bladder palpable?
  - Shifting dullness if distended
- Perform PR and carefully examine all hernial orifices and external genitalia

Investigations

Bloods
- FBC
  - Evidence of anaemia or sepsis, from haemoglobin and white cell count with differential respectively?
  - Be wary of white cell interpretation in the young and the extremely unwell; aberrant immune response may be a feature

- LFTs
  - Establish pattern of dysfunction (see p. 84–88)
  - Is there evidence of chronic (raised ALT) or acute (raised GGT) alcohol abuse?
- U&Es
  - Renal function and hydration status?
  - Electrolyte abnormalities may reflect both acute and chronic disease—crucial for assessment of sepsis and DKA
- Calcium
  - Important in pancreatitis assessment
  - May reflect chronic renal dysfunction or underlying malignancy
- Clotting profile is unlikely to be of use unless patient is known to be anticoagulated or there is concern over synthetic liver function
- Amylase
  - Useful in determining pancreatic causes of abdominal pain where levels are very high
  - Be suspicious of normal amylase with clinical picture of pancreatitis—late presenting patients may have normal levels
  - Also elevated in other causes of abdominal pain; useful in supporting the diagnosis of mesenteric ischaemia
- CRP
  - May point to an inflammatory cause for pain
  - Provides a useful baseline from which to assess progress or deterioration
- Blood cultures—appropriately taken before administration of antibiotics in septic patients
- Serum glucose
  - Important in assessment of the known diabetic patient and in pancreatitis
  - Hyperglycaemia is a cause of pain in its own right
- G&S
  - Prudent in abdominal presentations where there is potential for operation
  - If suspicious of AAA, discuss with senior whether crossmatching immediately may be more appropriate
- ABG sampling
  - Objective information on the degree and type of metabolic derangements
  - Allows directed therapy; sequential sampling provides evidence of response
  - Is an arterial line indicated?

Urine
- Urinalysis
  - Genitourinary sepsis as a cause for the pain?
  - Haematuria suggestive of renal tract pathology, but consider AAA or appendicitis
  - Ensure the sample is sent for C&S
- Urinary β-HCG for pregnancy—mandatory in female patients of reproductive age

Imaging
- Abdominal X-ray
  - Useful in the diagnosis of intestinal obstruction; may provide indication of the level of obstruction
  - May identify the presence of stones in renal colic
  - For most other causes of abdominal pain, lacks specificity and sensitivity—will this radiation dose aid management?
- Erect CXR
  - Good quality departmental film, taken after the patient has been sat up for 10 minutes. In the critically ill a lateral decubitus view is an alternative
  - May identify air under the diaphragm in a perforated viscus, along with pulmonary disease processes which may mimic abdominal pain
  - Often required by anaesthetist prior to operation
- Ultrasound
  - Increasing prominence in investigation of acute abdominal pain
  - Should be available in most surgical units
  - Allows identification of biliary disease, AAA, splenic pathology and to an extent pancreatic abnormalities. Renal tract and pelvic organs, including appendix and ovaries, may be assessed and it may be used to show free fluid and collections, assisting their drainage where appropriate
- CT scan
  - May provide valuable diagnostic and operative planning information in stable patients
  - Should not be considered in the unstable patient

Differential diagnosis

The conditions marked ❶ are those which are potentially rapidly life-threatening and likely to need surgical intervention or higher dependency care. Consider also that others, especially malignancy, may be presenting for the first time—a missed diagnosis can be life-threatening beyond the immediate situation.

- Gastric
  - Gastroenteritis
  - Dyspepsia/peptic ulcer disease
  - ❶ Perforated ulcer
  - Gastric malignancy
  - ❶ Hiatus hernia—gastric volvulus
- Small bowel
  - ❶ Intestinal obstruction (see p. 368–370)
  - ❶ Perforated ulcer
  - Mesenteric adenitis
  - ❶ Ischaemic bowel
  - Gastroenteritis
  - Inflammatory bowel disease (see p. 252–254)
  - Irritable bowel syndrome
  - Intussusception
  - Meckel's diverticulum
  - *Yersinia* infection
  - Pseudo-obstruction (see p. 368–370)

- Hepatobiliary
  - Hepatitis
  - ❶ Ascending cholangitis (see p. 256–257)
  - Cholecystitis
  - ❶ Perforation of gallbladder (ischaemic)
  - Biliary colic
  - ❶ Pancreatitis (see p.372–375)
  - Pancreatic malignancy
- Renal
  - Pyelonephritis (see p. 262–264)
  - Ureteric colic (see p. 266–268)
  - Renal malignancy
- Large bowel
  - Diverticulitis
  - ❶ Appendicitis (see p. 376–378)
  - Constipation
  - ❶ Ischaemic bowel
  - Inflammatory bowel disease (see p. 252–255)
  - ❶ Mechanical obstruction (see p. 368–370)
  - Pseudo-obstruction (see p. 368–370)
  - ❶ Sigmoid volvulus
  - Malignancy
- Vascular
  - ❶ Aortic aneurysm (see p. 364–366)
- Gynaecological/genitourinary
  - Urinary tract infection
  - Testicular torsion (see p. 280–281)
  - Epididymo-orchitis
  - ❶ Ectopic pregnancy
  - ❶ Ovarian torsion
  - Ovarian cyst
  - Mittelschmerz
  - Dysmenorrhoea
  - Pregnancy
  - Endometriosis
  - Pelvic inflammatory disease
- Other
  - ❶ Pulmonary embolism (see p. 200–203)
  - Lower lobe pneumonia (see p. 208–211)
  - ❶ Acute coronary syndrome (see p. 134–143)
  - ❶ Diabetic ketoacidosis (see p. 220–222)
  - ❶ Sickle cell crisis

Further reading

- *OHCM*, 7th edn. Oxford: Oxford University Press, p. 580.
- *Oxford Textbook of Medicine*, 4th edn, vol. 2. Oxford: Oxford University Press, p. 488.
- Andersson RE. Meta-analysis of the clinical and laboratory diagnosis of appendicitis. *Br J Surg* 2004; **91(1)**:28–37.
- Bugliosi TF, Meloy TD, Vukov LF. Acute abdominal pain in the elderly. *Ann Emerg Med* 1990; **19(12)**:1383–6.

- Cheung O, Regueiro MD. Inflammatory bowel disease emergencies. *Gastroenterol Clin North Am* 2003; **32(4)**:1269–88.
- De Dombal FT. Acute abdominal pain in the elderly. *J Clin Gastroenterol* 1994; **19(4)**:331–5.
- Ellis H, Calne RY, Watson CJE (2002). *Lecture Notes on General Surgery*, 10th edn. London: Blackwell Science.
- Gore RM *et al.* Helical CT in the evaluation of the acute abdomen. *Am J Roent* 2000; **174**:901–13.
- Jones DJ. ABC of colorectal diseases. Diverticular disease. *BMJ* 1992; **304(6839)**: 1435–7.
- Logan RP, Walker MM. ABC of the upper gastrointestinal tract: epidemiology and diagnosis of *Helicobacter pylori* infection. *BMJ* 2001; **323(7318)**:920–2.
- McLatchie GR, Leaper DJ (2002). *Oxford Handbook of Clinical Surgery*, 2nd edn. Oxford: Oxford University Press.
- Pace S, Burke TF. Intravenous morphine for early pain relief in patients with acute abdominal pain. *Acad Emerg Med* 1996; **3(12)**:1086–92.
- Reilly JM, Tilson MD. Incidence and etiology of abdominal aortic aneurysms. *Surg Clin North Am* 1989; **69(4)**:705–11.
- Russell RCG, Williams NS, Bulstrode CJK (eds) (2004). *Bailey & Love's Short Practice of Surgery*, 24th edn. London: Arnold.
- Schoetz DJ. Uncomplicated diverticulitis. Indications for surgery and surgical management. *Surg Clin North Am* 1993; **73(5)**:965–7.
- Vissers RJ, Abu-Laban RB, McHugh DF. Amylase and lipase in the emergency department evaluation of acute pancreatitis. *J Emerg Med* 1999; **17(6)**:1027–37.

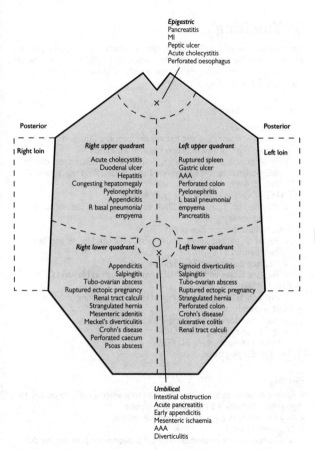

Epigastric
Pancreatitis
MI
Peptic ulcer
Acute cholecystitis
Perforated oesophagus

Posterior

Right loin

Posterior

Left loin

Right upper quadrant

Acute cholecystitis
Duodenal ulcer
Hepatitis
Congesting hepatomegaly
Pyelonephritis
Appendicitis
R basal pneumonia/
empyema

Left upper quadrant

Ruptured spleen
Gastric ulcer
AAA
Perforated colon
Pyelonephritis
L basal pneumonia/
empyema
Pancreatitis

Right lower quadrant

Appendicitis
Salpingitis
Tubo-ovarian abscess
Ruptured ectopic pregnancy
Renal tract calculi
Strangulated hernia
Mesenteric adenitis
Meckel's diverticulitis
Crohn's disease
Perforated caecum
Psoas abscess

Left lower quadrant

Sigmoid diverticulitis
Salpingitis
Tubo-ovarian abscess
Ruptured ectopic pregnancy
Strangulated hernia
Perforated colon
Crohn's disease/
ulcerative colitis
Renal tract calculi

Umbilical
Intestinal obstruction
Acute pancreatitis
Early appendicitis
Mesenteric ischaemia
AAA
Diverticulitis

Fig. 2.1 Causes of abdominal pain

ⓘ **Vomiting**

Vomiting is a complex reflex, which involves many neurological pathways, and therefore has a large number of causes. The initial treatment usually consists of treating the symptoms and effects of the vomiting, then investigating and treating the underlying cause.

Immediate management

- ABC assessment
  - If patient is vomiting and has impaired consciousness, it is vital to secure their airway to protect against aspiration
  - Patients with profuse vomiting (especially with diarrhoea) can be haemodynamically compromised and require fluid resuscitation (see p. 6–8)
- DEFG—Don't ever forget the glucose
  - May be high if patient has DKA, or may be low if patient has persistent vomiting
- Start IV fluid therapy (see p. 6–8)
  - Based on patient's fluid requirement, estimated losses and deficit (see below)
  - Replace deficit over 24–48 hours
  - Replace losses with 0.9% NaCl (vomit is high in Na^+ and Cl^-)
- Check ABGs
  - Hypochloraemic alkalosis indicates severe vomiting
- Start antiemetics
  - e.g. Metoclopramide, 10 mg TDS PO/IV
  - ± Cyclizine, 50 mg TDS PO/IV
  - ± Ondansetron, 4 mg BD PO/IV
- Treat underlying cause

History

- Recent-onset vomiting in an otherwise well adult is likely to be due to gastritis—but this is a diagnosis of exclusion
- Any contact with patients with gastroenteritis?
- Abdominal pain
  - Cramps are very common in gastritis, but severe pain may be due to intra-abdominal causes
  - Also consider inferior MI
- Chest pain—could this be an MI?
- Is the patient postoperative? Consider postoperative nausea and vomiting, paralytic ileus
- Headache, neck stiffness, visual disturbance, early morning vomiting—CNS cause (e.g. ↑ICP, meningitis, encephalitis, space-occupying lesion)
- LMP—is the patient pregnant?
- PMHx
  - Any history of possible cause (see below)
  - Check for history of DM—requires special treatment even if not the underlying cause (see p. 90–91)

- DHx
  - Antibiotics (e.g. erythromycin), opioids, digoxin, cytotoxic drugs
  - Illegal drug use (e.g. opioids)
  - Alcohol

Examination

- General examination
  - Assess the patient's hydration

Dehydration (% of body weight)	0–5% (Mild)	5–10% (Moderate)	>10% (Severe)
Mucous membranes	Wet	Dry	Very dry
Eyes	Normal	Sunken	Deeply sunken
Circulation	Normal	Tachycardic + cool extremities	Tachycardic + signs of hypovolaemia
Skin turgor	Normal	Slightly decreased	Markedly decreased
Urine output	Slightly reduced	Noticeably reduced	Severely reduced
Consciousness	Normal	Usually normal	Lethargy, irritability, coma

  - Check patient's weight, and calculate percentage loss if previous weight was known

    (Current weight/Previous weight) × 100 = Percentage dehydration

    (Percentage dehydration/100) × Previous weight (kg) = Deficit volume (litres)

- CVS
  - Check for signs of hypovolaemia—↑HR, ↓BP, ↓UO, ↑CRT
- RS
  - Look for Kussmaul's respiration—DKA, acidosis
  - Check for signs of aspiration (e.g. crepitations, particularly in right base)
- Abdomen
  - Any tenderness? (see p. 52–59)
  - NB. It is common to get rectus muscle tenderness with prolonged vomiting
  - Is there distension and absent/tinkling bowel sounds? Consider obstruction, paralytic ileus
- Neurological
  - Perform a full neurological examination—be suspicious of intracranial cause if there are any abnormalities
  - Check the fundi—suspect ↑ICP if there is papilloedema
  - Check for meningism (neck stiffness, photophobia, Kernig's sign)— meningitis, SAH
  - Check for nystagmus—labyrinthitis, Ménière's disease, cerebellar causes

Investigations
- FBC and CRP
  - Raised inflammatory markers may suggest an infective cause
  - ↑Hb can occur due to dehydration
- U&Es
  - Check for ↓Na$^+$ as a cause, and monitor whilst rehydrating
  - Monitor K$^+$—can drop due to losses in vomit
  - ↑Urea occurs with dehydration, but uraemia can cause vomiting
  - ↑Creatinine suggests renal impairment—could be cause or effect of vomiting
  - Chloride is lost in vomit, and ↓Cl$^-$ can exacerbate alkalosis
- Glucose
  - Raised in DKA, may be low in persistent vomiting
- ABGs
  - Metabolic hypochloraemic alkalosis indicates severe dehydration
- LFTs
  - Can be deranged in cholecystitis
- Bone profile
  - Check for ↑Ca^{2+} as a cause
- Amylase
  - Check for pancreatitis
- Cortisol
  - Could this be Addisonian crisis?
- Urine microscopy and C&S
  - Could this be a UTI?
- Urine/plasma βHCG
  - Is the patient pregnant?
- ECG
  - Check for evidence of myocardial ischaemia/infarction
- Erect CXR
  - Check for consolidation (aspiration pneumonitis) and for infradiaphragmatic free gas (perforation)
- AXR
  - Check for dilated loops/perforation if obstruction or ileus is suspected
- LP
  - If meningitis, encephalitis or SAH are suspected
  - Contraindicated if ↑ICP present
- CT head
  - Indicated if ↑ICP present—may detect underlying cause

Causes
- Gastrointestinal
  - Gastritis/gastroenteritis
  - Peptic ulcer disease
  - Intestinal obstruction/paralytic ileus (see p. 368–370)
  - Acute cholecystitis (see p. 380–382)
  - Acute pancreatitis (see p. 370–373)
- CNS
  - Meningitis/encephalitis (see p. 328–334)

- Migraine
- ↑ICP
- Ménière's disease
- Labyrinthitis/vestibulitis
- Cerebellar disease
- Metabolic/endocrine
  - DKA (see p. 220–222)
  - Hyponatraemia (see p. 388–390)
  - Hypercalcaemia (see p. 404–406)
  - Uraemia (see p. 270–275)
  - Addisonian crisis
- Drugs
  - Alcohol
  - Antibiotics (e.g. erythromycin)
  - Opioids
  - NSAIDs
  - Cytotoxics
  - Digoxin
- Psychiatric
  - Self-induced
  - Psychogenic
  - Bulimia nervosa
- Other
  - Acute MI (see p. 134–143)
  - UTI
  - Pregnancy
  - Autonomic neuropathy

Further reading

- *OHCM*, 7th edn. Oxford: Oxford University Press, p. 74, 232.
- *Oxford Textbook of Medicine*, 4th edn, vol. 2. Oxford: Oxford University Press, p. 488.
- *Oxford Handbook Gastroenterology and Hepatology*, 1st edn. Oxford: Oxford University Press, p. 89.

⑦ **Sudden weakness**

Sudden weakness is a common presenting complaint. Most will be due to cerebrovascular causes, but it is important to be vigilant in identifying and treating other important causes. Always be aware of any patients who present 'off legs'—are they generally unwell, or do they have lower limb weakness due to neurological disease?

Immediate management

- ABC assessment
  - Make sure that the airway is secure in any obtunded patients
  - Spinal shock can occur in spinal cord problems, leading to a distributive hypovolaemia—this may require fluid resuscitation
- DEFG—Don't ever forget the glucose
  - Hypoglycaemia can cause various neurological symptoms, so should always be ruled out
- Keep patient NBM if there are any concerns about swallowing
- Catheterize if patient is in urinary retention
- If patient is immobile, nurse on a low-pressure mattress, with particular attention paid to bowel and bladder care
  - Pressure sores can develop very quickly, and have serious adverse consequences if this is not done
- ⚠ Call for senior support if there is any evidence of spinal cord involvement—this needs urgent investigation and treatment
- Specific treatment depends on the underlying cause (see below)

History

- Distribution
  - Hemiplegia—this implies an intracranial cause, most likely stroke
  - Paraplegia/quadriplegia—this implies spinal cord involvement, and should be treated as an emergency
  - 'Glove and stocking'—this implies a peripheral neuropathy
- Associated neurological deficits
  - Dysphasia, homonymous hemianopia, inattention—consistent with intracranial causes
  - Urinary retention—consider spinal cord pathology
- Progression
  - ⚠ Rapidly progressing leg weakness requires immediate intervention to identify and treat spinal cord compression
  - Stroke generally has a sudden onset, but can progress in steps over a period of hours
- PMHx
  - Any history of malignancy increases the risk of spinal cord compression
  - History of epilepsy—Todd's paresis
  - History of rheumatoid arthritis—odontoid peg dislocation

- Risk factors for stroke: ↑BP, smoking, DM, cardiac disease (valvular, IHD, AF), peripheral vascular disease, previous TIAs, heavy alcohol consumption, coagulopathy, OCP use, ↑lipids
  - Any recent spinal surgery?
- DHx
  - Is the patient on any anticoagulants? Consider stopping/reversing if stroke is suspected
  - Has the patient taken an overdose?

Examination

- General
  - Is the patient cachexic/jaundiced? Consider underlying malignancy
- CVS
  - Murmurs—valvular heart disease, endocarditis
  - Pulse—is the patient in AF?
  - Check BP—increased risk of haemorrhagic stroke if raised
- Abdominal
  - Check for AAA
  - Check for hepatomegaly—may be due to metastases
- Neurological
  - Determine distribution of lesion (tone, power, reflexes, coordination, sensation)
  - Determine level of lesion if spinal cord problem is suspected
  - Check for associated neurological deficits—dysphasia, hemianopia, inattention, urinary retention
  - Check for saddle paraesthesia and check anal tone if spinal cord pathology suspected
  - Check for papilloedema which could indicate ↑ICP
  - Examine back for any evidence of trauma

Investigations

- MRI spine
  - This takes priority in any patient with a suspected spinal cord compression, and should be ordered urgently
- FBC, CRP, ESR
  - Is there any indication of an inflammatory cause?
  - Polycythaemia can predispose to stroke
- U&Es and glucose
  - Check for underlying electrolyte disturbances and hypoglycaemia
- LFTs
  - May be abnormal if there is metastatic disease
- B_{12} and folate
  - Screen for deficiency—may be underlying cause
- PSA
  - If markedly raised, may indicate source of underlying malignancy
- Syphilis serology
  - Screen for underlying cause
- ECG
  - Check for AF

- Echocardiography
  - Check for valvular disease, vegetations (endocarditis), atrial/mural thrombus
- CXR
  - Look for primary or secondary malignancy or TB
- Carotid Doppler
  - Check for carotid atheroscleroma
- CT head
  - May reveal underlying intracranial cause

Causes
- Intracranial
  - Stroke (see p. 312–316)
  - Intracranial bleed (see p. 318–327)
  - Space-occupying lesion
  - Migraine
  - Multiple sclerosis
  - Todd's paresis
  - Encephalitis
  - Cerebral abscess
  - Subacute pontine demyelination—secondary to rapid correction of hyponatraemia
  - Motor neurone disease
- Spinal cord
  - Spinal cord compression—metastatic malignancy, epidural abscess, disc prolapse, haematoma, intrinsic cord tumour, atlantoaxial subluxation (rheumatoid arthritis)
  - Trauma
  - Transverse myelitis
  - Spinal artery thrombosis
  - Cord vasculitis (polyarteritis nodosa, syphilis)
  - Subacute combined degeneration of the cord (B_{12} deficiency)
  - AAA (see p. 364–367)
- Peripheral nerves
  - Guillain–Barré syndrome
  - Myasthenia gravis
  - Tetanus
  - Botulism
  - Lead poisoning
- Other
  - Hypoglycaemia (see p. 226)
  - Overdose (see p. 408–421)

Further reading
- *OHCM*, 7th edn. Oxford: Oxford University Press, p. 439.

☼ Headache

Headache is a very common complaint in day-to-day life, and will often present to medical services if it is perceived to be severe. The vast majority of headaches are primary, and have a 'benign' cause, although they can be a cause of severe distress to a patient, so symptomatic treatment is important. This section will concentrate on identifying secondary headaches, which may have a more serious underlying pathology requiring intervention.

Immediate management

- ABC assessment
  - Patients with certain conditions may become obtunded, so will need to have their airway secured
  - Septic patients may require fluid resuscitation (see p. 6–8)
- If there is any suspicion of meningitis, start IV antibiotics immediately
  - e.g. cefotaxime, 2 g QDS IV
- Give adequate analgesia

History

- Onset of pain
  - 'Thunderclap' headache or description of a pain that feels like 'being hit on the back of the head' is classical of SAH
  - A chronic pain, which has been gradually getting worse, may suggest an intracranial space-occupying lesion
- Timing/triggers of pain
  - Pain worse in the morning, which is worse on stooping, coughing or performing a Valsalva manoeuvre is suggestive of ↑ICP
- Associated symptoms
  - Neck stiffness—consider meningitis or SAH
  - Photophobia, vomiting, ↓GCS—consider ↑ICP
  - Disturbance of higher cortical function, ataxia, clumsiness or weakness may indicate a sinister pathology
  - Petechial/purpuric rash occurs with meningococcal sepsis
  - Fever can directly cause headache, but may also indicate meningitis
  - Eye pain—acute glaucoma
- Is the patient pregnant? Consider pre-eclampsia
- Is there a history of foreign travel? Consider malaria
- DHx
  - Certain medications can cause headaches (e.g. nitrates, Ca^{2+} channel blockers)
  - Is the patient on anticoagulants? Important if intracranial haemorrhage is suspected

Examination

- General examination
  - Does the patient look severely unwell? Consider meningitis
  - Is there a petechial/purpuric rash? Consider meningococcal sepsis
  - Check teeth—dental caries can cause referred pain

- Face
  - Is there tenderness over a non-pulsatile, thickened temporal artery? Consider giant cell arteritis
  - Pain over sinuses may indicate sinusitis
- CVS
  - Check BP—is this malignant hypertension?
  - Check for any new murmurs—bacterial emboli from infective endocarditis can cause cerebral abscesses
  - ↑BP and ↓HR is a late sign of ↑ICP
- Neurological
  - Check for meningism (photophobia, neck stiffness, Kernig's sign)—meningitis, SAH
  - Check fundi—papilloedema (↑ICP), haemorrhages (malignant hypertension), Roth spots (infective endocarditis/cerebral abscess)
  - Any focal neurology should make you consider sinister underlying processes

Investigations

- FBC, CRP, ESR
  - Check for raised inflammatory markers indicating infective/inflammatory cause
  - ↑↑ESR in temporal arteritis
  - Check for ↓platelets—risk of haemorrhage
- Coagulation screen
  - Coagulopathy increases risk of haemorrhage
- U&Es and bone profile
  - Is there an underlying electrolyte disturbance?
- LFTs
  - Can be raised if there is metastatic malignancy
- LP
  - Indicated if meningitis, encephalitis or SAH is suspected
  - ⚠ Contraindicated if ↑ICP
- CT head
  - Useful for checking for intracranial pathology
  - Does have limited sensitivity for SAH

Causes

Primary
- Tension headache
- Migraine
- Cluster headache
- Exertional

Secondary
- SAH (see p. 318–322)
- Meningitis (see p. 328–331)
  - Bacterial, viral, aseptic, TB
- Encephalitis (see p. 332–334)
- Intracranial bleed (see p. 324–327)
- Space-occupying lesion
- Benign intracranial hypertension

- Cerebral abscess
- Stroke (see p. 312–316)
- Malignant hypertension (see p. 102–106)
- Temporal arteritis (see p. 358–359)
- Sinusitis
- Glaucoma
- Venous sinus thrombosis
- Vertebral artery dissection
- Electrolyte disturbances
  - e.g. hyponatraemia, hypercalcaemia

Further reading
- *OHCM*, 7th edn. Oxford: Oxford University Press, p. 448, 768.
- *Oxford Textbook of Medicine*, 4th edn, vol. 3. Oxford: Oxford University Press, p. 993.

☠ **Reduced GCS**

The Glasgow coma scale (GCS) was originally designed for assessing head injuries, but it is valuable for monitoring patients with reduced consciousness. There are many causes for this, but they all imply that there is an underlying problem with brain function, and as such should be taken very seriously.

The Glasgow coma scale

It has been shown that there is a great degree of inter-observer variation when assessing GCS, so it is most useful at determining progress over time. You should always use the best response gained at the time, and document the total score, along with the constituent parts—e.g. 'GCS-15 (E-4, M-6, V-5)'.

Table 2.1 Glasgow coma scale

Eye opening	
Spontaneous	4
To speech	3
To pain	2
No response	1
Motor response	
Obeys commands	6
Localizes pain	5
Withdraws from pain	4
Flexion to pain (decorticate posturing)	3
Extension to pain (decerebrate posturing)	2
No response	1
Vocal response	
Oriented speech	5
Confused speech	4
Inappropriate words	3
Incomprehensible noises	2
No response	1

Immediate management

- ABC assessment
  - Airway obstruction becomes increasingly likely when GCS ≤8. It is vitally important to maintain a patent airway (see p. 2–5)
    ☎ Call for senior/anaesthetic support if you have any difficulties
  - Give high-flow O_2 via a non-rebreath mask. Check the patients SpO_2 and ABGs (looking for ↓PaO_2)—hypoxia is an important cause and should be treated immediately

- If patient's airway and/or breathing are compromised they are likely to need intubation and ventilation. ☎ Call ITU early
  - Check perfusion (HR, BP, CRT) and treat with IV fluid boluses if compromised (see p. 6–8)—cerebral hypoperfusion will cause reduced conscious level
- DEFG—Don't ever forget the glucose
  - Another commonly missed cause of reduced GCS is hypoglycaemia (see p. 226–228 (Endocrine chapter))
- Perform a secondary survey, looking especially for any evidence of head injury (bruises, Battle's sign, haemotympanum)
  - ⚠ Alcohol consumption may cause ↓GCS, but does not rule out head injury or other cause
- If no obvious cause can be found immediately, or there is any suspicion of head injury, urgent CT scanning will be indicated
- Once the patient is stable (i.e. ABC are satisfactory), management consists of finding the underlying cause and treating it

History

The patient is unlikely to be able to give a good history, but it is important to get as much information from corroborative sources as possible (e.g. relatives, bystanders, paramedics).
- Any history of head trauma?
- Has the patient taken any drugs? This includes alcohol, illegal drugs or overdoses
- Does the patient suffer from DM? Hypoglycaemia in particular can cause reduced consciousness
- Any risk factors for intracranial bleed? Consider hypertension, arteriopathy, coagulopathy/anticoagulant medications, previous stroke
- Look at drug chart if assessing an inpatient—have they been oversedated/overmedicated (e.g. benzodiazepines, opioids)

Examination

Often, the only clues successive of causes will come from examination and laboratory tests, so be thorough.
- General examination
  - Does the patient have a medic alert bracelet indicating a medical problem?
  - Look for any obvious injuries, particularly to the head
  - Does the patient smell of alcohol? This may be the cause of the ↓GCS, but does not exclude other causes, so keep looking
  - Are there any track marks on the arms indicating IV drug use?
  - Is the patient septic? Have a low threshold for starting antibiotics
- CVS
  - Assess circulatory adequacy (HR, BP, CRT)
  - Carotid bruits raise the possibility of cerebrovascular disease
  - NB. ↓HR and ↑BP can indicate raised intracranial pressure

- RS
  - Check for clinical signs of respiratory problems which can cause severe hypoxia, e.g. pneumothorax (see p. 204–207), acute severe asthma (see p. 196–198), pleural effusion/haemothorax (see p. 216–218), atelectasis/pneumonia (see p. 208–211), PE (see p. 200–203)
  - A low RR should lead to consideration of opioid overdose
- Abdomen
  - Acute abdominal causes can result in shock, leading to cerebral hypoperfusion
  - Is the patient peritonitic?
  - Any indications of ruptured/leaking AAA (see p. 364–367)?
  - ☎ Call surgeons urgently if acute abdominal cause is suspected
- Neurological
  - Pinpoint pupils should lead to suspicion of opioid overdose
  - Unilateral dilated, unreactive pupil strongly suggests intracranial cause
  - Bilaterally fixed, dilated pupils indicate a poor prognosis
  - Check tone bilaterally—a difference will again make you suspicious of an intracranial cause

Investigations
- ABGs
  - Check for acid/base disorder, hypoxia or hypercapnia
- FBC, CRP, coagulation profile
  - Raised inflammatory markers should suggest infection
  - Severe anaemia can affect conscious level
  - Coagulopathy can precipitate or complicate intracranial haemorrhage
- Glucose
  - Hypoglycaemia, HONK and DKA (check urine for ketones) can all alter conscious level
- U&Es, calcium, phosphate, magnesium
  - Electrolyte disturbance can cause severe problems with conscious level
- Paracetamol and salicylate levels
  - Could this be an overdose?
- Blood alcohol level
- Urine toxicology
- TFT
  - Thyroid problems can rarely cause ↓GCS (e.g. myxoedema coma)
- CXR
  - Is there any pulmonary pathology which could be responsible for the hypoxia?
  - Is there a septic focus?
- CT head
  - Often the investigation of choice if no obvious cause is found. Will not necessarily reveal all intracranial problems (e.g. SAH)
- LP
  - Can be diagnostic if meningitis/encephalitis is suspected
  - ⚠ Contraindicated if any suspicion of raised intracranial pressure

- EEG
  - Often not available immediately, EEG can give some clues as to the underlying cause (e.g. encephalitis, status epilepticus) and sometimes about the prognosis

Causes

- Metabolic disturbance
  - Drug overdose—e.g. benzodiazepines (see p. 418–419), opioids (see p. 420–421), aspirin (see p. 412–413)
  - Hypoxia (see p. 36–39), hypoglycaemia (see p. 426–430)
  - HONK (see p. 224–225)
  - DKA (see p. 220–222)
  - Electrolyte disturbance (see p. 388–406)
  - Uraemia
  - Hepatic failure (see p. 246–251)
  - Hypothermia
  - Myxoedema coma (see p. 236–237)
- Cerebrovascular causes
  - SAH (see p. 318–322)
  - Intracerebral haemorrhage (see p. 312–316)
  - Brainstem infarction
  - Venous sinus thrombosis (see p. 338–339)
- Head injury/trauma
  - Extradural haemorrhage (see p. 324–325)
  - Subdural haemorrhage (see p. 326–327)
  - Cerebral contusion
- Infection
  - SIRS/sepsis (see p. 304–306)
  - Meningitis (see p. 328–331)
  - Encephalitis (see p. 332–334)
  - Intracranial abscess
- Other
  - Epilepsy—post-ictal (see p. 76–79) or status epilepticus (see p. 340)
  - Intracranial space-occupying lesion
  - Thiamine deficiency

Further reading

- *OHCM*, 7th edn. Oxford: Oxford University Press, p. 477, 774.
- *Oxford Textbook of Medicine*, 4th edn, vol. 3. Oxford: Oxford University Press, p. 988.

① Seizures

The presentation of apparent seizure can be very varied, and can be due to a large number of causes, but for the purposes of this book generalized seizures will be discussed. A true generalized seizure occurs due to abnormal electrical activity in the brain, causing loss of consciousness, often with abnormal motor activity. Other problems can present quite similarly (e.g. syncope), so careful history-taking is required to differentiate these from true seizures.

Immediate management

- ABC assessment
  - The airway may be compromised if the patient has a ↓GCS, particularly in the post-ictal period. Airway management can be difficult during a seizure due to hypertonia of the jaw, so airway opening manoeuvres and nasopharyngeal airways are particularly useful
  - ⚠ Never insert your fingers into the mouth of a seizing patient
  - Give high-flow O_2 via a non-rebreath mask if the patient is currently seizing—this will help to reduce cerebral hypoxia
  - DEFG—don't ever forget the glucose: hypoglycaemia is an easily treated cause of seizures (see p. 226–229)
- If the patient is having repeated seizures without regaining consciousness between them, or if a seizure has lasted longer than ~10 minutes, then they should be treated for status epilepticus (see p. 340)
- Further management relies on finding the underlying cause, and treating it as appropriate

History

Patients may be unable to give a history initially, so corroborative history can be vital. If the patient has recovered from their seizure episode, a detailed history should be elicited. A useful way of taking the history is to look at what happened before, during and after the episode.

Before

- Does the patient have a known seizure disorder (e.g. epilepsy)?
  - If so, what is the normal pattern for their seizures—this is significant, as, if the pattern is different in this episode, this should raise suspicion of a different cause
  - Has the patient recently changed antiepileptics, or have they not been able to take them (e.g. vomiting)?
- Is there any other significant PMHx (e.g. DM)?
- Has there been any recent head injury?
- Did the patient experience an 'aura' prior to the episode? e.g. strange smells, visual disturbance—this strongly suggests a seizure
  - 'Dizziness' and darkening vision often precede syncope

- What was the patient doing before the episode?
  - Precipitating factors for seizures include hyperventilation, drug use, tiredness/sleep deprivation, flickering lights
  - Syncope can be brought on by standing up quickly (postural hypotension) or emotional triggers (e.g. seeing blood)

During

- A patient who has had a generalized seizure will not remember the episode
  - If the patient remembers hitting the ground when falling over, this is likely to be due to syncope
- A corroborative history will be needed to determine events
- A classic tonic–clonic seizure will have two parts
  - Tonic phase: the patient will become hypertonic, often falling to the ground if standing. It is not uncommon for the patient to have a respiratory arrest with cyanosis at this point
  - Clonic phase: the patient will start having symmetrical jerking movements, which crescendo in intensity, then gradually become less as the seizure ends
- Patients can have jerking episodes during attacks of syncope, particularly if they are kept in a head-up position
- Was the seizure initially focal (e.g. involving one limb), with secondary generalization? This may indicate a more focal neurological problem
- Colour changes can be significant—cyanosis often occurs during seizures, whereas pallor is associated more with syncope
- A patient will not react to any stimuli during a generalized seizure
- Tongue-biting and urinary incontinence are common in generalized seizures, but can also occur with syncope

After

- Following a generalized seizure, patients will be post-ictal (compared to a relatively fast recovery following an episode of syncope)
  - They are likely to be very sleepy
  - They may be quite confused, and often have disoriented speech
  - This usually lasts for >30 minutes
- What is the first thing the patient remembers following the episode? There will often be some anterograde amnesia following a seizure
- It is common for there to be some transient neurological deficit following a seizure, but if this is persistent, then it should be investigated

Examination

- General
  - Are there any obvious head injuries (bruises, Battle's sign, haemotympanum)?
  - Is there a petechial/purpuric rash which may indicate meningococcal sepsis?
  - Is there any bruising/bleeding suggestive of coagulopathy—↑risk of intracranial haemorrhage
  - Check carefully for any evidence of head trauma

- CVS
  - Check lying and standing BP; a large postural drop will support a diagnosis of syncope
  - Any murmur suggesting aortic stenosis should be taken seriously (if this was syncope, it indicates critical stenosis)
- Neurological examination
  - Perform a detailed cranial and peripheral nervous system examination
  - Focal neurology may be present post-ictally, but should still raise suspicions that this may not be a primary seizure disorder
  - Check for neck stiffness and Kernig's sign—could this be meningitis/SAH?

Investigations

- FBC and CRP
  - ↑WCC and ↑CRP may indicate infective/inflammatory cause
- Coagulation screen
  - Check for coagulopathy—↑risk of intracranial bleed
- U&Es, bone profile and glucose
  - Check for electrolyte disturbance
- LFTs
  - Check for indication of liver failure
- ABGs
  - Check for hypoxia or acid/base disturbance
- Prolactin level
  - Useful for confirming a seizure—level is raised 3–4 × normal shortly after a seizure
- ECG
  - Look for arrhythmia, and in particular at the QT interval
- Brain imaging
  - Arrange for an urgent CT/MRI of the head if there is any suspicion of bleeding
  - Is also useful for detecting any structural brain pathology (e.g. space-occupying lesions)
- LP
  - Indicated if there is a suspicion of CNS infection or SAH
  - ⚠ Rule out ↑ICP before performing
- EEG
  - Is useful for detecting epileptic foci, but can be normal if patient is not currently fitting
  - EEG can be useful acutely in diagnosing encephalitis (otherwise it is usually a non-urgent investigation)

Causes

- Primary seizure disorder—either one-off episode or epilepsy
- Cardiac syncope
  - Vasovagal syncope
  - Postural hypotension
  - Arrhythmia (see p. 164–186)

- Micturition syncope
- Cough syncope
- Respiratory
  - Hypoxia (see p. 36–39)
  - Hypercapnia—e.g. over-administration of O_2 in patients with type 2 respiratory failure
- Metabolic
  - Hypoglycaemia (see p. 226–229)
  - Hyponatraemia (see p. 388–390)
  - Hypocalcaemia (see p. 400–402)
  - Acid/base disturbance (see p. 422–424)
  - Other electrolyte imbalances (see p. 388–406)
  - Hepatic encephalopathy (see p. 246–251)
  - Inborn errors of metabolism (rare)
- Intracranial
  - Stroke (see p. 312–316)
  - Head injury
  - Intracranial haemorrhage (see p. 318–327)
  - Infection—e.g. meningitis, encephalitis (see p. 328–334)
  - Cerebral oedema/raised intracranial pressure
  - Space-occupying lesion
  - Basilar migraine
- Other
  - Psychogenic/pseudoseizures
  - Alcohol withdrawal/delirium tremens (see p. 258–260)
  - Malignant hypertension (see p. 102–106)
  - Adverse drug reaction
  - SLE encephalitis
  - Multiple sclerosis
  - Creutzfeldt–Jakob disease
  - Alzheimer's disease

Further reading
- *OHCM*, 7th edn. Oxford: Oxford University Press, p. 482, 808.
- *Oxford Textbook of Medicine*, 4th edn, vol. 3, Oxford: Oxford University Press, p. 1001.

⊙ **Reduced urine output**

This is a very common problem for a doctor to be called about in hospital. There are many causes to consider, but most are amenable to simple treatment. Urine output in an adult should be >0.5 ml/kg/hour. Oliguria is defined as passing less than 400 ml of urine in 24 hours and anuria is the failure to pass any urine.

Immediate management

- ABC assessment
  - The patient may require fluid resuscitation if they are haemodynamically compromised (see p. 6–8)
- Consider catheterization if the patient does not already have a catheter
  - They may relieve an obstruction (if present) and will allow more accurate hourly measurement of urine output
- Ensure that strict fluid balance charts are kept, and that the patient is weighed daily
- Treat the underlying cause
  - Fluid therapy for pre-renal causes
  - Catheterization/urological consultation for post-renal causes
  - Renal failure (see p. 270–275)
- After any intervention, it is very important to reassess the urine output to see if it has been sucessful

History

- Check fluid balance charts and weights for previous days
  - An overall negative fluid balance/weight loss indicates a pre-renal cause
  - An overall positive balance/weight gain indicates fluid retention
  - Have ongoing fluid losses been neglected when calculating fluid requirement (e.g. drain losses, vomiting, etc.)?
- Anuria will suggest an obstructive cause, whereas oliguria will imply a pre-renal or renal cause
- Has the patient recently undergone surgery, trauma or been severely unwell? This is likely to indicate a pre-renal cause (or rarely SIADH)
- Does the patient have a background of renal failure or risk factors for this? (see p. 270–275)
- Is the patient on any medications which may cause ARF?

Examination

- General examination
  - Does the patient look unwell? They may be septic (see p. 304–306)
  - Assess the patient's hydration status (see p. 61)
- CVS
  - Check for signs of hypovolaemia—dry skin and tongue, ↑HR, ↓BP (with large postural drop), ↑CRT
  - Look for evidence of fluid overload—peripheral/sacral oedema, bibasal fine crepitations, ↑JVP

- Abdominal
  - Is there a palpable bladder? A bladder scan can be of use if this is difficult to discern

Investigations

Extensive investigation is not usually required in simple cases, which are most often due to pre-renal causes. Further investigation should be undertaken depending on the suspected cause.

- U&Es
  - ↑Na and ↑urea will imply dehydration
  - ↑Urea and ↑creatinine will indicate acute renal failure

Causes

- Pre-renal (most common)
  - Reduced effective arterial blood volume—hypovolaemia, sepsis, cardiac failure, liver failure
  - Reduced renal artery flow—renal artery stenosis, renal emboli, AAA
- Renal (see p. 270–275)
- Post-renal (see p. 266–268)

Further reading

- *OHCM*, 7th edn. Oxford: Oxford University Press, p. 66.
- *Oxford Textbook of Medicine*, 4th edn, vol. 3, Oxford: Oxford University Press, p. 231.

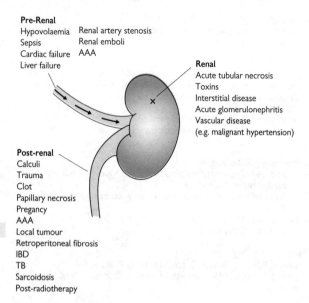

Pre-Renal
Hypovolaemia   Renal artery stenosis
Sepsis   Renal emboli
Cardiac failure AAA
Liver failure

Renal
Acute tubular necrosis
Toxins
Interstitial disease
Acute glomerulonephritis
Vascular disease
(e.g. malignant hypertension)

Post-renal
Calculi
Trauma
Clot
Papillary necrosis
Pregancy
AAA
Local tumour
Retroperitoneal fibrosis
IBD
TB
Sarcoidosis
Post-radiotherapy

Fig. 2.2 Causes of reduced urine output

⑦ Jaundice

The yellow discolouration of the skin and sclera seen when serum bilirubin levels are >51 µmol/l, jaundice may not necessarily be a presenting complaint, but an incidental finding on clinical examination. The causes are manifold and often not immediately life-threatening, but its association with rapidly decompensating conditions must be borne in mind.

Immediate management

- ABC
  - Increased risk of airway compromise in encephalopathy
  - IV fluid boluses for shock should be colloid rather than saline to avoid precipitating ascites
- Take blood cultures before any antimicrobial treatment given
- If patient appears to be septic (cholestasis predisposes to ascending cholangitis; see p. 256–257), start antibiotics
  - e.g. gentamlcin, 5 mg/kg IV OD (avoid in renal impairment)
  - *or* cefuroxime, 1.5 g IV TDS
  - *and* metronidazole, 500 mg TDS
- Common bile duct stones can cause jaundice and pancreatitis; consider this in the unwell patient

History

- RUQ pain, particularly after meals (can be confused with dyspepsia)—gallstone disease
- Pale stools and dark urine suggests cholestasis
- Paracetamol use or abuse—accidental/deliberate overdose?
- Foreign travel? Consider hepatitis A or B, less commonly amoebiasis
- Sexual history? Consider hepatitis B or C
- Recent anaesthesia? Jaundice is more commonly associated with inhalational agents rather than surgery itself
- Malignancy
  - Direct history
  - Altered bowel habit
  - PR bleeding
  - Anaemia
  - Post-menstrual bleeding
  - Weight loss
- Steatorrhoea—may indicate obstructive jaundice
- Family history
  - Gilbert's syndrome most common familial jaundice (3% of population)
  - Rarer forms include Crigler–Najjar (types 1 & 2), Dubin–Johnson and Rotor's syndromes
- Drugs
  - Check side-effect profile of all medicines on chart in BNF
  - Detailed alcohol history is especially important—remember to ask about previous drinking patterns as well as current ones

- Do not forget to start heavy alcohol users on appropriate treatment when admitting them (see p. 258–260)
  - Has the patient ever used any recreational IV drugs? Consider viral hepatitis B and C (and consider risk stratification for HIV infection)
- Risk factors for gallstones (5 Fs)
  - Fat, female, fair, fertile, forty

Examination
- General examination—check for stigmata of chronic liver disease
  - Pyrexial?
  - Personal care and nutritional status—suggestive of alcohol problem
  - Hands—palmar erythema, clubbing, leuconychia, liver flap
  - Trunk—spider naevi, gynaecomastia
  - Face—xanthelasma, rhinophyma
  - Bruising may indicate coagulopathy
  - Haemosiderin deposits and 'tanned' appearance may indicate haemochromatosis
- Abdomen
  - RUQ tenderness—cholangitis?
  - Epigastric pain should always be assessed for pancreatitis
  - Is there a palpable gallbladder? (rare but significant)—Courvoisier's law states that 'in the presence of jaundice, if the gallbladder is palpable, the cause is unlikely to be a stone'
  - Caput medusa may indicate portal hypertension
  - Ascites may be due to hypoalbuminaemia (a feature of chronic liver disease) or malignancy

Investigations
- LFTs
  - Differential analysis of bilirubin shows an increased unconjugated bilirubin in pre-hepatic jaundice, and a raised conjugated bilirubin in post-hepatic or hepatocellular jaundice
  - Significantly raised transaminases (AST or ALT) and GGT may indicate hepatocellular cause or intrahepatic obstruction
  - Markedly raised alkaline phosphatase suggests an obstructive cause
  - Hypoalbuminaemia—reduced liver synthetic function?
- Coagulation
  - Prolonged PT also suggestive of impaired liver synthetic function
  - If bleeding, this can be corrected with FFP (discuss with senior or haematology on call)
- FBC, film and CRP
  - ↓Hb can have many causes in the context of jaundice, including haemolysis, bleeding from tumour, anaemia of chronic disease
  - ↑Hb may indicate haemochromatosis
  - ↑MCV is common with long-term high alcohol intake
  - ↑Reticulocytes occur with haemolysis
  - A blood film will often demonstrate the presence of haemolysis
  - Direct Coombs' test for autoimmune haemolysis

- Urine dipstick
  - ↑Urobilinogen indicates pre-hepatic cause (↑enteric bilirubin excretion)
  - ↑Bilirubin and ↓urobilinogen indicate post-hepatic cause (↓enteric bilirubin excretion)
- Abdominal USS
  - Can demonstrate obstruction of the intrahepatic or extrahepatic bile ducts, and will often show the cause (e.g. gallstones, tumour)
- Specific blood tests
  - Viral serology—hepatitis viruses, EBV, CMV
  - Ferritin—raised in haemochromatosis
  - Autoantibodies (including anti-mitochondrial, anti-smooth muscle, ANA, anti-liver kidney microsomal)—autoimmune hepatitis
  - Serum ceruloplasmin and copper—Wilson's disease
  - Alpha-1 antitrypsin levels
- ERCP, PTC, MRCP—useful for imaging biliary tract
- Liver biopsy—discuss with hepatologist

Causes

Pre-hepatic

From excessive breakdown of red cells or haem-containing proteins. Results in predominantly unconjugated hyperbilirubinaemia.

- Fever/sepsis (see p. 304–306)
- Drugs
- Vigorous exercise—e.g. marathon running
- Extensive bruising
- Autoimmune haemolysis
- Rhabdomyolysis
- Mechanical haemolysis—prosthetic heart valves, vigorous exercise, thermal injury, microangiopathic haemolytic anaemia (e.g. DIC, thrombotic thrombocytopaenic purpura)
- Congenital blood disorders—e.g. thalassaemia, sickle cell disease, glucose-6-phosphate deficiency, pyruvate kinase deficiency, pyrimidine-5′-nucleotidase deficiency, hereditary spherocytosis or elliptocytosis
- Infections—malaria, *Clostridium perfringens* septicaemia

Hepatic

This will result in impaired excretion of bilirubin from the liver, either caused by liver cell damage, or intrahepatic cholestasis. Very high transaminases (>1000) can indicate this, but remember that a liver that has been extensively damaged cannot produce transaminases and so a low result does not exclude significant damage.

- Gilbert's syndrome
- Alcoholic liver disease
- Viral hepatitis (A,B,C, etc.)
- Bacterial hepatitis—miliary TB, widespread sepsis
- Drugs
- Haemochromatosis
- Wilson's disease

- Carcinoma—primary (rare), secondary, local infiltration (e.g. renal adenocarcinoma)
- Sarcoidosis
- Shock (reduced hepatic blood flow)
- Sclerosing cholangitis
- Autoimmune hepatitis
- Leptospirosis
- Alpha-1-antitrypsin deficiency
- Primary biliary cirrhosis
- Dubin–Johnson, Rotor's, Budd–Chiari syndromes

Post-hepatic

This is due to obstruction of the extrahepatic biliary tree (except for the cystic or pancreatic ducts). Characteristically, this will result in an ALP that is raised out of proportion to the transaminases. The classical clinical picture will be of pale stools and dark urine, and a urine dipstick showing ↓urobilinogen and ↑bilirubin.

- Gallstone disease
- Ascending cholangitis (see p. 256–257)
- Carcinoma—ampullary, pancreatic head, cholangiocarcinoma, metastases
- Traumatic biliary strictures—e.g. after surgery or after ERCP
- Parasitic infection
- Cystic fibrosis

Further reading

- *OHCM*, 7th edn. Oxford: Oxford University Press, p. 242.
- *Oxford Textbook of Medicine*, 4th edn, vol. 2. Oxford: Oxford University Press, p. 710.
- *Oxford Handbook Gastroenterology and Hepatology*, 1st edn, Oxford: Oxford University Press, p. 103.

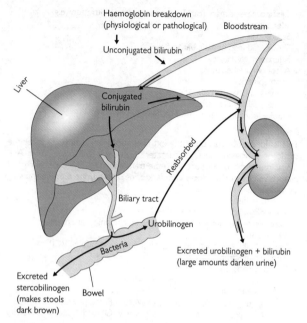

Fig. 2.3 Bilirubin processing and jaundice

The ill diabetic patient

Initial assessment of any unwell patient with diabetes should always include consideration and treatment of diabetic emergencies—hypoglycaemia (see p. 226–229), DKA (see p. 220–222) or HONK (see p. 224–225).

Subsequently, they will require special consideration if they are admitted, particularly if they are unable to eat. Failure to establish a plan for managing this can result in severe complications, i.e. hypoglycaemia, DKA or HONK.

Type 1 diabetes

These patients are unable to produce endogenous insulin, so require administration of exogenous insulin. Lack of insulin will cause:
• Hyperglycaemia
  • The patient will no longer be storing glucose as glycogen or fat
• Dehydration
  • Hyperglycaemia will cause loss of glucose into the urine, which will cause diuresis through osmotic pressure
  • This will manifest as polydipsia and polyuria, along with signs of dehydration
  • The urine dipstick will be positive for glucose
• Ketoacidosis
  • Inability to utilize glucose will lead to metabolism of fat to provide energy
  • The breakdown products of fat include ketones, an excess of which will lead to a metabolic acidosis (DKA)
  • The easiest way to monitor production of ketones is to dip the urine regularly and test for their presence

It is clear that these patients will require administration of insulin even if they are not eating. This does leave one problem—giving insulin to someone who is not eating will lead to hypoglycaemia.

This means that any patient with type 1 DM who is not eating (for any reason) will require an IV insulin and glucose infusion.

Your hospital should have a protocol for using insulin and glucose infusions.

⚠ Never run insulin through a different cannula to the dextrose. If the cannula supplying the dextrose fails, this can rapidly lead to severe hypoglycaemia.

Type 2 diabetes

These patients have a relative insensitivity to insulin, so they are at lower risk of becoming ketotic. Illness or other physiological stresses (e.g. surgery) will cause complications owing to release of cortisol, catecholamines and other stress hormones, leading to catabolism and hyperglycaemia. This can cause significant complications, and lead to a longer stay in hospital.

If a patient is unable to eat, then oral hypoglycaemic agents should be stopped. BMs should be monitored frequently, and IV insulin and dextrose should be started if there is inadequate glycaemic control.

Further reading
- *OHCM*, 7th edn. Oxford: Oxford University Press, p. 190.
- *Oxford Textbook of Medicine*, 4th edn, vol. 2. Oxford: Oxford University Press, p. 317.

① **Falls in hospital**

Falls are a very common occurrence in hospital; it is estimated that there will be ~24 per week in an average hospital. Most will result in little or no harm, but there is the potential for serious complications. Prevention is better than cure, so it is important to identify risk factors in any patient admitted to hospital, so that these may be minimised.

Initial management

- ABC assessment
  - Is the patient unconscious?
  - Is this an acute medical emergency?—e.g. cardiac arrest, status epilepticus
  - Has the patient collapsed owing to hypotensive shock? They may require fluid resuscitation (see p. 6–8)
  - Check the pulse—is there a tachycardia (see p. 172–286) or bradycardia? (see p. 164–170)
- Consider checking the BM if there is no obvious cause for the fall—could this be a hypoglycaemic episode?
- Check for evidence of severe head injury
  - ❶ Worrying symptoms—confusion, amnesia, vomiting, ↓GCS, depressed skull fractures, blood/CSF rhinorrhoea/otorrhoea, Battle's sign, haemotympanum (see p. 324–327)
  - Commence neurological observations at least hourly if there is any suspicion of head injury
- Check for evidence of bony trauma
  - Hip fracture: pain (can be difficult to elicit in a confused patient), shortened externally rotated leg (see p. 350–352)
  - Any bony tenderness anywhere
  - Check for scaphoid tenderness—common if the patient has fallen onto an outstretched hand
- Submit an incident report form detailing the circumstances of the episode, and if there is anything which can be done to prevent it from happening again

History

- Circumstances of the fall
  - Did the patient trip? If so, on what?
  - Was it a faint? Does the patient remember hitting the ground (likely to be due to syncope) or not (possibly a fit, or amnesia associated with head injury)?
  - Did the patient lose consciousness? May be a fit, syncope or severe head injury
- Associated symptoms
  - Dizziness, light-headedness, nausea, peripheral visual loss, pallor, sweating—consistent with syncope/presyncope
  - Palpitations—could this be an arrhythmia?
  - Aura, neurological symptoms—could this be a fit?

- PMHx
  - Has the patient had many falls previously? They will require intervention if this is so
  - Any history of conditions predisposing to falls?—e.g. Parkinson's disease and other movement disorders, hypotension, carotid sinus hypersensitivity, visual impairment, stroke, dementia
  - Does the patient have diabetes? Could this be hypoglycaemia?
  - Are they at high risk if they do fall?—e.g. osteoporosis, on warfarin
- DHx
  - Is the patient on any medications which may increase the risk of falls?—e.g. hypnotics, antihypertensives, antipsychotics, hypoglycaemics
  - Is the patient on any anticoagulants? These increase the risk of haemorrhage
  - Review the patient's medications, and consider altering/stopping any which may predispose to falls, or increase the risk of harm when falling

Examination

- General examination
  - Does the patient have any sign of movement disorders?— e.g. Parkinson's disease, hemiplegia
  - Thoroughly examine the patient for any external signs of trauma
  - Does the patient smell of alcohol?
  - Perform a MMSE—is the patient delirious?
- CVS
  - Assess the circulation: HR, BP, CRT—is the patient hypovolaemic?
  - Check the pulse rate and rhythm—is there an arrhythmia?
  - Check the lying and standing BP—is there postural hypotension?
- RS
  - Are there any signs of CO_2 retention?—tremor, warm peripheries, bounding pulses, injected conjunctivae
  - Check the SpO_2—is the patient hypoxic?
- Abdominal
  - Check for tenderness—has there been any abdominal trauma?
  - If the patient is confused/delirious, perform a PR to check for constipation
- Neurological
  - Perform a thorough examination if there is any suspicion of neurological causes or sequelae
  - If there was any head trauma, check for signs of skull fracture (see above)

Investigations

- FBC and CRP
  - Is the patient anaemic?
  - Raised inflammatory markers may make you consider delirium seriously (although they may be normal in delirium)
- Coagulation
  - Screen for coagulopathy, which may exacerbate the consequence of a fall

- U&Es and bone profile
  - Is an electrolyte disturbance the cause?
- Troponins
  - Check these at 12 hours after the fall, if suspicious of silent MI
- ABGs
  - Check if suspicious of hypercapnia or hypoxia
- ECG
  - Is there an arrhythmia?
  - Are there any ischaemic changes?
- Urine dipstick/microscopy + C&S
  - Check if the patient appears delirious/confused
- X-ray
  - Indicated if there is a suspicion of bony injury
  - Skull X-rays are not routinely used if suspicious of a skull fracture—CT is the first line investigation in this circumstance
- CT head
  - Indicated urgently if there is a suspicion of serious head injury
- Falls team referral
  - Indicated if the patient is at high risk of falls
  - They may organize further specialist investigations—e.g. tilt-table testing

Causes/risk factors

Intrinsic

- Personality and lifestyle
  - Activities, attitudes to risk, independence and receptiveness to advice
- Age-related changes
  - Changes in mobility, strength, flexibility and eyesight—occur even in healthy old age
- Illness and injury
  - Stroke, arthritis, dementia, cardiac disease, carotid sinus hypersensitivity, acquired brain injury, delirium, Parkinson's disease, dehydration, disordered blood chemistry, hypoglycaemia

Extrinsic factors

- Medication
  - Hypnotics, sedatives, analgesia, antihypertensives (and other drugs which lower BP), medication with Parkinsonian side-effects (e.g. typical antipsychotics, metoclopramide), alcohol, illicit drugs
- Environment
  - Poor lighting, wet floors, loose carpets, cables, steps, poor footwear, lack of mobility aids

Further reading

- *OHCM*, 7th edn. Oxford: Oxford University Press, p. 60, 452.
- *Oxford Textbook of Medicine*, 4th edn, vol. 3. Oxford: Oxford University Press, p. 1381.
- NHS National Patient Safety Agency. 'The third report from the Patient Safety Observatory: Slips, trips and falls in hospital.' www.npsa.nhs.uk
- National Institute of Clinical Excellence guideline: Falls (CG21). www.nice.nhs.uk

☹ **Hypotension**

Hypotension can be defined as a drop in blood pressure from a previously normal level. 'Normal' BP ranges from 90/60 to 130/80, so using absolute values can be misleading. That said, a systolic BP <100 warrants close attention. Hypotension can be life-threatening, so it is important to treat it promptly, and find the underlying cause.

Immediate management

- ABC assessment
- High-flow O_2 via non-rebreath mask
- Gain IV access
  - Ideally two large-bore cannulae
  - Take bloods (see below)
- Give IV fluid boluses
  - e.g. 250 ml 0.9% NaCl or colloid
  - Assess response—HR, BP, CRT, JVP
  - Give further boluses if required and continually reassess
  - If haemorrhaging is obvious, transfuse with O negative or type-specific blood if available, whilst awaiting crossmatch
  - ⚠ Caution if underlying cardiac or renal disease is suspected. The patient will likely need a central venous line and CVP monitoring on ITU. ☎ Contact seniors urgently
- Catheterize and monitor urine output
  - Should be >0.5 ml/kg/h
  - Keep strict input/output charts
- Cardiac monitor, SpO_2 monitor, BP monitor
- Full history and clinical examination to determine and treat cause
- Does this patient need urgent assessment for transfer to ITU?

History

Try to find out the underlying cause. Hypotension can cause cerebral hypoperfusion leading to confusion or coma, so often it is difficult to obtain a full history from the patient. Corroborative histories and thorough examination of the case notes can be vital.

- Duration
  - Does this coincide with recent medication changes or other intervention?
- What is this patient's baseline BP?
  - Some patients will have longstanding ↓BP, so will not need any immediate treatment
- Associated symptoms
  - Chest pain (IHD/ACS, tamponade, pneumothorax/haemothorax, PE, $2°$ to hypotension)
  - Palpitations (arrhythmia, $2°$ to hypotension)
  - Dizziness/collapse/confusion (hypoglycaemia, indicates cerebral hypoperfusion)
  - Temperature (hypothermia, sepsis)

- Abdominal pain (intra-abdominal cause, mesenteric ischaemia 2° to hypotension)
- Recent trauma/surgery
  - Visible blood loss/intraoperative loss
  - Occult blood/fluid loss (drains, internal blood loss, third space loss, long bone fracture)
  - Spinal trauma/anaesthetic (neurogenic shock)
- Any other fluid losses
  - Vomiting, diarrhoea, polyuria, fistulae
- Medications (particularly if newly introduced)
  - Antihypertensives, diuretics, opioids, benzodiazepines
  - Anaphylactic reaction
- PMHx to elicit risk factors for various causes
  - IHD, DM, DVT, renal failure, allergy, coagulopathy

Examination

Clinical evaluation of hypotension is vital in guiding treatment. Only by assessing clinical signs of hypotension can you judge whether treatment is working, and if any further therapy is required. It is also important to perform a full examination to elicit any causes.

General

- Pale, sweaty appearance and cool peripheries indicate hypovolaemia
  - Check central CRT (i.e. over sternum)—should be <2 seconds
  - Warm peripheries may be present in septic/distributive shock
- Raised temperature can indicate sepsis
- Any evidence of trauma
  - Check back as well

CVS

- HR
  - Tachycardia is often the first indicator of shock
  - Present in tachyarrhythmias
  - HR can be normal if on β blockers
  - Bradycardia can be underlying cause, but is also a preterminal sign
- Pulses
  - Radial pulse, if palpable, is a rough indicator of systolic BP >100
  - Radio–radial/radio–femoral delay could indicate aortic dissection
  - Central pulse (e.g. carotid) volume can give impression of cardiac output
- JVP
  - Raised in cardiogenic shock/fluid overload (⚠ be very cautious with fluid resuscitation), also raised in tamponade and tension pneumothorax
  - Low in hypovolaemia (i.e. difficult to elicit even with hepatojugular reflex)—useful in assessing clinical response
- BP
  - Ensure that the BP machine has been calibrated and that the correct cuff size is being used
  - Lying and standing BP can be very useful—large postural drop occurs with hypovolaemia

- Heart sounds
  - New murmur in context of ACS may indicate VSD/papillary muscle rupture
  - ❶ Muffled heart sounds can be present in cardiac tamponade (part of Beck's triad, see p. 152–155)

RS
- Tracheal deviation
  - ❶ Can indicate tension pneumothorax (see p. 204–207)
- Chest trauma
  - Flail segments, rib tenderness, bruising, surgical emphysema, penetrating injury
- Percussion note
  - Hyper-resonant in pneumothorax (difficult to elicit)
  - Dull in haemothorax, pleural effusion, consolidation or pulmonary oedema
- Auscultation
  - Bibasal fine crepitations are suggestive of pulmonary oedema
  - Localized coarse crepitations may indicate infection
  - Reduced/absent air entry suggests pneumothorax/haemothorax or infection

Abdominal
- Discoloration/bruising
  - ❶ AAA rupture
  - Cullen's/Grey Turner's sign in acute pancreatitis
  - Trauma
- Tenderness
  - Localized—visceral trauma (e.g. liver, spleen), infection (e.g. appendicitis), mesenteric ischaemia
  - Peritonism—intra-abdominal bleed, septic/chemical peritonitis (visceral rupture)
- Bowel sounds
  - Tinkling/absent—obstruction/ileus (fluid loss from vomiting)
- Monitor urine output
  - Indicates renal perfusion

Neurological
- Check AVPU/GCS
  - Indicates cerebral perfusion
- Any indication of head injury
- Spinal cord injury
  - Spinal shock

Investigations
- Serial BP, cardiac and SpO_2 monitoring
- Urine output and strict fluid balance
- ECG
  - Tachyarrhythmia (see p. 172–186), ischaemic change (see p. 134–143), bradycardia (see p. 164–170)
- CXR
  - Consolidation, pulmonary oedema, pneumothorax/haemothorax

- ABGs with lactate (see p. 422–424)
  - Underlying metabolic/respiratory cause
  - Lactic acidosis may indicate organ hypoperfusion
- FBC
  - ↑WCC—infection
  - ↓Hb/Hct—blood loss (NB. can be normal for hours following acute bleed)
  - ↓Plt—cause of bleeding
- Coagulation screen
- U&Es
  - ↑Urea—dehydration, GI bleed, renal failure (with ↑creatinine)
  - Check electrolytes and correct if necessary
  - Monitor and adjust IV fluid accordingly
- Glucose
- LFTs, AXR, amylase, CRP, troponins if clinical picture warrants them
- Further imaging (USS, CT)—if internal bleeding is suspected

Causes

BP is the product of peripheral vascular resistance and cardiac output. Cardiac output is the product of stroke volume and heart rate. Therefore:

BP = peripheral vascular resistance × stroke volume × heart rate

Hence, a reduction of any of these factors will involve a compensatory increase in the others to maintain BP. When these compensatory mechanisms are overwhelmed, the BP will fall.

Hypovolaemia—↓stroke volume
- Blood loss
  - External—trauma, haematemesis (see p. 44–46), PR bleed (see p. 48–50)
  - Internal—chest, abdomen, pelvis, long bone fracture, GI bleed
  - Intraoperative
- External fluid loss
  - Vomiting (see p. 60–63)
  - Diarrhoea
  - Polyuria—hyperglycaemia/DKA (see p. 220–225), nephrotic syndrome (see p. 276–279), diabetes insipidus
  - Burns/erythroderma (see p. 360–362)
- Internal (third space) fluid loss
  - Capillary leak—SIRS/sepsis (see p. 304–306), anaphylaxis (see p. 192–194)
  - Hypoalbuminaemia—malnutrition, liver failure (see p. 246–251), nephrotic syndrome (see p. 276–279)

Cardiogenic shock—↓stroke volume and/or ↓HR
- Coronary disease—ACS (see p. 134–143), acute heart failure (see p. 144–146)
- Arrhythmia
  - Tachyarrhythmia—SVT/AF, AVNRT, AVRT, VT (see p. 172–186)
  - Bradyarrhythmia—sinus node disease, heart block (see p. 164–170)
- Cardiac tamponade (see p. 152–155)
- Acute valve lesion—papillary muscle rupture/acute VSD 2° to ACS

- Sepsis—depressed myocardial contractility (see p. 304–306)
- Pulmonary embolism (see p. 200–203)
- Tension pneumothorax (see p. 204–207)
- Cardiomyopathy/myocarditis
- Hypothermia

Distributive shock—↓peripheral vascular resistance

- Sepsis (causes vasodilatation and capillary leak), especially with toxic shock syndrome (endotoxin-mediated)
- Anaphylaxis
- Neurogenic/spinal shock (spinal trauma, spinal anaesthetic)
- Hypothermia

Further reading

- *OHCM*, 7th edn. Oxford: Oxford University Press, p. 68, 778.
- *Oxford Textbook of Medicine*, 4th edn, vol. 2. Oxford: Oxford University Press, p. 1219.
- *Oxrord Handbook of Emergencies in Cardiology*, 1st edn. Oxford: Oxford University Press, p. 4.
- *Advanced Life Support Manual*, 4th edn. Resuscitation Council (UK), 2000.
- Annane D, Bellissant E, Cavaillon JM. Septic shock. *Lancet* 2005; **365(9453)**:63–78.
- Dellinger RP *et al*. Surviving sepsis campaign—guidelines for management of severe sepsis and septic shock. *Crit Care Med* 2004; **32(3)**:858–73.
- Shafi S, Kauder DR. Fluid resuscitation and blood replacement in patients with polytrauma. *Clinical Orthop Rel Res* 2004, **422**:37–42.

☼ Hypertensive emergency

Definition

Also known as accelerated or malignant hypertension, this is a rare condition which can occur with any of the causes of hypertension. It is defined as a severely raised BP in association with evidence of end organ dysfunction. The mortality rate at 1 year, if this condition is untreated, is over 90%. If the patient is pregnant, call the obstetric team urgently—pre-eclampsia is an obstetric emergency.

Presentation

The absolute BP level is not necessarily as important as the end organ damage, but the patient will generally have a systolic BP >160 mmHg and/or a diastolic BP >100 mmHg.

The systems most usually affected are the CNS, kidneys and CVS. This effect will manifest as any of:

- Hypertensive encephalopathy
    - Headache, seizures, visual disturbance, altered consciousness/confusion, focal neurological signs
- Hypertensive retinopathy
    - Flame haemorrhages, cotton wool spots, papilloedema
- Chest pain—myocardial ischaemia/infarction
- SOB—acute heart failure (see p. 144–146)
- Back pain—aortic dissection (see p. 160–162)
- Renal disease
    - Significant proteinuria, renal impairment
- Epistaxis
- Hyphaema

Immediate management

- ABC
    - Resuscitation is not usually necessary, but several manifestations involve inherently insecure airways, respiratory compromise or risk of circulatory compromise
    - If a seizure is in progress, immediate senior support should be sought
    - Check BP manually, and in both arms—>20 mmHg difference may indicate aortic dissection (see p. 160–162)

- ❶ *If encephalopathic*
- Request urgent senior support
- The patient will need to be admitted to a critical care/ITU ward
- Arterial access and invasive BP monitoring will be required
- Aim to reduce diastolic BP to ~110 over 4 hours
    - Will likely require IV antihypertensives
    - Seek advice from cardiologists/intensivists as to which agents to use

If not encephalopathic
- Provide a quiet bed for patient and re-evaluate BP
  - Relaxation can significantly reduce BP
- Is the patient in any distress?
  - Is there adequate analgesia?
- Gradually reduce BP
  - The choice of agent, and route of administration will depend on the nature of the end organ failure
  - Seek senior advice—detailed information on the patient's condition will be required; ensure that you provide this
  - ⚠ BP should not be lowered to normal levels initially, as organ autoregulation will be disturbed, and this may lead to ischaemia and infarction
  - BP should be monitored regularly during treatment
  - ⚠ Do not use sublingual nifedipine—it can lead to uncontrollable and dangerously fast fall in BP

Further management
- Check for and treat any underlying pathology which may be the cause (see below)
- Long-term antihypertensive therapy should be started, and monitored closely as an outpatient
- Risk factors (e.g. smoking, poor diet, obesity) should be discussed with the patient, and appropriate help offered (e.g. smoking cessation clinic, dietician input)
- Any end organ dysfunction (e.g. renal impairment) should be closely monitored following discharge

History

The most important details to elicit in the history concern any evidence of end organ damage and if there is an identifiable cause for the hypertension (if any).
- Are there any symptoms of end organ damage? (see above)
- Previous hypertension
  - Check duration and level of control—it will often be helpful to talk to the GP about this
- PMHx
  - Is there any past history of end organ damage? (e.g. previous stroke, renal impairment)
  - Significant illnesses to ask about include: DM, thyroid disease, Cushing's (idiopathic or iatrogenic), SLE, cardiovascular and renal disease
- DHx
  - Is the patient currently on any antihypertensives, and have they been taking them as prescribed?
  - Has the patient been using any over-the-counter medicines which may raise BP? (e.g. sympathomimetics)
  - Has the patient been taking any illegal drugs? (e.g. cocaine, amphetamines)

Examination

- General examination
  - Is the patient generally unwell?
  - Does the body habitus or appearance suggest underlying pathology? (e.g. Cushing's, Grave's disease)
- Eyes
  - Any gross changes? (scleral haemorrhages, hyphaema)
  - Perform fundoscopy looking for flame haemorrhages, cotton wool haemorrhages and papilloedema
- Cardiovascular
  - Check manual BP—both arms and supine/standing
  - Is there evidence of heart failure? (↑JVP, peripheral oedema, bibasal crepitations, 3rd/4th heart sound)
- Full neurological examination—look for any evidence of hypertensive encephalopathy
- Abdomen—check for any masses or bruits suggestive of AAA

Investigations

- U&Es
  - Is there any renal impairment? eGFR may be useful
  - Mild hypokalaemia may indicate secondary (or rarely primary) hypoaldosteronism
- FBC
  - Check for microangiopathic anaemia
- BNP
  - If suspicious of heart failure
- Endocrine tests
  - TFTs, random cortisol, 24-hour urine catecholamines, pregnancy test—likely to be negative, but useful to rule out
  - Renin and aldosterone levels if hypokalaemic—look for Conn's syndrome
- Autoantibodies
  - Is there vasculitis affecting the kidneys?
- Urine dipstick
  - Check for proteinuria (without features of UTI)
  - If unsure, check 24-hour urine albumin
- Urine toxicology
  - With patient's consent, to check for illegal drugs (patient may not necessarily know what they have taken)
- ECG
  - Check for ischaemic changes or evidence of L ventricular hypertrophy
- Renal USS
  - Should be performed in all patients
  - There should be a low threshold for further investigation (e.g. renal angiography) if any evidence of renal artery stenosis
- CXR
  - Can demonstrate pulmonary oedema or cardiomegaly if suspicious of heart failure
  - Widened mediastinum is consistent with aortic dissection

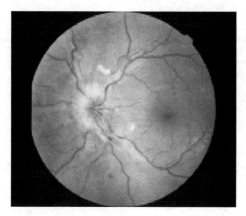

Fig. 2.4 Hypertensive retinal findings. Ocular fundus in hypertension, showing papilloedema, exudates, and a few haemorrhages

- CT head
  - Indicated if there is any evidence of hypertensive encephalopathy
- CT thorax, TOE, aortic angiography
  - Indicated if suspicious of aortic dissection—discuss with radiologist

Causes

The majority of cases will be caused by an unexplained rise in BP in a patient with chronic essential hypertension. Secondary causes include:
- Renal parenchymal disease
  - e.g. reflux nephropathy, glomerulonephritis—accounts for 80% of secondary causes
- Systemic disorders with renal involvement
  - SLE, DM, vasculitis
- Renovascular disease
  - Renal artery stenosis, polyarteritis nodosa
- Endocrine
  - Thyrotoxicosis, phaeochromocytoma, Cushing's syndrome/disease, Conn's syndrome
- Drugs
  - Illegal—cocaine, amphetamines, phencyclidine
  - Ciclosporin, oral contraceptive pills
  - MAOIs with tricyclic antidepressants, antihistamines, or tyramine-containing food
- CNS trauma or spinal cord disorders, such as Guillain–Barré syndrome
- Coarctation/dissection of the aorta
- Pre-eclampsia/eclampsia
- Postoperative hypertension

Further reading
- *OHCM*, 7th edn. Oxford: Oxford University Press, p. 124.
- *Oxford Textbook of Medicine*, 4th edn, vol. 2. Oxford: Oxford University Press, p. 1195.
- *Oxford Handbook of Emergencies in Cardiology*, 1st edn. Oxford: Oxford University Press, p. 278.

ⓘ **Delirium**

An acute onset mental state characterised by altered consciousness, disturbance of cognition, perceptual abnormalities with a fluctuating course. It is frequently regarded as a problem of the elderly in hospital but, on general medical wards, 10–20% of patients will exhibit some symptoms of delirium. Mortality of patients with delirium ranges from 6–18%.

Immediate management

- Assess ABC
  - Confusion can be a sign of serious systemic illness
  - Important causes to detect and treat early are: hypoxia, hypotension and hypoglycaemia
- Reassure patient and try to orientate them as much as possible
  - Ensure the patient is close to the nurses' station in a lit area, preferably with a clock in sight
- Does the patient require sedation?
  - Confused patients can be extremely disruptive and difficult to manage, particularly on wards used to more medically stable patients. It is not uncommon to be called to prescribe sedation rather than to assess a confused patient; this should, however, be a last resort
  - Use a single drug initially, e.g. haloperidol, 1 mg IM, titrate to effect
- Investigations and physical examination may be the only information on which to base initial clinical decisions

History

The patient may be able to give some history; explore any delusions or disorganized thoughts. Speak to relatives, carers or anyone who may know the patient's normal level of function; ensure that this is genuinely an acute episode. Be aware that acute-on-chronic confusion can often be the only symptom of underlying illness.

- Onset, duration and nature of confusion
  - Delirium typically has a fluctuating course, worsening at night—'sun-downing'
- Symptoms of physical illness suggesting an underlying cause
  - e.g. fever, pain, dysuria, constipation
  - Has the patient had any surgery recently?
- Premorbid condition
  - Emotional or personality changes, sensory impairment
- Any history of recent head injury or falls?
- Alcohol and drug history
  - Beware of alcohol withdrawal in the patient who becomes confused several days into their admission
  - Could this be Wernicke–Korsakoff's syndrome? (will require IV vitamin B_1)
  - Many drugs (particularly stimulants) can cause acute psychosis

- PMHx
  - DM—is this hyper/hypoglycaemia?
  - Epilepsy—could this patient be post-ictal?
  - Previous episodes of confusion, and what they were caused by
  - Past psychiatric history—could there be a psychiatric cause (e.g. mania)
- DHx
  - Benzodiazepines, opioids, corticosteroids, anticholinergics
- Food and fluid intake
  - Dehydration and hypernatraemia are well known causes of confusion, particularly in the elderly

Examination

- General examination
  - Take notice of signs such as odour suggestive of UTI or alcohol intoxication
- Check cognitive function and conscious level (MMSE and GCS)
  - MMSE is very useful as a tool for monitoring progress, so should be repeated at least daily for acutely confused patients
- Chest
  - Check for signs of chest infection, effusion, heart failure or endocarditis
- Abdomen
  - Is there any tenderness?
  - Check for masses—especially spleen, liver, bladder or faecal masses
  - Perform a PR—constipation is a very common cause of confusion
- Skin
  - Check for thrombophlebitis at cannula sites, cellulitis, ulcers, bruising from falls, gout and pressure sores
- Full neurological examination
  - Cranial nerves—look for evidence of increased intracranial pressure (papilloedema, false localising signs, i.e. 6th nerve palsy) and cerebral lesions (visual field defects, isolated cranial nerve lesions)
  - Assess language—aphasia can be mistaken for confusion
  - Peripheral nervous system—look for evidence of stroke (hemiplegia, unilateral sensory loss, sensory inattention). Meningitic signs should flag up the possibility of meningitis or SAH

Investigations

- FBC and CRP
  - Is there evidence of underlying infection, i.e. ↑WCC, ↑CRP
- U&Es, LFTs, glucose, bone profile
  - Any electrolyte disturbance can cause confusion, but hypoglycaemia, hypercalcaemia and sodium disturbances are the most common culprits
  - Deranged LFTs may raise suspicion of hepatic encephalopathy
- TFT
  - Particularly hyperthyroidism
- ABGs
  - Check for hypoxia and hypercapnia

- CXR if any chest signs present
- ECG
  - Could this be an unusual presentation of MI?
- Urine dipstick, microscopy and culture
  - UTI is a very common cause of confusion
- Blood alcohol level and toxicology screen

Causes

Intracranial

- Cerebrovascular events
  - TIA, stroke (see p. 312–316), bleeds (see p. 318–327)
- Infection
  - Meningitis (see p. 328–331), encephalitis (see p. 332–334), cerebral abscess
- Epilepsy and post-ictal states (see p. 76–79)
- Space-occupying lesions/metastases

Extracranial

- Infections (see p. 304–306)
  - Chest, UTI and soft tissue infections are common culprits
  - Any infection can cause confusion
- Constipation
- Inadequate nutrition
- Withdrawal from alcohol or benzodiazepines
- Pain from any cause (see p. 10–11)
- Electrolyte disturbance
  - Especially hypo/hypernatraemia (see p. 388–393), hypercalcaemia (see p. 404–406) and hypoglycaemia (see p. 226–229)
- Iatrogenic
  - Almost any medication may be the culprit; be particularly suspicious of newly started or recently changed drugs
- Social upheaval
  - e.g. move to a nursing home or hospital
- Postoperative complications
  - Anastomotic leaks, wound infections, pain
- Endocrine conditions (rare)
  - Hyperthyroidism, Cushing's disease

Further reading

- *OHCM*, 7th edn. Oxford: Oxford University Press, p. 476.
- *Oxford Textbook of Medicine*, 4th edn, vol. 3. Oxford: Oxford University Press, p. 1283.
- Burns A, Gallagley A, Byrne J. Delirium. *J Neurol Neurosurg Psych* 2004; **75**:362–7.
- Brown TM, Boyle MF. ABC of psychological medicine: delirium. BMJ 2002; **325(7365)**:644–7.
- Meagher DJ. Delirium: optimizing management. *BMJ* 2001; **322**:144–9.

⊙ **Raised INR**

The International Normalized Ratio (INR) is the ratio of time taken for blood to clot when compared to a control, and is mainly used to monitor warfarin therapy. For the purpose of this section, only patients on warfarin, not those with coagulation defects, are considered. A raised INR is defined as being one appreciably higher than the target for the treated condition (usually 2–3). Although generally asymptomatic, raised INR can present with:

• Spontaneous bleeding (haematemesis, epistaxis, PR bleed, etc.)
• Excessive bruising
• Intracranial haemorrhage
  • Around 14% of intracranial haemorrhages presenting to neurosurgical units are in patients established on warfarin. Although many will have an INR in the therapeutic range, several will have an excessive INR, unmasked only by this catastrophic presentation

Immediate management

• Assess ABC
  • IV access is especially important if there is evidence of active bleeding, as fluid, blood and reversal agents will need to be given
• Send bloods as detailed below
  • ⚠ Remember to send properly labelled G&S
• Reverse anticoagulation as detailed in table below
• Stop warfarin—record reason on drug/warfarin chart
• Try to staunch bleeding if possible
  • Apply pressure to wounds
  • Upper GI bleed (see p. 44–46)
  • Epistaxis

Table 2.1 British Society for Haematology guidelines

Clinical picture + INR	Treatment
Major bleeding + ↑INR	Vitamin K, 5–10 mg IV FFP/prothrombin complex concentrate ☎ Haematologist on call
INR >8 ± minor bleeding	*If in danger of bleeding* Vitamin K, 0.5 mg IV *or* Vitamin K, 5 mg PO (IV solution can be used PO) *For partial reversal* Vitamin K, 0.5–2.5 mg PO Review INR in 24 hours Repeat PO vitamin K if necessary
INR 6–8	Stop warfarin and monitor INR Restart warfarin when INR <5
INR >0.5 over target to 6	Stop or reduce warfarin Monitor INR

History
- DHx
  - How long has the patient been on warfarin?
  - What is the indication? This may have implications for reversal (e.g. prosthetic heart valve)
  - Was this an overdose? If so, was it accidental or deliberate?
  - Has the patient started any other medications recently? This particularly applies to liver enzyme inducers/inhibitors
- Any history of bleeding
  - Bruising
  - Epistaxis
  - Haematemesis, melaena, PR bleed
  - Menorrhagia/postmenopausal bleeding
  - Haematuria
  - Joint pain—haemarthroses
  - Haemoptysis
- Are there any symptoms of anaemia?
  - Lethargy, worsening angina/heart failure, SOB
- Recent trauma
  - Particularly of head injury
- Any PMHx which predisposes to bleeding?
  - Peptic ulcer disease
  - Oesophageal varices
  - Bowel cancer
  - Previous epistaxis
- Risk factors for liver disease
  - Alcohol, hepatitis, malignancy, haemochromatosis, Wilson's disease, etc.

Examination
- Is there evidence of sepsis?
  - Associated coagulopathy can be worsened by warfarin
- Cardiovascular
  - Check that the patient is haemodynamically stable—HR, BP, CRT
  - Evidence of chronic anaemia (nail changes, palm creases, pale conjunctiva, glossitis/angular stomatitis)
- GI
  - Abdominal tenderness—be especially wary of LUQ pain with a history of trauma, investigate for splenic bleeding
  - PR—malaena, fresh blood
  - Stigmata of liver disease—hepatomegaly, jaundice, spider naevi, ascites
- Skin
  - Is there any obvious bruising?
- Musculoskeletal
  - Joint pain + effusion—could there be a haemarthrosis (call orthopaedic surgeon)
  - Long bone fracture may cause a significant bleed

- Neurological
  - Confusion/↓GCS—intracranial bleed, hepatic encephalopathy
  - Cranial and peripheral nerve examination—any evidence of intracranial bleed?

Investigations

- INR
  - Rapid reversal can occur in as little as 15 minutes with maximum treatment
- G&S
  - Required for blood, FFP and clotting factor transfusion
  - Do not waste time by labelling sample incorrectly—the lab will refuse to process it
- FBC + coagulation screen
  - Check for ↓Hb—may remain normal for several hours after an acute bleed
  - PT will be raised if on warfarin
  - Raised APTT will indicate problem with intrinsic pathway (i.e. not associated with warfarin)
- U&Es
  - ↑Urea can indicate GI bleed
- LFTs
  - Deranged liver function can indicate reason for ↑INR
- Investigate bleeding as necessary
  - CT head if suspicious of intracranial bleed
  - OGD if upper GI bleed
  - Colonoscopy/sigmoidoscopy if PR bleed or chronic anaemia with no other cause found (warfarin can unmask malignancy)

Causes

- Overdose—accidental or deliberate
- Drug interactions
  - Many drugs interact with warfarin
  - Always use care when prescribing to patients on warfarin
- Low dietary intake of vitamin K
- Diarrhoea
- Genetically reduced metabolism (P450 2C9)
- High alcohol intake
- Malignancy

Further reading

- *OHCM*, 7th edn. Oxford: Oxford University Press, p. 334.
- *Oxford Textbook of Medicine*, 4th edn, vol. 2. Oxford: Oxford University Press, p. 1151.
- Hanley JP. Warfarin reversal. *J Clin Pathol* 2004; **57(11)**:1132–9.
- Hylek EM et al. Acetaminophen and other risk factors for excessive warfarin anticoagulation. *JAMA* 1998; **279**:657–62.
- Guidelines on oral anticoagulation: third edition. *Br J Haematol* 1998; **101**:374.

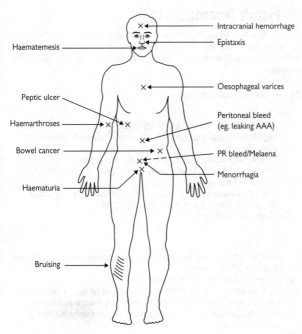

Fig. 2.5 Raised INR. Bleeding sites

⑦ **Frank haematuria**

This is defined as the passage of blood in urine in sufficient quantity to be visible to the naked eye. It can occasionally cause significant bleeding, leading to haemodynamic compromise, and can signify serious underlying pathology.

Immediate management

- ABC
  - Assess for and treat signs of hypovolaemia
  - High-flow oxygen via non-rebreath mask if haemodynamically compromised
  - Gain IV access and take bloods as detailed below
  - Consider IV fluid boluses if patient is shocked
- Urinary catheterization
  - Use a three-way catheter if not contraindicated (e.g. suggestion of urethral trauma) and start saline irrigation
- ☎ Liaise with urologists

History

Be careful to differentiate between true haematuria (with or without blood clots) and PV/PR bleed.
- Where does blood appear in stream?
  - Initial bleeding suggests urethral bleeding flushed out by urination
  - Terminal bleeding is more likely to be from prostate or bladder
  - Blood throughout stream (complete) is usually due to bladder, ureteric or renal causes
- Pain
  - Painless lesions are more suspicious of malignancy
  - Loin or iliac fossa pain suggests renal pathology
  - Lower urinary tract symptoms indicate a bladder problem
- Trauma
  - Any history of trauma to the renal tract?
  - Has the patient been catheterized recently?
- Is there a history of coagulopathy?
  - e.g. anticoagulant use, easy bruising, bleeding gums, epistaxis
  - If so, are they bleeding elsewhere? (e.g. intracranially)
- PMHx
  - Has the patient had a recent Streptococcal infection (sore throat, cellulitis, pneumonia, scarlet fever)—consider post-Streptococcal glomerulonephritis
  - Is there any previous renal disease or urological problem that could account for this?—e.g. prostatic disease, renal cancer
  - Are there any systemic diseases?—e.g. vasculitic disorders, TB, malignancy
- FHx—this is particularly significant for polycystic kidney disease

Examination
- General appearance
  - Cachexia should raise suspicion of malignant process, chronic renal failure or glomerular disease
- Abdomen
  - Loin tenderness should increase suspicion of infection
  - Is there any organomegaly? Palpable kidney should be investigated further for malignancy, and a palpable bladder suggests urinary retention
- Penis
  - Are there signs of trauma or ulcers as causing the bleeding?
- PR
  - Smooth enlarged prostate suggests benign prostatic hypertrophy, whilst a craggy prostate may be malignant

Investigations
- Urine dipstick
  - Blood—infection, malignancy (haemolysed blood indicates bleeding from high in the renal tract, whereas red cells indicate bleeding from lower down)
  - Protein—infection, glomerulonephritis
  - Nitrates/leucocytes—infection
- MSU for microscopy and C&S
- FBC
  - ↓Hb can be acute or chronic
  - ↑WCC can indicate infection. Very high counts may suggest pyelonephritis (see p. 262–264)
- U&Es
  - ↑Urea + ↑creatinine can indicate renal failure, but are only raised if there is a >50% loss of functioning nephron mass
- CRP
  - Elevated in glomerular disease and infection. Useful baseline for assessing response to treatment
- Coagulation screen + INR (if on warfarin)
  - May explain bleeding
  - Always investigate further as it may reveal underlying disease
- LFTs
  - May explain underlying coagulopathy or suggest metastases
- Renal USS
  - Check for stones, ureteric obstruction or renal masses/dilatation
- Further imaging (e.g. IVU)
  - Should be performed under the guidance of a urologist
- Cystoscopy
  - This should be considered in all cases to rule out bladder cancer

Causes
- Cancer
  - Bladder, prostate, kidney or ureter
- Calculi anywhere in urinary tract (see p. 266–268)

- Trauma
  - Can be to kidneys, pelvis or urethra
  - Catheterization or operations on renal tract
- Nephrological causes
  - e.g. IgA nephropathy, glomerulonephritis, vasculitis, AV malformations
- Coagulation defects
  - Anticoagulants, e.g. warfarin (see p. 112–115)
  - Thrombocytopenia (see p. 294–296)
- Renal artery occlusion or renal vein thrombosis
- Sickle cell anaemia/trait
- Infection anywhere in urinary tract
- Causes of red urine with no blood
  - Myoglobinuria—can indicate rhabdomyolysis (dipstick will be positive for blood)
  - Diet, e.g. beetroot, aniline dyes
  - Drugs, e.g. rifampicin, phenindione, phenolphthalein
  - Porphyria (rare)—urine darkens on standing

Further reading

- *OHCM*, 7th edn. Oxford: Oxford University Press, p. 278.
- *Oxford Textbook of Medicine*, 4th edn, vol. 3. Oxford: Oxford University Press, p. 235.

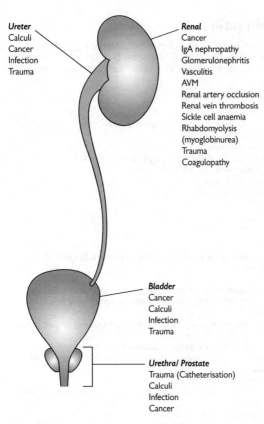

Ureter
Calculi
Cancer
Infection
Trauma

Renal
Cancer
IgA nephropathy
Glomerulonephritis
Vasculitis
AVM
Renal artery occlusion
Renal vein thrombosis
Sickle cell anaemia
Rhabdomyolysis
(myoglobinurea)
Trauma
Coagulopathy

Bladder
Cancer
Calculi
Infection
Trauma

Urethral Prostate
Trauma (Catheterisation)
Calculi
Infection
Cancer

Fig. 2.6 Causes of frank haematuria

ⓘ **Loin pain**

This is defined as pain perceived over the posterior region of the trunk, but lateral to the erector spinae and below the 12th rib. It is important to differentiate this from lower back, lumbosacral and gluteal pain.

Immediate management

- ABC assessment
- High-flow O_2 via non-rebreath mask if unwell
- IV access and bloods (see below)
  - Consider IV fluid boluses
- Give empirical IV antibiotics if patient appears septic
  - e.g. cefuroxime, 1.5 g TDS
- Monitor urine output
- Analgesia (see p. 10–11)
- Keep NBM

History

- Severity
  - Assess this regularly and ensure that the patient has adequate analgesia
- Onset
  - Sudden onset (within minutes) suggests ureteric obstruction; slower onset may indicate kidney, renal pelvis or non-urinary cause
- Character
  - Renal calculi often cause severe, colicky pain causing patient to roll around the bed
  - Lying very still may indicate peritoneal inflammation
- Radiation to the groin, testes, labia or urethral meatus suggests urinary tract pathology
- Timing (continuous vs. colicky)
  - Colicky pain is often due to obstruction of hollow viscus, e.g. renal calculi in ureter
- Alleviating and exacerbating factors
  - Pain on movement and deep inspiration suggests musculoskeletal origin
- Associated features—nausea, vomiting, pyrexia, rigors
  - Be aware of possibility of atypical presentation of an acute abdomen
  - Urinary symptoms—urgency, increased frequency, dysuria, oliguria, change in colour (cloudy, darker, haematuria) and offensive smell all suggest pyelonephritis, calculi or urinary tract obstruction
- Age
  - 35–45 is the peak age for renal calculi
  - Elderly—is there a possibility of malignancy?
- Any history of arteriopathy? Always consider abdominal aortic aneurysm (AAA) if this is the first presentation of loin pain (10% of AAAs present with loin/back pain)

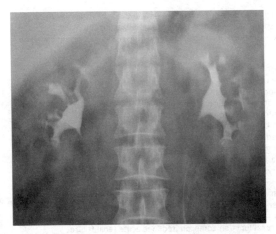

Fig. 2.7 IVU with calculus in right proximal calyx, leading to clubbing and dilatation

- Recent history of strenuous activity—could this be muscle strain?
- Previous history of urological problems—calculi can often be recurrent
- Are there any risk factors for calculi?
  - Infection
  - Hypercalciuria ± hypercalcaemia
  - Gout or excessive excretion of uric acid
  - Oliguria
  - Hyperoxaluria
  - Renal tract malformation
  - Family history (doubles risk)
- Symptoms of malignancy
  - Weight loss, lethargy, frank haematuria
- Consider the possibility of sickle cell anaemia, especially in people of African, Hispanic, Saudi Arabian or Mediterranean descent

Examination
- General appearance
  - Pale and sweaty—is the patient shocked? Are they pyrexial? Are they looking unwell and lying still (peritonitic)?
- Respiratory
  - SOB, low SpO_2, pleuritic chest pain—PE, pneumonia and TB may cause referred pain
- Cardiovascular
  - Are there any indicators of arteriopathy (e.g. poor peripheral circulation); if so be very sure to check for an AAA
- Abdomen
  - Rigid abdomen and rebound/percussion tenderness indicate peritonitis. ☎ Urgent surgical review is required

- Any masses or organomegaly—could there be malignancy?
- Inspect back—are there any bruises indicating trauma?
- Other—Inspection and palpation may reveal shingles or lumbar spine pathology

Investigations

- Urine dipstick
  - Blood—Calculi (negative in 10%), infection, malignancy
  - Protein—Infection, glomerulonephritis
  - Nitrates/leucocytes—infection
- Urine culture and microscopy
  - Red cells—calculi, trauma
  - Organisms—infection
  - Casts—renal disease
  - Crystals—calculi
- FBC
  - Anaemia of chronic disease (e.g. malignancy, renal failure)
  - Very raised WCC should raise the suspicion of pyelonephritis
- U&Es
  - Is renal function compromised? See acute renal failure
- LFTs
  - May be deranged in sepsis or with metastatic cancer
- CRP
  - Elevated in glomerular disease and infection
- Clotting screen
- Bone profile
  - Hypercalcaemia is a risk factor for calculi, and can be raised in para-neoplastic syndromes. Hypocalcaemia can be caused by renal failure
- KUB X-ray (kidneys, ureters and bladder)
  - 90% of renal calculi are radio-opaque, though phleboliths can deceive. May also reveal a calcified AAA
- Abdominal USS
  - May reveal hydronephrosis, ureteric dilatation proximal to obstruction, renal masses and other intra-abdominal pathology
- CXR if there are chest symptoms, or if TB or metastatic disease is suspected
- CT abdomen

Causes

Most common

- Muscle strain—dull aching discomfort exacerbated by bending and lifting
- Pyelonephritis ± renal calculus—sudden onset, severe pain radiating anteriorly and to the groin ± tenderness over renal angle
  - Acute pyelonephritis—dull ache, very high temperature, rigors, vomiting, ↑WCC, pyuria (see p. 262–264)

Less common causes
- Renal infarction (unilateral flank pain + haematuria, fever, nausea, and vomiting, mean age of 65, history of risk factors for thromboembolism, e.g. atrial fibrillation, ↑WCC, ↓LDH)
- Ureteric obstruction caused by pelvi-ureteric junction obstruction or papillary necrosis 2° to analgesic abuse, recurrent pyelonephritis, urinary tract obstruction, TB, sickle cell disease, renal transplant rejection and DM
- Blood clots causing ureteric obstruction or colic 2° to renal biopsy, bleeding disorders, renal tumours or sickle cell disease
- Renal tumours
- Idiopathic loin pain haematuria syndrome (LPHS)
- Radiculitis or transverse process fracture of 10th, 11th or 12th ribs or lumbar spine (may mimic renal colic pain)

Uncommon
- Dissecting AAA (see p. 364–367)
- Glomerulonephritis
- Renal vein thrombosis
- Referred pain from chest, back or abdomen
- Shingles (dermatomal distribution of pain—may present before rash manifests)
- Retroperitoneal fibrosis (insidious onset of a dull pain which progressively becomes more severe)
- Polycystic kidney disease
- Adrenal tumours and haemorrhage (very rare)

Further reading
- *OHCM*, 7th edn. Oxford: Oxford University Press, p. 52.
- *Oxford Textbook of Medicine*, 4th edn, vol. 3. Oxford: Oxford University Press, p. 434.
- *Oxford Handbook of Urology*, 1st edn. Oxford: Oxford University Press, p. 20–21.

① **Sudden onset visual loss**

Definition

A marked reduction of vision, either in acuity or perception of light.

Immediate management

- ABC assessment
- Blood pressure and circulatory assessment (accelerated hypertension is a potential causative mechanism; see p. 102–106)
- Bloods—FBC, U&Es, ESR, lipid profile, glucose
- Gross inspection of eye
  - Check for corneal abrasions or cloudiness, red eye, frank haemorrhage
- Fundoscopy
  - Conditions such as retinal detachment are time-critical in their management. Be especially watchful for signs of retinal artery occlusion (pale disc with cherry-red macula) or papilloedema

  ❶ ☎ Ophthalmologist now—this may be a sight-saving measure!

- ⚠ Potential pitfalls to be mindful of include:
  - Failure to examine the other eye fully in unilateral symptoms
  - Use of mydriatic drops in acute eye emergencies, exacerbating acute angle closure glaucoma

---

History

- Establish the degree and nature of loss
  - Is it a total imperception of light or a partial loss? Many patients will describe any serious reduction in acuity as total loss
  - Is partial loss a reduction in acuity (e.g. blurring or fogginess) or the loss of central or peripheral fields? Establishing pattern of loss may localize the lesion (see Figure)
  - Are symptoms unilateral or bilateral? Unilateral suggests localized pathology (optic nerve or ocular)
- Is there associated pain?
  - Painful conditions in combination with red eye represent serious pathology
- Timing
  - 'Snap' onset often represents vascular pathology
- Does the patient use contact lenses?
  - Infective keratitis can cause extensive damage (especially with *Acanthamoeba* infection)
- Key symptoms include:
  - Headache
  - Jaw claudication, scalp tenderness (temporal arteritis)
  - Floaters and flashing lights (retinal damage, preceding retinal detachment)
  - Reduction in colour perception—'red desaturation'

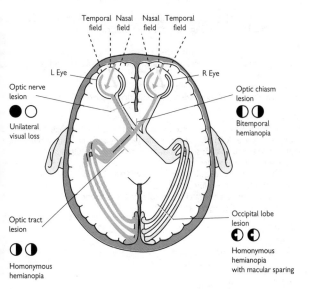

Fig. 2.8 Patterns of visual field loss

- Discomfort with eye movements (optic neuritis)
  - Previous neurological deficits separated in space and time (multiple sclerosis—optic neuritis)
- Key associations include:
  - Diabetes
  - Hypertension
  - Age-related maculopathy or other eye disease
  - Smoker
  - Arterial disease

Examination

- Vision
  - Formally assess visual acuity in each eye using a Snellen chart. If visualization of the largest letter is not possible then assess ability to count fingers, detect movement or discriminate between light and dark (increasingly poor acuity being demonstrated by these tests)
  - Ishihara colour perception—affected disproportionately to acuity in optic nerve pathology
- Neurology
  - Pupillary reflex, being sure to check for direct and consensual response (afferent vs. efferent lesions) and RAPD
  - Visual field assessment (by confrontation testing)

- Full cranial nerve and peripheral nerve assessment—is this deficit is isolated or part of a more global neurological process?
- Systemic
  - Lying/standing BP in both arms
  - Cardiovascular—murmurs, splinter haemorrhages, carotid artery bruits
  - Vasculitic rashes, joint deformity, etc.
  - Scalp and shoulder tenderness (temporal arteritis)

Investigations

Having made initial investigations in the immediate management, the following may be considered for reinforcement or exclusion of differentials. All will require discussion with team senior ± consultant.

- Carotid artery Doppler
- CT head (differentiates bleeding and ischaemic lesions, although infarcts will not be visible immediately)
- MRI head (for soft tissue changes such as those found in MS, smaller infarcts, optic chiasm tumours)

Causes

- Painful
  - Acute glaucoma
  - Temporal arteritis
  - Iritis
- Painless/minimally painful
  - Central or branch retinal vein occlusion
  - Retinal detachment
  - Amaurosis fugax (transient 'curtain descending over eye' due to ophthalmic artery occlusion)
  - Vitreous haemorrhage
  - Optic neuritis
  - Central or branch retinal artery occlusion (rare)
  - Optic nerve infarction (rare)
- Visual field loss
  - Stroke
  - Space-occupying lesion (e.g. bitemporal hemianopia with pituitary tumour)
- Gradual onset and partial loss
  - Age-related maculopathy
  - Cataracts
  - Glaucoma

Further reading

- *OHCM*, 7th edn. Oxford: Oxford University Press, p. 74.
- *Oxford Textbook of Medicine,* 4th edn, vol. 3. Oxford: Oxford University Press, p. 1255.

① **Diarrhoea**

Diarrhoea can be an extremely distressing symptom, but the vast majority of cases are self-limiting and don't cause serious illness. Some cases, however, can cause problems either due to dehydration or the inflammatory effects of the pathogen involved. This can be particularly problematic in vulnerable patients (e.g. the elderly).

Immediate management

- ABC assessment
  - Is the patient hypovolaemic? They may require IV fluid resuscitation (see p. 6–8)
  - The patient may be peritonitic if they have a perforated bowel
- Initiate rehydration
  - This can usually be achieved with oral rehydration therapy (ORT) solutions—via an NG tube if necessary
  - Patients may require IV fluid therapy if they have a ↓GCS or are vomiting profusely as well
  - Patient is likely to require supplemental K^+, as this is lost in diarrhoea
- Antibiotic therapy may be indicated if the patient is systemically unwell (e.g. high fever), has bloody diarrhoea, has had a prolonged course (>2 weeks) or *C. difficile* infection is suspected
  - e.g. ciprofloxacin, 500 mg BD PO *or* ciprofloxacin, 200–400 mg BD IV if PO route not tolerated
  - *if C. difficile infection is suspected:* metronidazole, 500 mg TDS PO (preferred route), and stop other antibiotics if possible
- Antidiarrhoeal agents can be of benefit
  - e.g. loperamide, 4 mg PO loading dose, *then* loperamide, 2 mg PO after each stool (max. 16 mg daily)
  - Avoid in patients with acute severe colitis
- Isolate the patient and initiate barrier nursing
  - Particular care should be taken with patients suffering from *C. difficile* infection, as the spores are resistant to alcohol hand rubs, so thorough handwashing is essential

History

- Details about diarrhoea
  - When did it start? Is it acute or chronic?
  - How often is the patient having diarrhoea, and how much are they producing? This will give an idea of fluid losses
  - Is there any blood or mucus in the stool? The presence of this will indicate acute colitis
- Food intake
  - Has the patient eaten any foodstuffs which may be the cause?— e.g. undercooked chicken or eggs, off meat, raw shellfish
  - Could the illness be related to a food vendor? This may have significant public health implications

- Contact history
  - Has the patient had contact with any others with diarrhoeal illness?
  - Is the patient resident somewhere where there have been cases of *C. difficile* infection?
- Sexual history
  - A history of rectal intercourse may implicate different pathogens
- Foreign travel
  - A returning traveller may have an atypical organism causing the infection
- PMHx
  - Any history of IBD/recurrent diarrhoea—could this be an exacerbation of IBD?
- DHx
  - Has the patient had any recent courses of antibiotics (particularly cefalosporins or clindamycin)? These substantially increase the risk of *C. difficile* infection

Examination

- General examination
  - Assess hydration status (see p. 61)
  - Is the patient cachexic? Consider malabsorption, malignancy
  - Any features of thyroid disease?
- Abdomen
  - Lower abdominal tenderness indicates large bowel inflammation
  - Peritonitis may indicate a bowel perforation
  - Faecal masses may be palpable if there is constipation with overflow
  - PR examination—look for faecal masses, rectal tumours and examine stool for blood/mucus

Investigations

- FBC and CRP
  - ↓Hb may occur with coeliac disease, colorectal carcinoma, ileal Crohn's disease or in haemolytic uraemic syndrome (HUS)
  - ↓Platelets occur in HUS
  - Raised inflammatory markers occur with infective causes, and IBD
- U&Es
  - ↑Na^+ and ↑urea occurs in dehydration
  - ↑Urea and ↑creatinine indicates acute renal failure
  - ↑Urea occurs with HUS
  - Monitor K^+ owing to large GI losses
- TFT
  - Check if there is a suspicion of thyrotoxicosis
- Anti-endomysial antibody/tissue transglutaminase (TTG)
  - Screen for coeliac disease if suspected
- Stool
  - Check for *C. difficile* toxin
  - Microscopy—look for polymorphs and parasites

- Direct immunofluorescence—can detect viral causes
- Bacterial and viral culture—can give definitive diagnosis of infective cause
- AXR/erect CXR
  - Check for toxic megacolon or perforation
- Sigmoidoscopy/colonoscopy
  - Rarely indicated, but can allow tissue diagnosis of colitis

Causes

- Gastroenteritis
  - Viral: rotavirus, Norwalk virus, astrovirus, adenovirus
  - Bacterial: *C. difficile*, *Salmonella* spp., *Shigella* spp., *Campylobacter* spp., *Escherichia coli*, *Yersinia* spp., *Clostridium perfringens*, *Staphylococcus aureus*, *Bacillus cereus*, *Listeria* spp., *Vibrio cholerae*
  - Parasitic: *E. histolytica*, *Entamoeba* spp
- Drug-induced
  - Antibiotics, proton pump inhibitors, cimetidine, propranolol, cytotoxic drugs, NSAIDs, digoxin, alcohol, laxatives
- IBD (see p. 252–255)
  - Ulcerative colitis
  - Crohn's disease
- Constipation with overflow diarrhoea
- Malabsorption
  - Coeliac disease, pancreatic insufficiency, bile salt malabsorption, short bowel syndrome
- Lactose intolerance
- Bacterial overgrowth
- Autonomic neuropathy (rare)
- Addison's disease (rare)
- Thyrotoxicosis (rare) (see p. 234–235)
- Ischaemic colitis (rare)
- Amyloidosis (rare)
- Tropical sprue (rare)
- Malignant (rare)
  - Colorectal carcinoma (unusual presentation)
  - VIPoma, gastrinoma, carcinoid syndrome, thyroid carcinoma (secretary)

Further reading

- *OHCM*, 7th edn. Oxford: Oxford University Press, p. 238.
- *Oxford Textbook of Medicine*, 4th edn, vol. 2. Oxford: Oxford University Press, p. 658.

Section 2

Cardiology

⊙ Acute coronary syndrome

Definition

The spectrum of myocardial ischaemic conditions comprising: ST elevation myocardial infarction (STEMI), non-ST elevation myocardial infarction (NSTEMI) and unstable angina (also known as troponin-negative acute coronary syndrome). Stable angina is not part of the acute coronary syndrome.

Myocardial infarction

Myocardial infarction (MI) describes death of myocardial tissue owing to lack of blood supply. It is divided into STEMI and NSTEMI, mainly because of the differing treatment of the presentation, which has a good evidence base.

Presentation

- Chest pain
  - Central, crushing, chest pain
  - Radiates to the neck, jaw or arm
  - Often more severe than previous anginal pain, and lasting longer
- Sympathetic symptoms
  - Massive ↑sympathetic tone—nausea, vomiting, sweating, cool peripheries and tachycardia
- Shortness of breath
- Acute heart failure (see p. 144–146)
- Cardiogenic shock
- Atypical presentation
  - No overt pain if diminished cardiac autonomic nervous supply (e.g. old age, DM, previous cardiac transplant)
  - Mainly sympathetic symptoms, but also syncope, SOB or general deterioration in health
  - Epigastric pain (especially with inferior MI)

Investigations

- ECG (see below)
- FBC, U&Es, glucose
  - ↓Hb will exacerbate ischaemia
  - ↑/↓K^+ will predispose to arrhythmia
  - ↑Glucose is indication for initiation of glycaemic control—use hospital protocol
- Troponins (I or T)
  - Only diagnostic 8–12 h after onset of pain
  - If raised, indicates a degree of myocardial damage
  - Elevated with ischaemia, myocarditis, renal failure
  - Remain elevated for up to 10 days
  - Troponin T may be elevated in chronic renal disease, troponin I less so
  - Other cardiac markers may also be of use (e.g. CKMB)
- INR if patient established on warfarin
- CXR—a widened mediastinum should raise the suspicion of aortic dissection (see p. 160–162)

☼ ST elevation myocardial infarction (STEMI)

Diagnosis

Based on thorough history and ECG findings. The outcome is improved in STEMIs treated with thrombolysis or primary angioplasty, usually within 12 h of the onset of symptoms. The following are the criteria used for administration of thrombolytics.

- Cardiac chest pain with an onset <12 h ago
- **Plus** any of the following ECG findings:
  - ≥2 mm ST elevation in two or more contiguous chest leads (V_1–V_6)
  - ≥1 mm ST elevation in two or more contiguous limb leads (II, III and aVF, or I and aVL)
  - Left bundle branch block
- If ECG indication of posterior MI (e.g. reciprocal ST depression in chest leads), ☎ discuss with senior

The criteria for primary angioplasty will vary between centres, dependent on its availability.

Immediate management

- ABC assessment
  - ⚠ Cardiogenic shock is very difficult to treat, and should be done so in consultation with seniors
- Sit patient up
- IV access
- Continuous cardiac monitoring
- 12-lead ECG
- M.O.N.A
  - **M**orphine, 5–10 mg IV *or* diamorphine, 2.5–5 mg IV, with antiemetic (e.g. metoclopramide, 10 mg IV)
  - **O**xygen—give high flow via non-rebreath mask
  - **N**itrates, 3–5 mg using buccal or sublingual GTN, 3–5 mg
  - **A**spirin, 300 mg PO
- Check criteria for thrombolysis (see above)
- Thrombolysis if not contraindicated (see below), with informed consent *or* arrange for primary angioplasty, if available
- If pain persists and the patient is not hypotensive
  - Consider GTN IV infusion (starting at 2 mg/h)
- Start a beta blocker
  - e.g. metoprolol, 5 mg IV × 3 doses over 15 min
  - *then after 15 min* metoprolol, 50 mg PO QDS (for 48 h before changing dose regimen)
  - ⚠ Check for contraindications, e.g. asthma, severe congestive cardiac failure, marked hypotension, bradycardia
- Check blood glucose
  - If BM >10, initiate glycaemic control—use hospital protocol
- Low molecular weight heparin
  - Regimen will depend on thrombolytic agent used

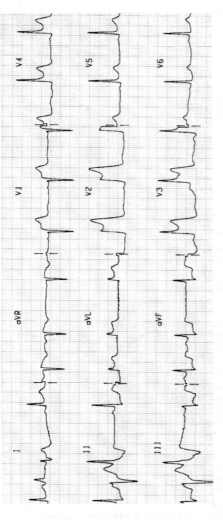

Fig. 3.1 ECG in acute anterolateral MI. There is marked ST segment elevation in leads V1-V4 and aVL. Reciprocal ST segment depression is present in leads II, III and aVF

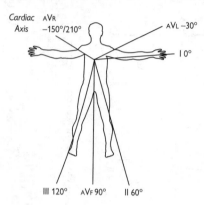

Fig. 3.2 Limb lead views

Thrombolysis

Thrombolysis has been shown to improve outcome in STEMI, but can also have adverse effects. For this reason, clear documentation of informed consent and exclusion of contraindications is vital.

Absolute contraindications
- Haemorrhagic stroke or stroke of unknown origin at any time
- Ischaemic stroke in preceding 6 months
- Central nervous system damage or neoplasms
- Recent major trauma/surgery/head injury (within preceding 3 weeks)
- Gastrointestinal bleeding within the last month
- Known bleeding disorder
- Aortic dissection

Relative contraindications
- Transient ischaemic attack (TIA) in preceding 6 months
- Oral anticoagulant therapy
- Pregnancy or within 1 week post-partum
- Non-compressible punctures
- Traumatic resuscitation
- Refractory hypertension (systolic BP >180 mmHg)
- Advanced liver disease
- Infective endocarditis
- Active peptic ulcer

Other considerations
- Check if previously thrombolysed with streptokinase, or previous Streptococcal infection
  - Use thrombolytic other than streptokinase (e.g. rTPA)
- During thrombolysis
  - Cardiac monitoring is essential
  - Resuscitation equipment (including defibrillator) must be available

- Reperfusion arrhythmias are common, and can cause VF cardiac arrest
- In this situation, VF cardiac arrest often has a good outcome
- Failed reperfusion can present with
  - Ongoing symptoms of angina, despite thrombolysis
  - ST segment elevation should decrease to <50% of peak by 60 min after administration of thrombolytic
  - Consider referring for immediate rescue angioplasty

☼ **Non-ST elevation myocardial infarction and unstable angina**

Non-ST elevation MI (NSTEMI)

Myocardial injury due to coronary artery occlusion or critical stenosis. The ECG does not fulfil the criteria for STEMI (hence neither for thrombolysis), and can be normal. Troponins are raised, indicating that there has been myocardial injury. The extent of the myocardial damage is frequently not as severe as in STEMIs, so revascularisation is often able to prevent further damage of the tissue distal to the obstruction.

Unstable angina

Chest pain due to myocardial ischaemia. It is differentiated from stable angina as it is worsening pain in terms of severity or duration. One definition is of >15–20 min of typical ischaemic pain, or more than two episodes lasting >5 min at rest. As there is usually no infarction of the tissue distal to the stenosis, revascularisation can save the tissue from an impending MI.

Diagnosis

This is primarily a clinical diagnosis, and history is vitally important. ECG findings can aid diagnosis, although they may be normal. Troponins at 12 h will aid differentiation between NSTEMI (where they will be raised) and unstable angina.

ECG findings with myocardial ischaemia:
- ST segment changes
  - ST depression—myocardial ischaemia (may also be reciprocal changes in posterior MI)
  - ST elevation—indicates myocardial infarction (see STEMI, p. 136–139)
  - ST segments can normalize as ST depression becomes elevation—check ECG evolution every 2–4 h
- Q-waves
  - Pathological Q-waves—>40 ms (1 mm) duration and >0.02 mV (2 mm) deep, or >25% the height of the following R-wave
  - Suggest transmural infarction

Immediate management

- ABC assessment
  - ⚠ Cardiogenic shock can be very difficult to treat, and should be done so in consultation with seniors
- Sit patient up
- IV access
- Continuous cardiac monitoring
- 12-lead ECG
- M.O.N.A
  - **M**orphine, 5–10 mg IV or diamorphine, 2.5–5 mg IV with antiemetic (e.g. metoclopramide, 10 mg IV)
  - **O**xygen—give high flow via non-rebreath mask

- • **N**itrates, 3–5 mg—buccal or sublingual GTN, 3–5 mg
  - • **A**spirin, 300 mg PO
- Clopidogrel, 300 mg PO
- Low molecular weight heparin
  - e.g. enoxaparin, 1 mg/kg SC BD
- Give glycoprotein IIb/IIIa inhibitors in high-risk patients
  - Age >65 years
  - Co-morbidity (especially DM)
  - Cardiac pain lasting >15 min at rest
  - ST segment depression on admission or during pain
  - T-wave inversion
  - Impaired LV function (either before or after admission)
  - ↑CRP
  - ↑Troponin
  - e.g. Eptifibatide, 180 µg/kg loading dose
  - *Then* maintenance dose: eptifibatide, 2 µg/kg/min to continue for up to 72 h (96 h if PCI has been performed)
- If pain persists and the patient is not hypotensive, consider an IV GTN infusion (starting at 2 mg/h)
- Start a beta blocker
  - e.g. metoprolol, 5 mg IV × 3 doses over 15 min
  - *Then after 15 min* start maintenance metoprolol, 50 mg PO QDS (for 48 h before changing dose regimen)
  - ⚠ Check for contraindications, e.g. asthma, severe congestive cardiac failure, marked hypotension, bradycardia
- Check blood glucose
  - If BM >10, initiate glycaemic control—use hospital protocol

Post-MI complications

- Acute heart failure (see p. 144–146)
- Cardiogenic shock
- Arrhythmias
  - Usually ventricular—i.e. VT (see p. 184–186)
  - AV nodal infarction (usually with inferior MIs) can result in complete heart block (see p. 164–166)
  - ❶ Can result in cardiac arrest (see Inside cover)
- Cardiac tamponade (see p. 152–155)
- Ventricular septal defect (VSD)
  - Features of L→R shunt, new loud pansystolic murmur, pulmonary congestion
  - ❶ Urgent diagnosis (echo) and surgical referral is vital
- Papillary muscle rupture
  - Acute pulmonary oedema + new pansystolic murmur
  - ❶ Like VSD—also requires urgent diagnosis (echo) and surgical referral
- Mural thrombus
  - Will require anticoagulation with LMWH then warfarin
  - Can result in stroke (see p. 312–316)
- Pericarditis (see p. 148–151)

Further management

Following acute treatment, the plan for secondary prevention should follow on seamlessly.
- Cardiac rehabilitation programme
- Lifestyle advice
  - Smoking cessation, dietary modification, exercise
- Low-dose aspirin
- β blocker
- ACE inhibitor
- Statin
- For patients with NSTEMI
  - Clopidogrel 75 mg OD should be continued for 1 year
- Risk stratification
  - Patients should have their risk of further coronary disease stratified, and arrangements should be made for inpatient/outpatient percutaneous coronary intervention

Further reading

- *OHCM*, 7th edn. Oxford: Oxford University Press, p. 104.
- *Oxford Textbook of Medicine*, 4th edn, vol. 2. Oxford: Oxford University Press, p. 906.
- *Oxford Handbook of Emergencies in Cardiology*, 1st edn. Oxford: Oxford University Press, p. 45.
- Van Der Werff et al. Management of acute myocardial infarction in patients presenting with ST-segment elevation. *Eur Heart J* 2003; **24**:28–66.
- Bertrand ME et al. Management of acute coronary syndromes in patients presenting *without* persistent ST-segment elevation. *Eur Heart J* 2002; **23**:1809–40.
- Guidance on the use of glycoprotein IIb/IIIa inhibitors in the treatment of acute coronary syndromes. *NICE Guideline*, Sept 2002. www.nice.org.uk
- Clopidogrel in the treatment of non-ST-segment-elevation acute coronary syndrome. *NICE Guideline*, July 2004. www.nice.org.uk
- Fibrinolytic Therapy Trialists' (FTT) Collaborative Group. Indications for fibrinolytic therapy in suspected acute myocardial infarction: collaborative overview of early mortality and major morbidity results of all randomized trials of more than 1000 patients. *Lancet* 1994; **343**:311–22.
- Antiplatelet Trialists' Collaboration. Collaborative overview of randomised trials of antiplatelet therapy I: prevention of death, myocardial infarction, and stroke by prolonged antiplatelet therapy in various categories of people. *BMJ* 1994; **308**:81–106.
- Freemantle N, Cleland J, Young P et al. Beta blockade after myocardial infarction: systematic review and meta regression analysis. *BMJ* 1999; **318**:1730–7.
- Théroux P, Welsh RC. Meta-analysis of randomized trials comparing enoxaparin versus unfractionated heparin as adjunctive therapy to fibrinolysis in ST-elevation acute myocardial infarction. *Am J Cardiol* 2003; **91**:860–4.

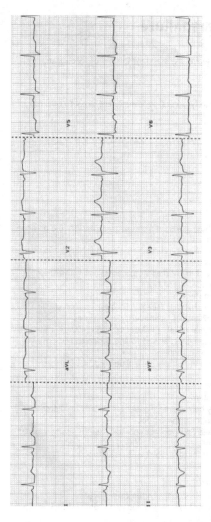

Fig. 3.3 ECG during chest pain. ST segment depression in leads I, V5 and V6 with T wave inversion in leads II, III and aVF is suggestive of ischaemia in the inferolateral territory

⊙ Acute heart failure

Definition

New or markedly worsening signs and symptoms of inadequate systolic or diastolic heart function.

Presentation

Truly unilateral failure rarely occurs, so features are likely to be a mix of
- Shortness of breath
- Fatigue
- Pitting oedema
- Ascites
- Hypotension
- $\downarrow$SpO$_2$

Immediate management

- ABC assessment
  - ⚠ Cardiogenic shock is very difficult to treat, and should be done so in consultation with seniors
  - Give high flow O$_2$ via non-rebreath mask; aim for SpO$_2$>95%
- If distressed or in pain
  - Give diamorphine, 3 mg IV (repeat as necessary) with antiemetic (e.g. metoclopramide, 10 mg IV)
- Assess heart rate and rhythm
  - Treat underlying arrhythmia (see p. 164–186)
- If mean arterial BP >70 mmHg, consider giving nitrates
  - e.g. GTN—sublingual tablets (300 µg) or spray (400 µg) PRN
  - *or* GTN—IV infusion, Start at 5 mg/h and titrate to response— close BP monitoring is required
  - ⚠ Contraindicated in outflow obstruction, e.g. severe aortic stenosis
- If overload is likely, start diuretics
  - Furosemide, 20–50 mg IV
  - Larger doses may be required if patient is already on diuretics
- Catheterize and monitor urine output
- If clinical condition and SpO$_2$ do not improve, call for senior support and consider inotropes
  - e.g. dobutamine IV infusion. Start at 2 µg/kg/min

Further management

- ☎ Manage cases in conjunction with the cardiologists
- Treat possible causes as they become apparent; rate and rhythm control, antimicrobials, etc
- Ongoing control of fluid balance is better managed by challenge-response than continual infusion
- If serial ABGs or invasive monitoring are likely, consider radial artery catheterization

- Anticoagulation is not shown to have specific benefit in heart failure (though it does in some causes of it, such as ACS), but reduces overall risk of co-morbidity

Investigations
- FBC, CRP
  - ↑WCC + ↑CRP indicate infection
  - Anaemia can exacerbate or precipitate heart failure
- U&Es
  - ↑/↓K^+ may cause arrhythmia
  - ↑Urea and ↑creatinine—renal impairment is a possible cause
- BNP
  - Levels >500 will confirm the diagnosis, whereas levels <100 should make you question it
- Troponins
  - Taken 12 h after the onset of symptoms, if significantly raised will indicate an ischaemic cause or myocarditis
  - Levels may be more mildly raised in heart failure
- ABGs/central VBG
  - Metabolic acidosis + ↑lactate indicate organ hypoperfusion in extremely compromised patients
  - Low mixed venous oxygen saturation also indicates organ hypoperfusion
- D-dimer if indicated by Well's score and PE suspected (see p. 188–190)
- INR if patient established on anticoagulation
- CXR
  - Helpful in excluding other causes of SOB (e.g. pneumonia)
  - Useful in assessing the extent of pulmonary oedema
  - Will also provide clues such as heart size and shape
- ECG
  - Look for ischaemic changes, arrhythmia, strain patterns, axis deviation, heart block
- Transthoracic echocardiogram
  - Useful for fluid assessment and inotrope use
  - Can assess systolic pulmonary pressures, IVC size and give an idea of ventricular size and function
  - Can detect regional wall motion abnormalities

Causes
- Decompensation of existing chronic heart failure
- Acute coronary syndromes (see p. 134–143)
- Arrhythmias (see p. 164–186)
- Heart valve, muscle or pericardial disease (see p. 148–151)
- Aortic dissection (see p. 160–162)
- Cardiac tamponade (see p. 152–155)
- Infection—especially pneumonia (see p. 208–211) or septicaemia (see p. 304–306)
- Drug or alcohol abuse
- Iatrogenic—drugs or surgery
- Traumatic brain injury

- Volume overload
- Renal impairment
- Non-compliance with existing treatment for heart failure
- Asthma (see p. 196–198)
- High-output syndromes (e.g. thyrotoxicosis, anaemia, shunt syndromes, septicaemia)
- Phaeochromocytoma (rare) (see p. 242–243)

Further reading

- *Ohcm*, 7th edn. Oxford: Oxford University Press, p. 120.
- *Oxford Textbook of Medicine*, 4th edn, vol. 2. Oxford: Oxford University Press, p. 832.
- *Oxford Handbook of Emergencies in Cardiology*, 1st edn. Oxford: Oxford University Press, p. 67.
- Nieminen M S, Böhm M et al. Executive summary of the guidelines on the diagnosis and treatment of acute heart failure. *Eur Heart J* 2005; **26(4)**:384–416.

ⓘ **Acute pericarditis**

Definition

Inflammation of the pericardium. In some cases it is associated with a pericardial effusion, which can be fibrinous, serous, haemorrhagic or purulent, depending on the underlying pathology. If the effusion becomes large, it may seriously impair ventricular function (therefore cardiac output), and is defined as cardiac tamponade (see p. 152–155).

Presentation

History
- Chest pain
  - Typically retrosternal pain, with 'sharp' character (cf. 'dull/crushing' ischaemic pain)
  - Worse on lying flat/deep inspiration—improves on sitting up
  - Onset commonly over hours, but it can occasionally be sudden
- SOB
- Recent cardiac interventions? e.g. Surgery, cardiac catheterization
- Recent history of viral illness?
  - Most idiopathic cases are thought to have a viral aetiology
- Recent MI? Characteristically occurs within two time periods:
  - A few days after the MI—often after a large infarction
  - 2–8 weeks after the MI—Dressler's syndrome
- PMHx
  - History of renal impairment may be significant—uraemia
  - Autoimmune disease can cause pericarditis—e.g. rheumatoid arthritis, SLE
  - Possibility of TB? Consider contacts, foreign travel, etc
- Is there any history of malignancy? Consider malignant pericarditis

Examination
- May be normal
- Tachycardia
- ⚠ Look for features of Beck's triad, indicating cardiac tamponade (see p. 152–155)
  - Hypotension
  - Distended neck veins
  - Muffled heart sounds
- Pericardial friction rub is pathognomonic of pericarditis
  - Best heard at lower left sternal edge, using the diaphragm of the stethoscope
  - 'Like feet crunching in snow'
  - Can be very difficult to hear, or may be confused with a murmur

ECG
The ECG may show ST segment elevation, therefore may be confused with acute MI. Thrombolysis in pericarditis can be dangerous, as it may precipitate bleeding into the pericardium, thus worsening the situation. Likewise, failure to thrombolyse an actual MI may lead to a poor outcome. If you have any doubts, speak to your seniors or an experienced cardiologist.

- Is normal in 10% of cases
- 'Saddle-shaped' ST segment elevation
  - Distribution may not correspond to coronary artery territory, helping to differentiate from MI
- Non-specific T-wave inversion may be present
- PR depression is highly specific for pericarditis
- ↓QRS amplitude may suggest pericardial effusion (compare with previous ECG)

Immediate management

- ABC assessment
- Pericarditis with a pericardial effusion will not usually be life-threatening, unless a pericardial effusion is large enough to cause cardiac tamponade
- Look for signs of cardiac tamponade
  - Severe SOB
  - Hypotension
  - Reduced pulse pressure—systolic minus diastolic BP
  - Pulsus paradoxus—drop in systolic BP of >10 mmHg on inspiration
  - Neck vein distension, Kussmaul's sign—JVP rises on inspiration
  - Muffled heart sounds
- ▶▶ If any of these are present, manage as per cardiac tamponade (see p. 152–155).

Further management

- Give adequate analgesia. NSAIDs are often very effective, and usually the only treatment required
  - e.g. diclofenac, 50 mg PO TDS (check for contraindications)
  - Give with paracetamol, 1 g PO QDS
- Consider antibiotics if bacterial cause or rheumatic fever is suspected
- Immunosuppressant agents (e.g. colchicine, steroids) may be of value in certain circumstances
  - Under direction of a cardiologist
- Diagnostic/therapeutic pericardiocentesis may be indicated
  - Done under ultrasound guidance
- Surgical procedures such as creation of a pericardial window or pericardectomy may be indicated with significant or recurrent effusion

Investigations

- ECG—see above
- FBC, CRP, blood culture
  - Check for raised inflammatory markers suggesting infective cause
- U&Es
  - Is the patient uraemic?
- TFT
  - Check for hypothyroidism
- ASOT
  - Rheumatic fever may rarely be the cause

- Autoantibodies
  - Could this be autoimmune disease?
- Paired viral titres
  - May identify viral culprit—but often will not
- Troponins
  - May be elevated in pericarditis, when a degree of myocarditis is also present
  - Will not differentiate from acute MI
- Echocardiography
  - Will demonstrate a pericardial effusion, if present
  - Regional wall movement abnormalities may help in differentiating from MI
- CXR
  - Classically 'globular' or 'pear-shaped' heart shadow
- Pericardiocentesis
  - Fluid should be sent for protein level, Gram stain, LDH, cytology, culture and Ziehl–Nielsen staining

Causes
- Idiopathic—most common, often thought to be caused by undiagnosed viral infection
- Viral, e.g. Coxsackie, EBV, influenza, HIV
- Post MI—acute or subacute (Dressler's syndrome)
- Following cardiac surgery
- Bacterial—local or haematogenous spread, post-surgical/penetrating trauma
- TB—have a high index of suspicion in patients with contact history, or from endemic areas
- Autoimmune, e.g. rheumatoid arthritis, SLE, scleroderma, rheumatic fever, sarcoidosis
- Uraemia
- Dialysis-associated pericarditis
- Hypothyroidism
- Aortic dissection (see p. 160–162)
- Neoplastic—often metastatic, but local spread of mesothelioma is another important cause
- Iatrogenic
  - Drugs (e.g. hypersensitivity to penicillin, cyclophosphamide, procainamide, phenytoin)
  - Radiotherapy
  - Post-surgical or following cardiac catheterization
- Oesophageal rupture
- Trauma—penetrating or non-penetrating

Further reading
- *OHCM*, 7th edn. Oxford: Oxford Unversity Press, p. 140.
- *Oxford Textbook of Medicine*, 4th edn, vol. 2. Oxford: Oxford Unversity Press, p. 1044.

- *OH Emergencies in Cardiology*, 1st edn. Oxford: Oxford Unversity Press, p. 181.
- Bernhard Maisch *et al.* Guidelines on the diagnosis and management of pericardial diseases, executive summary. *Eur Heart J* 2004; **25**: 587–610.

☢ **Cardiac tamponade**

Definition

Acute heart failure, secondary to a large or rapidly increasing pericardial effusion. This results in reduced ventricular filling during diastole, hence reduced cardiac output (therefore ↓BP) and central venous congestion. It can be immediately life-threatening, so rapid diagnosis and treatment can save lives.

Presentation

This can present with cardiac arrest (see Inside cover). Be especially suspicious if there has been any penetrating chest trauma.

History
- Chest pain
  - Often similar in character to pericarditis (see p. 148–151)
- SOB
- Dizziness and syncope
- Cough and dysphagia
- If insidious in onset, may initially present with symptoms of end organ ischaemia
  - e.g. Renal failure, mesenteric ischaemia

Examination
- Beck's triad
  - Distended neck veins
  - Hypotension
  - Muffled heart sounds
- Tachycardia
- Severe SOB—often with clear lung fields
- Reduced pulse pressure—systolic minus diastolic BP
- Pulsus paradoxus—drop in systolic BP of >10 mmHg on inspiration
- Neck vein distension
- Kussmaul's sign—JVP rises on inspiration
- Ewart's sign—dullness and bronchial breathing at left base

ECG
- Tachycardia is often the only sign
- Reduced QRS amplitudes may be seen (compare with previous ECGs)
- Changing QRS axis from beat-to-beat may be present, as the heart is swinging around in a large amount of pericardial fluid
- Changes consistent with pericarditis (see p. 148–151)

Immediate management

- ABC
  - If patient is obtunded, maintain a stable airway
  - Give high flow O_2 via a non-rebreath mask
  - Gain large bore IV access and give fluid boluses to increase cardiac preload (therefore ventricular filling), but do not delay definitive treatment

- - Continuous cardiac monitoring is required
- ☎ Call for senior support
- If patient is severely compromised, perform an emergency needle pericardiocentesis immediately (ensuring full arrest trolley is available)
  - Equipment: 20 ml syringe, 3-way tap, long 18G cannula (packs are available with all of the required equipment)
  - The patient must be on an ECG monitor during the procedure
  - Be as aseptic as circumstances allow
  - Put the patient at 45° if possible
  - Attach the syringe to the 3-way tap, and the 3-way tap to the cannula
  - Insert the needle 1 cm below and 1 cm to the left of the xiphisternum
  - Advance, aiming for the tip of the left scapula, continuously aspirating the syringe whilst observing the ECG tracing
  - Stop as soon as you aspirate any fluid, or if you see frequent ventricular ectopics or ST depression on the ECG (indicates you have hit the myocardium—withdraw)
  - Aspirate pericardial fluid using syringe and 3-way tap—taking off as little as 20 ml can cause marked clinical improvement
  - The needle can be removed, and the cannula left in situ with the end stopped off if a reaccumulation is likely
  - ⚠ Complications include: coronary artery laceration, penetration of the ventricle (with bleeding into the pericardium), ventricular arrhythmia (± cardiac arrest), pneumothorax, puncturing of the aorta, oesophagus or peritoneum—this procedure should only be performed in an emergency
- All patients will require urgent referral to cardiologist or cardiothoracic surgeon for more definitive treatment

Further management
- Insertion of a central line may be indicated to monitor for reaccumulation
  - CVP >12–14 cmH$_2$O is usually present in tamponade
- For more stable patients, pericardiocentesis is best performed under ultrasound guidance, or in a cardiac catheter lab with access to X-ray monitoring
  - This is less likely to result in the needle being placed in the wrong place, so substantially reduces the risk of the procedure
- Some patients will require surgical intervention if subject to recurrent tamponade
- Manage pain as for pericarditis (see p. 148–151)

Further investigations
- ECG—see above
- FBC, CRP, blood culture
  - Check for raised inflammatory markers suggesting infective cause

- U&Es
  - Is the patient uraemic?
- TFT
  - Check for hypothyroidism
- ASOT
  - Rheumatic fever may rarely be the cause
- Autoantibodies
  - Could this be autoimmune disease?
- Paired viral titres
  - May identify viral culprit—but often will not
- Troponins
  - May be elevated in pericarditis, when a degree of myocarditis is also present
  - Will not differentiate from acute MI
- Echocardiography
  - Will demonstrate a pericardial effusion, if present
  - Regional wall movement abnormalities may help in differentiating from MI
- CXR
  - Classically 'globular' or 'pear-shaped' heart shadow
- Pericardiocentesis
  - Fluid should be sent for protein level, Gram stain, LDH, cytology, culture and Ziehl–Nielsen staining
  - Heavily bloodstained pericardial fluid will not clot—this is useful in assessing whether fluid aspirated is from the ventricle or from the pericardium (although in massive haemopericardium due to ventricular wall rupture, the blood will clot)
- CT or MRI
  - These can be useful in assessing the pericardial anatomy

Causes

- Pericarditis with large pericardial effusion (see p. 148–151 for causes)
- Malignant deposits causing bleeding are one of the most common causes of tamponade in hospital
- Trauma—particularly penetrating chest injury most commonly, but also with deceleration injuries
- Post MI—ventricular rupture
- Following cardiac surgery (typically 1 day to 6 weeks)
- Aortic dissection (see p. 160–162)
- Iatrogenic
  - After dialysis
  - Post-surgical
  - Cardiac catheterization
  - Central line insertion
  - Pacemaker insertion
  - Sternal bone marrow biopsy
  - Pericardiocentesis
  - Intracardiac injections

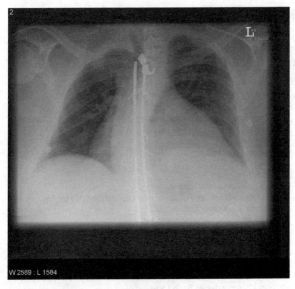

Fig. 3.4 CXR of globular heart in tamponade

Further reading
- *OCHM,* 7th edn. Oxford: Oxford University Press, p. 140, 761, 788.
- *Oxford Textbook of Medicine,* 4th edn, vol 2. Oxford: Oxford University Press, p. 1044.
- *OH Emergencies in Cardiology,* 1st edn. Oxford: Oxford University Press, p. 184.

① Infective endocarditis

Definition

An infection of the intracardiac structures. It carries a high mortality rate (15–20%), and can be non-specific in presentation and hard to diagnose.

Presentation

Infective endocarditis can present in a variety of ways, most of which are quite non-specific.

- Subacute (over months) or acute (over weeks)
  - Fever
  - Night sweats
  - Tiredness and lethargy
  - Weight loss
  - Worsening heart failure
- Hyper-acute (over hours/days)
  - Presents with features of acute heart failure (see p. 144–146), owing to acute valve regurgitation
- Stroke or focal neurological complaint
  - Up to 20% of cases can present with this, due to bacterial emboli
- Incidental new murmur
- Glomerulonephritis/vasculitis—immune-mediated
- On examination
  - Petechiae, splinter haemorrhages, Osler's nodes, Janeway lesions, retinal haemorrhages/Roth spots

Be particularly suspicious in individuals with any of the following problems:
- Structural heart disease
  - Congenital (e.g. VSD), acquired valve lesions, prosthetic valves
- Increased susceptibility to infection
  - e.g. Immunosuppression, DM, old age, dental problems, long-term alcohol abuse
- Recurrent bacteraemia
  - e.g. IV drug use, inflammatory bowel disease, colorectal carcinoma

Immediate management

- ABC assessment
  - Patients can be potentially unwell from acute heart failure (see p. 144–146) or sepsis (see p. 304–306)
- Gain IV access
  - Take initial blood cultures—obtain a good sized sample (e.g. 10 ml) and be careful to avoid contamination (use aseptic technique)

If acutely unwell, start empirical antibiotic therapy

- ☎ Discuss with microbiologist and cardiologist
- Suggested regimen for 'blind' treatment
  - Flucloxacillin, 2 g IV QDS (if >85 kg, give six times daily)
  - *and* gentamicin, 1 mg/kg TDS (monitor blood levels)

- If penicillin-allergic, MRSA-positive or if patient has prosthetic valve, use:
  - vancomycin, 1 g IV BD (monitor blood levels; half dose if patient >65 years)
  - *and* rifampicin, 600 mg BD
  - *and* gentamicin, 1 mg/kg TDS (monitor blood levels)
- The regimen will vary depending on the suspected source
- Patients with prosthetic valves should be converted from warfarin to IV heparin as urgent surgical intervention is often necessary
- ☎ Call cardiothoracic surgeon if acute valve incompetence or prosthetic valve infection is suspected

Further management

- ☎ Cases should be managed in close conjunction with a cardiologist
- If patient is not unwell, antibiotics can be delayed for several days to wait for blood culture results
- The antibiotic therapy is likely to last for 4–6 weeks, so early consideration should be given to long-term venous access
- Many patients with prosthetic valves will need to have the valves replaced to eradicate the infection

Investigations

- Blood cultures
  - Take 3–6 sets from different sites, preferably >1 h apart
  - Obtain good sized samples (e.g. 10 ml)
  - Use aseptic technique to avoid contamination, as it can make results very difficult to interpret
- Echocardiography
  - Should be performed if there is a high clinical suspicion. The combination of transthoracic and transoesophageal echocardiography has a high negative predictive value for endocarditis (95%)
  - ⚠ Transthoracic echocardiography alone is not enough to exclude endocarditis
- FBC
  - May show anaemia if subacute onset; ↑WCC will suggest infection
- ESR, CRP
  - Non-specific, but raised in 90% of cases
- U&Es
  - Check renal function—baseline level required if patient is being treated with gentamicin for several weeks
- Send serology for atypical organisms
- Urine dipstick and microscopy
  - Blood, protein and casts will indicate glomerulonephritis
- Repeat ECGs
  - Lengthening PR interval may indicate aortic root abscess
- If prosthetic valve is removed, it should be sent for C&S and PCR for likely organisms

Diagnosis

This is based on the modified Duke criteria. Clinical diagnosis is confirmed if there are:

- two major criteria *or* one major and three minor criteria, *or* if there are five minor criteria

Major criteria

- Two separate blood cultures growing organisms typical of endocarditis
- Persistently positive blood cultures with consistent organisms taken >12 h apart *or* ≥three positive cultures, with first and last taken >1 h apart
- Positive serology or PCR for causes of culture-negative endocarditis (e.g. Q fever, *Coxiella burnettii*)
- Echocardiogram findings
  - Vegetations
  - Abscess
  - New partial dehiscence of prosthetic valve
  - New valve regurgitation

Minor criteria

- Predisposing risk factors (see above)
- Temp >38°C
- Vascular phenomena
  - Arterial emboli
  - Septic pulmonary infarcts
  - Mycotic aneurysm
  - Intracranial or conjunctival haemorrhage
  - Janeway lesions
  - Splinter haemorrhages
  - Splenomegaly
  - Newly diagnosed clubbing
- Immunological phenomena
  - Glomerulonephritis
  - Osler's nodes
  - Roth spots
  - Positive rheumatoid factor
  - ESR >1.5 × normal
  - CRP >100
- Suggestive microbiological evidence not meeting major criteria
- Suggestive echocardiogram findings not meeting major criteria
- Supportive findings on echocardiography

Complications

- Cardiac
  - Abscesses
  - Valve rupture, perforation or regurgitation
  - Ventricular septal defect
  - Heart failure (see p. 144–146)
  - Heart block (see p. 164–166)
  - Recurrent endocarditis

- Non-cardiac
  - Systemic emboli—can lead to strokes, peripheral artery occlusion, and renal infarctions. The emboli may also develop into abscesses where they deposit
  - Mycotic aneurysms—can lead to SAH (see p. 318–322) if in cerebral artery
  - Renal failure
  - Septic shock (see p. 304–306)

Further reading

- *OHCM*, 7th edn. Oxford: Oxford University Press, p. 136.
- *Oxford Textbook of Medicine*, 4th edn, vol. 2. Oxford: Oxford University Press, p. 1056.
- *OH Emergencies in Cardiology*, 1st edn. Oxford: Oxford University Press, p. 96.

:☠: **Aortic dissection**

Definition

A tear in the tunica intima of the aorta that allows blood to penetrate into the tunica media, stripping it from the tunica adventitia. This may cause aortic rupture (commonly fatal), compromise of the blood supply to major branches, aortic root dilatation (with aortic regurgitation) or cardiac tamponade.

The Stanford classification defines aortic dissection involving the ascending aorta as type A, and that involving the descending aorta as type B. Type A aortic dissection is a surgical emergency, with a very high mortality rate.

Presentation

History

- Chest pain
  - Characteristically very severe pain of near instantaneous onset, felt in the anterior chest and radiating to between the scapulae
  - Classically tearing or ripping in nature, but may be described as sharp, stabbing or pulsatile
- SOB
- Syncope
- Acute heart failure—acute aortic regurgitation
- Collapse
- Stroke
- Abdominal pain—due to mesenteric or renal ischaemia

Examination

- △ There may be no clinical signs
- Shocked patient, with ↔ or ↑BP
  - ↓BP should make you consider tamponade
- Pulmonary oedema—due to acute aortic regurgitation
- Absent or reduced pulses (only 20% of patients)
- Difference of >10 mmHg in systolic BP between both arms
- Left pleural effusion is occasionally seen

Immediate management

- ABC
  - The patient is likely to be very ill
  - Secure the airway if the patient is obtunded
  - Give high flow O_2 via a non-rebreath mask
  - Cannulate with two large bore cannulae, and send blood for urgent crossmatch
- ☎ Call for senior support and involve the cardiothoracic surgeons early
- Give opioid analgesia with antiemetic
  - e.g. diamorphine, 2.5–5 mg IV
  - *and* metoclopramide, 10 mg IV

- Aim to maintain a systolic BP of 100–120 mmHg
  - e.g. esmolol, 500 µg/kg IV, then infuse at 50–200 µg/kg/min (titrate to response)
  - ± Nitroprusside, 0.5–1.5 µg/kg/min IV infusion, increased by 0.5 µg/kg/min every 5 min, titrated to response (max 8 µg/kg/min)
  - or Isosorbide dinitrate, 2–10 mg/h IV infusion and nifedipine, 5–20 mg PO (if β blockers contraindicated)
  - ⚠ Less rapid reduction of BP may be required if the patient is oliguric or has any neurological symptoms
- Consider cardiac tamponade if the patient is hypotensive
  - ⚠ Pericardiocentesis should not be performed prior to surgery, as it may precipitate collapse
- Arrange urgent diagnostic imaging.

Further management

- Type A aortic dissections should be considered for immediate surgery
  - Hourly death rate is ~1–2%
  - Surgical mortality rate is 10–15%
- Type B aortic dissections can often be managed medically, aiming to maintain the systolic BP <130 mmHg
  - Surgery may be indicated if there is proximal extension, increasing aortic enlargement or ischaemia owing to compromised blood supply from major branches
  - The surgical mortality rate is slightly higher than for type A
- Monitor the BP in both arms to avoid pseudohypotension

Investigations

- CXR
  - Normal in 10% of cases
  - Widened mediastinum is seen in 90% of cases
  - Left-sided pleural effusions are sometimes seen with type B dissections
  - 'Calcium sign' suggests type A dissection—separation of the intimal calcification in the aortic knob by >1 cm
- ECG
  - Non-specific ST and T wave changes are common
  - Inferior MI may be caused by dissection compromising the right coronary blood flow (more commonly than the left)
  - Left ventricular hypertrophy may suggest longstanding hypertension
- CT/MRI scan
  - Will diagnose dissection with a very high degree of accuracy, and will differentiate between type A and type B
- Echocardiography
  - Not sensitive or specific for looking at dissection, but will give information about aortic regurgitation and tamponade

Complications
- Type A
  - Aortic rupture
  - MI
  - Cardiac tamponade
  - Aortic regurgitation
  - Stroke
- Type B
  - Aortic rupture
  - Renal ischaemia/infarction
  - Mesenteric ischaemia
  - Leg ischaemia

Causes
- Hypertension
- Pregnancy
- Cocaine use
- Associated with bicuspid aortic valve
- Connective tissue disorders
- Congenital conditions (e.g. Marfan's syndrome, Turner syndrome, Ehlers–Danlos syndrome)
- Complication of cardiac catheterization

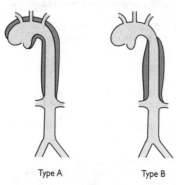

Type A   Type B

Fig. 3.5 Stanford classification

Further reading
- *OHCM*, 7th edn. Oxford: Oxford University Press, p. 586.
- *Oxford Textbook of Medicine*, 4th edn, vol. 2. Oxford: Oxford University Press, p. 1105.
- *OH Emergencies in Cardiology*, 1st edn. Oxford: Oxford University Press, p. 169.

☼ Bradycardia

Definition

Bradycardia is defined as a heart rate of less <60/min. It can often be a normal variant, with most people having this at some point during the day. If it is inappropriate, it is important to treat those who have heart rates which are slow enough to cause haemodynamic compromise, or who are at risk of becoming asystolic.

Presentation

- Incidental finding on examination
- Fatigue
- SOB on exertion or at rest
- Presyncope/syncope
- ❶ Cardiogenic shock

Adverse signs

- Systolic BP <90
- Heart rate <40
- Ventricular arrhythmias requiring suppression
- Heart failure

Immediate management

- ABC assessment
  - Give high flow O$_2$ via non-rebreath mask
  - Gain IV access
  - Continuous cardiac monitoring required

If adverse signs present

- Give atropine, 0.5 mg IV
- Assess response
  - If inadequate, repeat atropine dose and reassess
  - Continue repeating atropine up to a maximum total of 3 mg (six doses)

If there is still an inadequate response

- ⚠ Call for senior support
- Start transcutaneous pacing
  - If equipment is not immediately available, percussive pacing may be enough to keep the patient stable for a short period
- or Consider adrenaline infusion
  - Start with: adrenaline, 2 µg/min IV
  - Titrate to response
  - This should only be done on a high dependency unit

Further management

- Establish if patient has a high risk of becoming asystolic:
  - Recent asystole
  - Möbitz type II AV block

- Complete heart block with broad QRS complexes (>120 ms)
  - Ventricular pause >3 s
- If there are any of the above:
  - ☎ Call for senior support
  - Give atropine as above
- Patients who have had adverse signs, or are at risk of asystole will likely require transvenous pacing urgently, probably followed by permanent pacemaker insertion depending on the cause and liklihood of resolution
- Stop any drugs which may be responsible—e.g. β blockers, calcium channel antagonists, digoxin
- Patients without adverse signs or at high risk of asystole should be monitored, and a cardiology referral requested

Investigations

- 12-lead ECG
  - Sinus bradycardia—rate <60/min, every P-wave followed by a QRS complex
  - Sinus arrest—occasional asystole, with no electrical activity seen until the next P-wave. Pauses are significant if >3s
  - Junctional bradycardia—retrograde P-waves (negative in II, III and aVF) before, during or after QRS complex (which is usually narrow, but can be broad)
  - First degree AV block—every P-wave followed by QRS complex, but PR interval is >200 ms (1 large square)
  - Möbitz type I AV block (Wenckebach)—gradually increasing PR interval, until a P-wave is not followed by a QRS complex
  - Möbitz type II AV block—constant PR interval, with a fixed number of P-waves followed by a QRS complex before one isn't
  - Third degree (complete) heart block—constant P-wave rate and constant R–R interval, with no association between the two—the QRS complex may be broad or narrow
- Ambulatory ECG
  - If patient is having transient episodes of bradycardia, can reveal underlying rhythm disturbance
  - Frequency or nature of episodes can help determine need for permanent pacemaker
- U&Es, glucose, Ca^{2+}, PO_4^{2-}, Mg^{2+}
  - Electrolyte disturbance can cause bradycardia
- TFTs
  - Hypothyroidism can cause bradycardia
- Troponins
  - Complete heart block can be a complication of MI (particularly inferior MI)
- BP
  - ↑BP in an obtunded patient with bradycardia should make you look for ↑ICP
- BMI
  - Sinus bradycardia is common in anorexia nervosa or starvation

Causes
- Physiological—particularly sinus bradycardia in athletic people and in the elderly
- Ischaemic heart disease—especially inferior MI
- Drugs—e.g. β-blockers, calcium channel antagonists, digoxin, antiarrhythmics, lithium
- Sinus node disease
- Myocarditis
- Anorexia nervosa/starvation
- Decompensating shock
- ↑ICP
- Hypoglycaemia
- Hypothermia
- Hypothyroidism
- Carotid sinus hypersensitivity

Further reading
- *OHCM*, 7th edn. Oxford: Oxford University Press, p. 110.
- *Oxford Textbook of Medicine,* 4th edn, vol. 2. Oxford: Oxford University Press, p. 976.
- *OH Emergencies in Cardiology,* 1st edn. Oxford: Oxford University Press, p. 126.

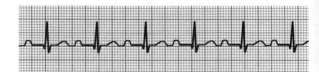

Fig. 3.6 Ist degree AV block. The PR interval is greater than 200 ms (1 large square). There is a QRS after every P wave

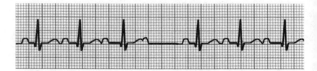

Fig. 3.7 Möbitz type I AV block (Wenkeback). The PR interval lengthens after each successive P wave until finally one P wave is not conducted

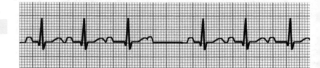

Fig. 3.8 Möbitz type II AV block. P waves fail to conduct to the ventricle in a fixed ratio without preceding lengthening or variation in the PR interval

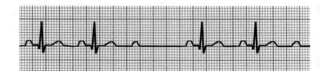

Fig. 3.9 Complete (third degree) AV block. All P waves fail to conduct to the ventricle, resulting in a slow, dissociated ventricular escape rhythm. QRS complexes may be narrow or wide depending upon the site of the escape rhythm origin

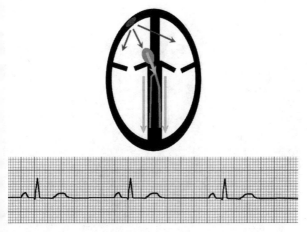

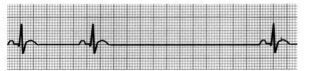

Fig. 3.10 Sinus bradycardia. The P wave and QRS have a constant relationship but the rates slower than 60 bpm (R–R interval of more than 5 large squares). Black arrows indicate a compulsory part of the rhythm/circuit, grey arrows indicate bystander (non-participating) pathways

Fig. 3.11 Sinus arrest. The P waves slows or stop suddenly, resulting in a pause. Significant pauses are those >3 seconds, particularly when the patient is awake

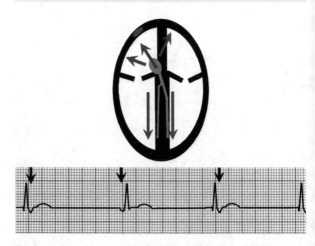

Fig. 3.12 Junctional bradycardia. If the sinus node pacemaker fails, the AV junction is next in line in the pacemaker hierarchy. P waves originate from the AV node area and are therefore negative in leads II, III and aVF. They occur just before, during or after the QRS (arrows), depending upon which point in the AV junction they originate. There is a QRS complex, usually narrow, for every P wave. Black arrows indicate a compulsory part of the rhythm/circuit, grey arrows indicate bystander (non-participating) pathways

⚠ **Supraventricular tachycardia (SVT)**

Definition

SVT is an increased heart rate (>100 bpm), where the electrical activity originates above the ventricular level. For the purposes of emergency management, this encompasses narrow complex tachycardias (QRS duration <120 ms). This definition also includes sinus tachycardia, which is usually a physiological response to stress, but this chapter primarily deals with abnormal electrical activity in the heart causing the tachycardia.

Broad complex tachycardias should be dealt with as ventricular tachycardias (see p. 184–186). Atrial fibrillation is dealt with separately (see p. 178–182).

Presentation

- Fatigue
- Light-headedness
- Dyspnoea
- Rapid palpitations
- Syncope/presyncope (rare)
- ⚠ Cardiogenic shock
  - Can occur if there is pre-existing poor LV function

⚠ *Adverse signs*

- Systolic BP <90
- Chest pain
- Heart failure
- Heart rate >200

Initial management

- ABC assessment
  - Give high flow O_2 via a non-rebreath mask
- 12-lead ECG to confirm diagnosis (exclude physiological causes if sinus tachycardia)
- Attach cardiac monitor
- Large bore IV access into large proximal vein
- Vagal manoeuvres (e.g. Valsalva manoeuvre, carotid sinus massage)
- Give adenosine
  - Adenosine, 6 mg IV rapid bolus injection into a large proximal vein, followed by large flush
- If unsuccessful:
  - Adenosine, 12 mg IV rapid bolus injection followed by large flush
  - Repeat every 1–2 min up to three times until successful
  - You will often see seniors giving larger doses than this
- ☎ Call for senior support

If adverse signs present

- Sedation/general anaesthetic
- Synchronized DC cardioversion
  - 100 J: 200 J: 360 J (or biphasic equivalents)

- ⚠ Ensure machine is set to give **synchronized** shock. There may be a delay after pressing the button before the shock is delivered—be very careful
- If unsuccessful, consider amiodarone before repeating shocks
  - Amiodarone, 300 mg IV over 10–20 min
  - Repeat shocks
  - *then* amiodarone, 900 mg IV over 24 h

Further management

If no adverse signs

- AV nodal blocking drugs
  - Amiodarone, 300 mg IV over 20–60 min *then* 900 mg IV over 24 h
  - *or* Esmolol, 40 mg IV over 1 min, then infuse at 4 mg/min (IV injection can be repeated and infusion can be increased gradually up to 12 mg/min)
  - *or* Verapamil, 5–10 mg IV (contraindicated if on β blockers)
  - *or* Digoxin, 500 µg IV over 30 min (maximum twice)

Investigations

- FBC, U&Es, glucose, Ca^{2+}, Mg^{2+}, TFTs, CRP
  - ↓Hb, infection, electrolyte derangement and hypothyroidism/hyperthyroidism can all cause SVT
- 12-lead ECG
  - Sinus tachycardia—normal P-wave before every QRS
  - Atrial tachycardia—abnormal P-wave before every QRS
  - Atrial flutter—'saw tooth' P-waves (atrial rate ≈ 300/min) with AV block (often 2:1 ∴ ventricular rate = 150/min)
  - AF—absent P-waves, irregularly irregular R–R interval
  - Junctional tachycardia—absent (lost in QRS) or retrograde (after QRS) P-waves
  - Check for ischaemic changes (see p. 134–143)
  - Short PR interval and delta wave in Wolff–Parkinson–White syndrome (resting ECG—not during tachycardia)
  - It is important to take an ECG recording whilst performing vagal manoeuvres or giving adenosine as it may reveal underlying atrial rhythm

Causes

- Physiological (i.e. sinus tachycardia)
  - Treat the underlying cause, e.g. hypovolaemia, sepsis, cardiac failure, PE
- Cardiac
  - Ischaemic heart disease, LV aneurysm, mitral valve disease, cardiomyopathy, pericarditis, myocarditis, aberrant conduction pathways
- Metabolic or endocrine causes
  - K^+/Ca^{2+}/Mg^{2+} derangement, acidosis, hypoxia, hypercapnia, thyroid disease, phaeochromocytoma
- Drugs
  - β_2 agonists, digoxin, L-dopa, tricyclic antidepressants, adriamycin, doxorubicin, caffeine, alcohol

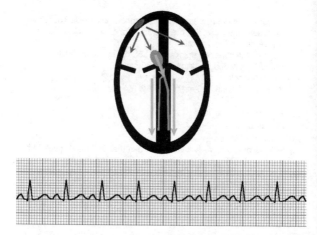

Fig. 3.13 Sinus tachycardia. The P wave is a normal shape and axis and precedes each QRS with a normal PR interval. There are often subtle variations in the heart rate. Black arrows indicate a compulsory part of the rhythm/circuit, grey arrows indicate bystander (non-participating) pathways

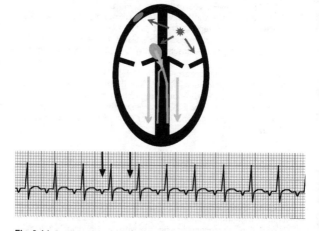

Fig. 3.14 Atrial tachycardia. A focal, automatic tachycardia producing a discrete P wave, although the shape is usually different from the P wave shape seen during sinus rhythm. Usually 1:1 AV conduction unless a very rapid atrial rate or drugs have been given. May have subtle variations in heart rate. Black arrows indicate a compulsory part of the rhythm/circuit, grey arrows indicate bystander (non-participating) pathways

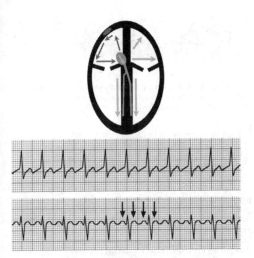

Fig. 3.15 Atrial flutter. Regular QRS complexes, typically at 150 bpm. Rapid, regular atrial activity usually between 280 and 320 bpm (one flutter wave every large square). During 2:1 AV conduction alternate flutter waves may be hidden in QRS com-plexes. Lead V1 is often a good lead for spotting atrial activity (arrows). In typical flutter the flutter waves are negative in leads II, III and aVF (sawtooth pattern). Black arrows indicate a compulsory part of the rhythm/circuit, grey arrows indicate bystander (non-participating) pathways

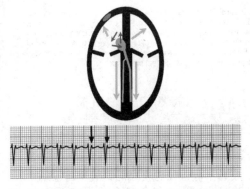

Fig. 3.16 AV nodal reentrant tachycardia. A rapid, regular tachycardia. Usually narrow complex (unless bundle branch aberrancy occurs). Retrograde P wave occur during the QRS complex and are difficult to see, although typically appear as a 'pseudo-R wave' in lead V1 (arrows). Black arrows indicate a compulsory part of the rhythm/circuit, grey arrows indicate bystander (non-participating) pathways

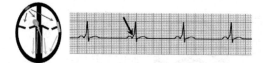

Sinus rhythm and pre-excitation. There is a short PR interval and delta wave at the beginning of the QRS (arrow). Black arrows indicate a compulsory part of the rhythm/circuit, grey arrows indicate bystander (non-participating) pathways

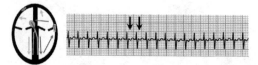

Orthodromic tachycardia. A rapid, regular rhythm. The circuit goes from atrium to ventricle through the AV node and bundle branches so the delta wave disappears and the QRS is narrow (unless there is bundle branch block aberrancy); then from ventricle to atrium through the accessory pathway. The retrograde P wave occurs after the QRS (arrows). Black arrows indicate a compulsory part of the rhythm/circuit, grey arrows indicate bystander (non-participating) pathways

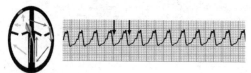

Antidromic tachycardia. Much less common. A rapid, regular rhythm. The circuit goes from atrium to ventricle through the accessory pathway so the ventricle is totally pre-excited and the QRS is very wide; then from ventricle to atrium through the bundle branches and AV node. The retrograde P wave occurs at the end of the QRS (arrows). Black arrows indicate a compulsory part of the rhythm/circuit, grey arrows indicate bystander (non-participating) pathways

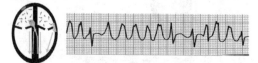

Pre-excited AF. AF is conducted to the ventricles through a combination of the AV node (narrow complexes) and the accessory pathway (wide, pre-excited com-plexes). The accessory pathway tends to dominate producing a very rapid ventricular rate. Black arrows indicate a compulsory part of the rhythm/circuit, grey arrows indicate bystander (non-participating) pathways

Fig. 3.17

ⓘ **Atrial fibrillation**

Definition

Chaotic atrial electrical activity, resulting in ineffective atrial contraction and random depolarization of the AV, causing an irregularly irregular ventricular rate. The ventricular response can be quite rapid, leading to problematic tachycardia. AF is dealt with separately here, as treatment differs from the management of SVT because of the potential to have atrial thrombi, which can cause systemic embolism (e.g. stroke).

Presentation

- Incidentally noted on examination
- Fatigue
- Dyspnoea
- Rapid palpitations—will feel irregular
- Syncope/presyncope (rare)
- ❶ Cardiogenic shock
  - Can occur if there is pre-existing poor LV function, or in Wolff–Parkinson–White syndrome with 1:1 AV conduction through an aberrant pathway

ECG

The ECG will show an irregularly irregular R–R interval, with no P-waves and an irregular baseline. This is diagnostic of AF (the exception being AF with complete heart block, where the rate will be regular at around 40/min).

Risk stratification

The treatment of AF is dependent on the clinical picture, as there is a substantial risk of stroke if cardioverting the patient (either electrically or chemically). This has to be balanced against the risk of the underlying arrhythmia to the patient.

High risk

- Heart rate >150/min
- Ongoing chest pain
- Critically compromised perfusion (↓BP, ↑CRT, ↓GCS)

Intermediate risk

- Heart rate 100–150/min
- SOB

Low risk

- Heart rate <100/min
- Mild symptoms or asymptomatic
- Well perfused

Determining the onset of symptoms is very important. Previous ECGs can also be of great help in determining this. The risk of thrombus formation is lower if the onset was <48 h ago but, if in any doubt, assume that it was >48 h ago.

Immediate management

- Assess ABC
  - Give high flow O_2 via non-rebreath mask
  - Gain IV access into a large peripheral vein
- 12-lead ECG to confirm diagnosis and ventricular rate
- Stratify risk (see above)

High risk

- ☎ Call for senior support
- Give heparin
  - Heparin, 5000–10 000 units IV
- Sedation/general anaesthetic
- Synchronized DC cardioversion
  - 100 J: 200 J: 360 J (or biphasic equivalents)
- If unsuccessful, consider amiodarone before repeating shocks
  - Amiodarone, 300 mg IV over 10–20 min
  - Repeat shock
  - *then* amiodarone, 900 mg IV over 24 h

Intermediate risk

- ☎ Call for senior support
- Assess whether the patient is poorly perfused or if there is known structural heart disease

Poor perfusion ± structural heart disease—onset <24 h ago
- Treat as for high risk

Poor perfusion ± structural heart disease—onset >24 h ago
- Give amiodarone
  - Amiodarone, 300 mg IV over 20–60 min *then* 900 mg IV over 24 h
- Start anticoagulation
  - e.g. Warfarin, 10 mg PO OD (monitor INR and adjust dose as necessary; target is 2–3)
  - LMWH, e.g. Tinzaparin, 175 units/kg SC OD (until INR is >2 for 2 consecutive days)
- Electrical cardioversion may be attempted in 3–4 weeks

Well perfused with no structural heart disease—onset <24 h ago
- Give heparin
  - Heparin, 5000–10 000 units IV
- Attempt chemical cardioversion
  - e.g. flecainide, 100–150 mg IV over 30 min
  - or amiodarone, 300 mg IV over 20–60 min *then* 900 mg IV over 24 h
- If not successful, consider DC cardioversion
  - Sedation/general anaesthetic
  - Synchronized DC cardioversion—100 J: 200 J: 360 J (or biphasic equivalents)

Well perfused with no structural heart disease—onset >24 h ago
- Initiate rate control
  - e.g. Metoprolol, 25–100 mg PO TDS
  - *or* Verapamil, 40–120 mg PO TDS (contraindicated if on β blockers)
  - *or* Diltiazem, 60–120 mg PO TDS (contraindicated if on β-blockers)
  - *or* Digoxin, 500 μg PO 12-hourly × 3 doses, then 62.5–250 μg PO OD
- *or* consider anticoagulation with LMWH and warfarin for 3–4 weeks followed by DC cardioversion

Low risk
Onset <24 h ago
- Give heparin
  - Heparin 5000–10 000 units IV
- Attempt chemical cardioversion
  - e.g. Flecainide 100–150 mg IV over 30 min
  - *or* amiodarone, 300 mg IV over 20–60 min *then* 900 mg IV over 24 h
- *and/or* consider DC cardioversion
  - Sedation/general anaesthetic
  - Synchronized DC cardioversion—100 J: 200 J: 360 J (or biphasic equivalents)

Onset >24 h ago
- Commence anticoagulation with LMWH and warfarin
- Consider DC cardioversion once anticoagulated for 3–4 weeks

Further management
- Rarely, patients with Wolff–Parkinson–White syndrome can get rapid conduction of AF into the ventricle through the accessory pathway. This is called pre-excited AF, and it can cause severe symptoms
  - ECG will show rapid, irregular, broad complex tachycardia
  - ☎ Call cardiologist urgently
  - Give heparin, 5000–10 000 units IV
  - Treat with flecainide, 2 mg/kg (max 150 mg) IV over 10–15 min
  - *or* consider DC cardioversion under sedation/anaesthesia (as under high risk)
  - ⚠ Avoid digoxin, verapamil and adenosine (or other drugs which cause AV nodal block)
  - All patients with Wolff–Parkinson–White syndrome who develop AF should see a cardiologist before being discharged
- Patients who remain in AF will need further management
  - Anticoagulation with warfarin (if not contraindicated)
  - Regular rate control medication if initially tachycardic
- For patients with paroxysmal AF, targeted RF ablation can reduce recurrence

Investigations
- FBC, U&Es, glucose, Ca^{2+}, Mg^{2+}, TFTs, CRP
  - ↓Hb, infection, electrolyte derangement and hypothyroidism/hyperthyroidism can all precipitate AF
- Echocardiography
  - Useful if valve lesion suspected—mitral valve disease can cause AF
  - Transoesophageal echocardiography can detect atrial thrombi, so allows cardioversion after a much shorter period of anticoagulation if no thrombus is seen

Causes
- Ischaemic heart disease
- Idiopathic
- Hypertension
- Mitral valve disease
- Cardiomyopathy
- Acute infection
- Hyperthyroidism
- Post-cardiac surgery

Further reading
- *OHCM*, 7th edn. Oxford: Oxford University Press, p. 116.
- *Oxford Textbook of Medicine,* 4th edn, vol. 2. Oxford: Oxford University Press, p. 986.
- *OH Emergencies in Cardiology,* 1st edn. Oxford: Oxford University Press, p. 140.
- Resuscitation Council (UK) guidelines 2005
- Valentin Fuster *et al.* ACC/AHA/ESC Guidelines for the management of patients with atrial fibrillation, executive summary. *Eur Heart J* 2006 **27**:1979–2030.

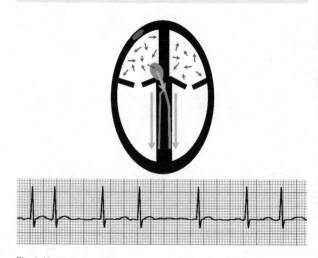

Fig. 3.18 AF. Irregular QRS complexes. No obvious discrete P wave activity, although it is not unusual to see more organized activity in lead V1 with sharp bumps every 4–6 small squares. Black arrows indicate a compulsory part of the rhythm/circuit, grey arrows indicate bystander (non-participating) pathways

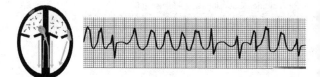

Fig. 3.19 Pre-excited AF. AF is conducted to the ventricles through a combination of the AV node (narrow complexes) and the accessory pathway (wide, pre-excited com-plexes). The accessory pathway tends to dominate producing a very rapid ventricular rate. Black arrows indicate a compulsory part of the rhythm/circuit, grey arrows indicate bystander (non-participating) pathways

:O: **Ventricular tachycardia**

Definition

Increased heart rate (>100) where the electrical activity arises from the ventricular level. For the purposes of emergency management, all broad complex tachycardias (QRS duration >120 ms) should be assumed to be VT. VT is very common following cardiac ischaemia, particularly during thrombolysis (reperfusion arrhythmia).

Presentation

In general, VT tends to present more dramatically than SVT.
- Rapid palpitations
- Syncope/presyncope
- Dyspnoea
- ❶ Cardiogenic shock
- ❶ Cardiac arrest (see Inside cover)

❶ *Adverse signs*
- Systolic BP <90 mmHg
- Chest pain
- Heart failure
- Heart rate >150/min

Initial management
- ABC
  - Give high flow O_2 via a non-rebreath mask
- Large bore IV access into large proximal vein—take blood for urgent U&Es
- Attach cardiac monitor
- 12-lead ECG

If adverse signs present
- ☎ Call for senior support
- Sedation/general anaesthetic (if time)
- Synchronized DC cardioversion
  - 100J: 200J: 360J (or biphasic equivalent)
- If ↓potassium, give IV potassium and magnesium
  - Potassium chloride, max 60 mmol IV infusion at max 30 mmol/h
  - Magnesium sulphate 8 mmol over 10–15 min, with the option of repeating once
  - ⚠ Patient must be on cardiac monitor whilst giving these
- If unsuccessful, consider amiodarone before repeating shocks
  - Amiodarone, 300 mg IV over 10–20 min
  - Repeat shock
  - *then* amiodarone, 900 mg IV over 24 h
- Further cardioversion as required

No adverse signs
- If ↓potassium, give IV potassium and magnesium
  - Potassium chloride, max 60 mmol IV infusion at max 30 mmol/h
  - Magnesium sulphate 8 mmol over 10–15 min, with the option of repeating once

- ⚠ Patient must be on cardiac monitor whilst giving these
- Attempt chemical cardioversion
  - Amiodarone, 300 mg IV over 20–60 min *then* 900 mg over 24 h
- ☎ Call for senior support
- Sedation/general anaesthetic
- Synchronized DC cardioversion
  - 100J: 200J: 360J (or biphasic equivalent)
- Repeat DC cardioversion

Further management
- Torsades de pointes
  - ⚠ Expert input required
  - Give 50% magnesium sulphate, 5 ml IV over 15 min
  - Consider overdrive pacing
  - Consider stopping antiarrhythmics
- For refractory VT consider:
  - Additional pharmacological agents, e.g. amiodarone, lidocaine, procainamide, sotolol
  - Overdrive pacing
  - Patients may require aortic balloon pump, percutaneous coronary intervention or coronary artery bypass graft
- Correct any underlying electrolyte disturbance (see p. 388–406)
- If there is a risk of recurrence, consideration should be given to inserting an implantable cardioverter/defibrillator (ICD)

Investigations
- U&Es, Ca^{2+}, Mg^{2+}
  - Electrolyte derangement may be the cause
- Troponins (repeat after 12 h)
  - A rise may indicate ischaemic insult
- 12–lead ECG
  - VT—broad QRS complexes, QRS concordance (i.e. all +ve or –ve) in chest leads, L axis deviation, AV dissociation, fusion or capture beats, RSr† in V_1, QRS complex in V_6
  - Torsades de pointes—VT with a rotating axis (can be confused with VF)
  - Check for ischaemic changes (see p. 134–143)
  - In sinus rhythm, QT_c should be less than 420 ms

  $$QT_c = QT/\sqrt{(R–R \text{ interval in secs})}$$

- Echocardiography
  - This can help to assess any damage to the heart

Causes
- Ischaemia/infarction, previous cardiac surgery
- Metabolic
  - K^+/Ca^{2+}/Mg^{2+} derangement, acidosis, hypoxia, hypercapnia
- Prolonged QTc interval (torsades de pointes)
  - Electrolyte disturbance (see above), congenital, drugs (sotolol, quinidine, antihistamines, macrolide antibiotics, amiodarone, pheno-thiazines, tricyclic antidepressants, cisapride
  - ⚠ Risk of sudden cardiac death

- Differential diagnosis
  - SVT with aberrant conduction pathway (e.g. SVT + LBBB), antidromic tachycardia in Wolff–Parkinson–White syndrome

Further reading

- *OHCM*, 7th edn. Oxford: Oxford University Press, p. 114, 790.
- *Oxford Textbook of Medicine*, 4th edn, vol. 2. Oxford: Oxford University Press, p. 992.
- *Oxford Handbook of Emergencies in Cardiology*, 1st edn. Oxford: Oxford University Press, p. 156.
- Resuscitation Council (UK) Guidelines 2005
- Zipes DP *et al.* ACC/AHA/ESC Guidelines for management of patients with ventricular arrhythmia and the prevention of sudden cardiac death, executive summary. *Eur Heart J* 2006; **27**:2099–140.

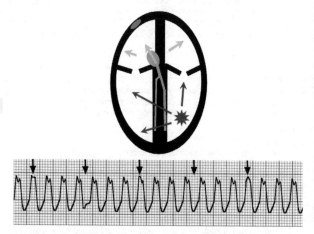

Fig. 3.20 Monomorphic ventricular tachycardia. A regular, wide complex tachycardia. The QRS shape is constant although may be distorted by the independent P wave activity if there is visible AV dissociation (arrows). Black arrows indicate a compul-sory part of the rhythm/circuit, grey arrows indicate bystander (non-participating) pathways

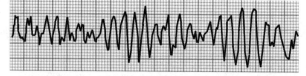

Fig. 3.21 Torsade de Pointes. An irregular, broad complex tachycardia. The QRS axis twists around the baseline

⑦ **Deep vein thrombosis (DVT)**

Definition

A blood clot that forms in one of the deep veins, usually in the leg. This is dangerous as the thrombus may embolise, resulting in pulmonary embolism.

Presentation

- May be asymptomatic
- Unilateral leg swelling ± pain
- Mild pyrexia and persistent tachycardia
- Pulmonary embolism (see p. 200–203)

Immediate management

- ABC
  - DVT in itself does not normally cause severe illness
  - If the patient is tachycardic or tachypnoeic, suspect PE (see p. 200–203)
- Assess DVT probability using Wells' score (see below)

High probability

- Start anticoagulation
  - LMWH, e.g. tinzaparin, 175 units/kg SC OD (until INR is >2 for 2 consecutive days)
  - Warfarin, 10 mg PO OD (monitor INR and adjust dose as necessary; target is 2–3)

Intermediate probability

- Start anticoagulation with LMWH
  - e.g. Tinzaparin, 175 units/kg SC OD
- Arrange for diagnostic imaging (see below)
- If DVT is confirmed commence warfarin (see above)
- Stop anticoagulation if DVT not present

Low probability

- Measure D-dimer
  - If normal, then DVT can be excluded
  - If raised, treat as intermediate probability

Further management

- Oral anticoagulation should be continued for 3 months in all patients, then reassessed
  - Anticoagulation should be continued if there are risk factors for further DVTs, e.g. idiopathic, premature or familial presentation; thrombophilias; malignancy; chronic infection; inflammatory bowel disease; nephrotic syndrome; thromboembolic pulmonary hypertension

- If oral anticoagulation is contraindicated, the patient should be referred for consideration of a vena cava filter to prevent PE
  - Contraindications to warfarin include: peptic ulcer disease, severe hypertension, bacterial endocarditis, high risk of falls/head injury, pregnancy
  - If any of these conditions are present, expert input is required to assess the risk/benefit of the management plan

Wells' score for DVT probability

Active cancer (treatment ongoing, or within 6 months or palliative)	+1
Paralysis or recent plaster immobilization of the lower extremities	+1
Recently bedridden for >3 days or major surgery <4 weeks ago	+1
Localized tenderness along the distribution of the deep venous system	+1
Entire leg swelling	+1
Calf swelling >3 cm compared to the asymptomatic leg	+1
Pitting oedema (greater in the symptomatic leg)	+1
Previous documented DVT	+1
Collateral superficial veins (non-varicose)	+1
Alternative diagnosis as likely or greater than that of DVT	−2

- Score ≥3—high probability (75%)
- Score 1–2—intermediate probability (17%)
- Score ≤0—low probability (3%)

Investigations
- Diagnostic imaging
  - Duplex Doppler USS is non-invasive and good at detecting DVTs, especially above the knee (if nothing found, consider rescan in 1 week if symptoms persist)
  - Ascending venogram is the gold standard, and can be used when USS is inconclusive
- ECG
  - Check for changes consistent with PE, e.g. sinus tachycardia, $S_1Q_3T_3$, right ventricular strain pattern
- Thrombophilia screen
  - Indicated if there is a family history of DVT/PE or if this is a recurrent problem

Causes
- Hypercoagulable state
  - Malignancy
  - Antiphospholipid syndrome
  - Myoproliferative disorder
  - Factor V leiden deficiency
  - Oral contraceptive pill use
  - Pregnancy

- Venous stasis
  - Immobility
  - Recent surgery
  - Pelvic mass (e.g. tumour)

Further reading
- *OHCM*, 7th edn. Oxford: Oxford University Press, p. 564.
- *Oxford Textbook of Medicine*, 4th edn, vol. 2. Oxford: Oxford University Press, p. 1137.

☠ Anaphylaxis

Definition

An immunologically mediated clinical syndrome with severe dermal and systemic manifestations.

Presentation

- Cardiovascular collapse
  - Hypotension, tachycardia, arrhythmias (occasionally)
  - This may be the sole feature of a reaction
- Skin manifestations
  - Rash (erythematous, urticarial, erythroderma) or pallor (due to hypotension)
- Bronchospasm
  - Can be transient or intractable
- Angioedema
  - Laryngeal oedema (stridor, respiratory distress), rhinitis, conjunctivitis
- Generalized symptoms
  - Nausea, vomiting, diarrhoea, abdominal cramps
- Less commonly
  - Pulmonary oedema
  - Convulsions
  - Loss of consciousness
  - Clotting abnormalities

Immediate management

- Assess ABC
  - ❶ If any evidence of airway obstruction, obtain assistance from someone experienced in airway management (i.e. anaesthetist) early
- Administer high flow O_2 via non-rebreath mask
- Stop administration of any likely provoking agent
- Lie patient flat with legs elevated if possible
- Administer adrenaline
  - Adrenaline, 0.5 mg IM (0.5 ml 1:1000 solution)
  - Repeat after 5 min if no improvement (see below)
- Fluid resuscitation with rapid infusion of intravenous crystalloid or colloid (1–2l)
- Administer parenteral antihistamine
  - Chlorphenamine, 10–20 mg IV or IM
- Administer steroid
  - Hydrocortisone, 100–300 mg IV or IM
- Nebulized salbutamol may be useful for those in whom bronchospasm which fails to respond to adrenaline is a prominent feature
- Early involvement of critical care staff is essential, particularly in those with severe refractory bronchospasm or airway compromise due to angioedema

⚠ Adrenaline (epinephrine)

- Intravenous adrenaline may be extremely hazardous. Its use should be restricted to those with specialist experience in the use of intravenous inotropic and vasopressor therapy, and to the treatment of those with profound hypotension resulting in immediate threat to life
  - 50–100 µg (0.5–1 ml 1:10 000 solution) over 1 minute, titrated to effect, is the recommended dose
  - ⚠ Undiluted adrenaline 1:1000 solution should never be given intravenously
- Patients taking tricyclic antidepressants or monoamine oxidase inhibitors (MAOIs) may exhibit an exaggerated response to adrenaline, and should receive 50% of standard doses, titrated to effect
- Patients taking beta blockers may require higher total doses of adrenaline to achieve a satisfactory response. Fluid resuscitation is particularly important in this subgroup of patients
- If hypotension does not respond to adrenaline, alternative vasopressor therapy may be useful (e.g. noradrenaline, metaraminol). This should only be undertaken in a critical care environment by experienced staff

Further management

- Send 10 ml clotted blood immediately after reaction has been treated and again after 1 and 6 hours, for assay of mast cell tryptase (highly specific for anaphylaxis)—notify lab and mark specimens 'urgent'
- Patients with even moderate reactions should be observed closely for 8–24 h owing to the possibility of recurrent symptoms
- A full history into the suspected reaction should be undertaken, with details of suspected provoking agents and time of exposure
- Referral to an allergist for follow-up investigation and determination of hypersensitivity. Include copies of drug charts and clinical notes
- Report any suspected anaphylactic reaction caused by medication to the MHRA/CSM via Yellow Card system (cards available in BNF, or report online at www.mhra.gov.uk)
- Where appropriate, advice should be given to the patient and their family regarding the use of warning bracelets and immediate home treatment of repeat reactions

Immunology of anaphylaxis

The syndrome is usually due to a type 1 hypersensitivity reaction which occurs in response to exposure to an allergen in individuals who have previously been exposed to it. This leads to IgE-mediated release of histamine and other vasoactive inflammatory substances.

Anaphylactoid reactions are clinically identical, and occur in non-sensitised individuals (i.e. IgE does not mediate the response). Substances implicated include food (especially peanuts), insect venom, drugs, allogenic blood and blood components, radiological contrast media, and, increasingly, latex. Immediate treatment of the syndrome is identical, regardless of underlying immunological mechanism. The key to successful treatment is early administration of adrenaline.

Further reading

- *OHCM*, 7th edn. Oxford: Oxford University Press, p. 780.
- *Oxford Textbook of Medicine*, 4th edn, vol. 1. Oxford: Oxford University Press, p. 147.
- Resuscitation Council (UK). The Emergency Medical Treatment of Anaphylactic Reactions for First Medical Responders and for Community Nurses (Revised May 2005). www.resus.org.uk/pages/reaction.htm
- Association of Anaesthetists of Great Britain and Ireland. Suspected Anaphylactic Reactions Associated With Anaesthesia (revised edition 2003). www.AAGBI.org/publications/guidelines/docs/anaphylaxis03.pdf

Respiratory

☠ Acute severe asthma

Definition

Worsening of asthma symptoms over a short period, which can be life-threatening and requires rapid assessment and treatment.

Presentation

Patients usually present with shortness of breath and a 'tight' chest. In most cases there will be a past history of asthma.

⚠ Absence of wheeze on clinical examination can be falsely reassuring, as in severe asthma the airflow through the bronchioles can be too low to produce audible wheeze.

Acute severe asthma can be of varying severity—it is important to determine its presence in order to start the appropriate treatment and when to consider referral to ICU.

Acute severe asthma

Any one of
- PEFR 33–50% best or predicted
- Respiratory rate ≥25
- Heart rate ≥110
- Inability to complete sentences in one breath

❶ Life-threatening asthma

Any one of the following in a patient with severe asthma
- PEFR <33% best or predicted
- SpO$_2$ <92% in air
- PaO$_2$ <8 kPa
- **Normal** PaCO$_2$ (4.6–6.0 kPa)
- Silent chest
- Cyanosis
- Feeble respiratory effort
- Bradycardia
- Dysrhythmia
- Hypotension
- Exhaustion
- Confusion
- Coma

❶ Near fatal asthma

- **Raised** PaCO$_2$ (>6 kPa) ± requiring mechanical ventilation with raised inflation pressures

Immediate management

- ABC—best assessment of gas exchange will be ABG (see p. 412–414) as soon as steps below are in place
- High flow O$_2$ via non-rebreath mask
- Monitor SpO$_2$ and maintain >92%
- Nebulized β$_2$ agonist
  - Salbutamol, 5 mg nebulized (ideally O$_2$ driven)—can be repeated at 15–30-min intervals as needed
  - *or* Continuous salbutamol nebulizer, 5–10 mg/h (requires appropriate nebulizer system) if inadequate response to initial treatment

- Nebulized anticholinergic
  - Ipratropium bromide, 0.5 mg nebulized 4–6-hourly
- Corticosteroids
  - Prednisolone, 40–50 mg OD
  - *or* Hydrocortisone, 100 mg IV QDS (if too breathless to take PO medication)
- Continuous re-assessment of the patient's condition is the most important aspect of treatment. If not improving
  - give more frequent salbutamol/ipratropium nebulizers
  - consider IV therapies (see 'further management')
  - timely referral maximizes benefit from ITU

Further management

IV therapies

Use only after consultation with senior medical staff. Cardiac monitoring and access to resuscitation equipment is required when administering any of the following medications.

- Magnesium sulphate, 1.2–2 g IV over 20 min—single dose
- Aminophylline
  - Loading dose, 5 mg/kg IV over 20 min (omit if on theophylline)
  - Maintenance, 0.5–0.7 mg/kg/h (check level daily)
- Salbutamol, 5 μg/min initially—continuous IV infusion
  - Adjust according to heart rate and response, 3–20 μg/min

Antibiotics

Infective aetiology of acute severe asthma is usually viral, so antibiotics are not routinely prescribed. Only give if there is evidence of bacterial infection.

Referral to ITU

Consider referral to ITU if

- Deteriorating PEFR
- Persisting or worsening hypoxia
- Hypercapnia or rising pCO_2 within normal range
- Falling pH (or increasingly negative base excess) on ABG
- Exhaustion, feeble respiration
- Drowsiness, confusion
- Coma or respiratory arrest

Investigation

- Peak expiratory flow rate
  - Useful in assessing initial response to treatment
  - Percentage of patient's previous best is most useful, but Nunn and Gregg nomogram can be used to calculate predicted value
  - Continue to measure and chart QDS before and after bronchodilators during hospital stay
- ABG
  - Type 1 respiratory failure—↓PaO_2 and ↓$PaCO_2$
  - ⚠ Normal or high $PaCO_2$ indicates life-threatening disease (decompensating)
  - Use this as rapid-access monitoring tool for K^+ levels (see below)

- U&Es
  - Salbutamol causes cellular uptake of K^+, monitor serum level and correct if low, being especially aware that hypokalaemia potentiates the arrhythmogenic effects of β agonists and aminophylline
- FBC/CRP—any evidence of infection?
- CXR—not usually indicated, but must be performed if suspecting associated pneumothorax

Causes
- Respiratory tract infections, usually viral
- Drugs, e.g. NSAIDS, β blockers
- Allergens, e.g. pollens, dust mites, occupational dust exposure, moulds
- Food sensitivities
- Smoke or respiratory irritant
- Psychological stress

Further reading
- *OHCM*, 7th edn. Oxford: Oxford University Press, p. 164–7.
- British Thoracic Society Guidelines (Asthma) 2004 + 2005 and 2007 update www.brit-thoracic.org.uk
- *Oxford Textbook of Medicine*. Section 17.4.4, vol. 2. Oxford: Oxford University Press, p. 1333.

Can the patient help you?

As a disease now frequently diagnosed in the very young, many patients will have lived with asthma as long as they can remember. If the patient is well enough, let them tell you what works for them; the patient feels empowered and you know what to expect. The patient who has had 54 similar admissions may well have a wealth of suggestions, and be less worried by his PEFR than you!

☠ **Pulmonary embolism**

Definition
The lodging of a clot, normally arising from leg or pelvic veins, in the pulmonary circulation.

Presentation
The classic presentation features are detailed below. The astute clinician should, however, be alert to more subtle presentations, especially when there is a history suggestive of venous thromboembolism (VTE) or recent surgery.

- Sudden onset shortness of breath
- Tachycardia, arrhythmia or cardiac arrest
- Hypotension
- Engorged neck veins
- Right ventricular gallop
- Pleuritic chest pain
- Raised JVP
- Cyanosis
- Haemoptysis
- Preceding leg pain
- History of previous VTE or risk factors for it (see later)

Immediate management
- ABC
  - Maximum flow FiO_2, rapid chest survey and ABG should all be first line steps
  - Have a very low threshold for applying cardiac monitoring. If the patient appears compromised in any aspect of their ABC, it should be considered mandatory. Remember that defibrillators can monitor if logistical issues arise
  - Resuscitation as per p. 2–5, remembering that clinical condition may deteriorate precipitously and therefore reliable IV access is essential
- Blood tests as detailed
- Focused history to assess clinical probability of PE (see later)
- ❶ Remember that a PE causing significant cardiorespiratory compromise is a peri-arrest situation. A senior must be called—if any delay is predicted and the patient remains compromised, an arrest call (or medical emergency team if locally available) is not inappropriate— ☎ 2222
- Suspected massive PE will need thrombolysis—before this is given, the consultant on call needs to assess the situation. Are there any absolute or relative contraindications? (see p. 138)
- ECG—the classic $S_1Q_3T_3$ is rare; more likely manifestations are non-specific ST changes or inverted T waves in V_1–V_4, reflecting right ventricular strain, right bundle branch block and tachycardia
- CXR—wedge infarcts, dilated pulmonary artery, pleural effusion or oligaemia of segment distal to occlusion. Most often normal

Assess clinical probability

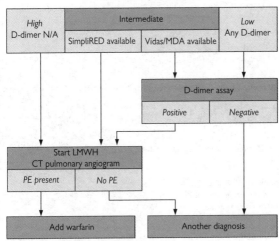

Fig. 4.1 Management of pulmonary embolism

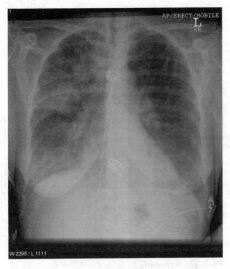

Fig. 4.2 X-ray of Pulmonary Embolism

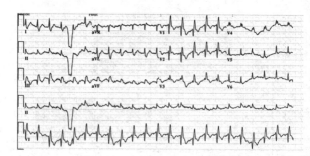

Fig. 4.3 Demonstrative $S_1Q_3T_3$ with right ventricular strain patient seen in PE ECG

Probability scoring in PE
Is there a clinical feature of PE?
One or more of:
- Breathlessness
- Tachypnoea
- Pleuritic chest pain
- Haemoptysis

A. *Absence of any other reasonable clinical explanation*

B. *Is a major risk factor present?*
- Surgery
  - Major abdominal/pelvic surgery
  - Hip/knee replacement
  - Postoperative ITU care
- Obstetrics
  - Late pregnancy
  - Caesarian section
  - Puerperium
- Lower limb problems
  - Fracture
  - Varicose veins
- Malignancy
  - Abdomen/pelvis
  - Advanced or metastatic disease
- Reduced mobility
  - Hospitalization
  - Institutional care
- Previous **proven** VTE

With a clinical feature of PE:
- If A&B are **both** true, risk is **high**
- If **either** A or B is true, risk is **intermediate**
- If neither A nor B is true, risk is **low**

Further management

Once risk is assessed, the algorithm shown (Fig. 4.1) should be used to guide management. Three blood tests exist, SimpliRED or Vidas/MDA, offering differing sensitivity and specificity. It is imperative, however, that D-dimer assays are only requested when indicated by best practice guidelines; they are frequently over-requested, and the information can complicate rather than clarify.

Pregnant patients must not be warfarinised—an acceptable alternative is LMWH to late pregnancy, substituted for unfractionated heparin nearer term for ease of reversal.

Further reading

- Miller et al. BTS guidelines for the management of suspected acute pulmonary embolism. *Thorax* 2003; **58**:470–84.
- *OHCM*, 7th edn. Oxford: Oxford University Press, p. 174–5.

☼ Pneumothorax

Definition

Air in the pleural cavity, between the chest wall and lung, leading to collapse of the lung with accompanying respiratory compromise. If air entering the pleural cavity cannot escape, the resulting positive pressure leads to a tension pneumothorax, a life-threatening condition requiring immediate treatment.

A pneumothorax can be:
- Primary spontaneous (no underlying cause, e.g. young smokers)
- Secondary spontaneous (pre-existing lung disease such as asthma or COPD, but no traumatic cause)
- Secondary traumatic/iatrogenic (e.g. central line insertion or RTA)

Presentation
- Pleuritic chest pain (usually sudden onset)
- Dyspnoea
- Anxiety or feeling of impending doom, malaise
- Cyanosis (particularly if pre-existing lung disease)
- Tachypnoea
- Tachycardia
- Hypoxia
- Reduced movement of chest wall on affected side
- Resonant percussion note on affected side
- Reduced breath sounds on affected side

It is essential to differentiate a tension pneumothorax from a simple pneumothorax. Consider tension pneumothorax if there is:
- An obvious cause of chest wound such as penetrating trauma to the chest, or a recent invasive procedure
- A disproportionately severe symptom profile for estimated size of pneumothorax
- Hypotension
- Elevated JVP
- Pulsus paradoxus (decrease in systolic BP on inspiration—very difficult to establish by palpation but easy with a sphygmomanometer)
- Cyanosis
- Tracheal deviation (away from pneumothorax—late sign, respiratory arrest is imminent)
- Abdominal distension
- Reduced consciousness/increased confusion
- Rapidly increasing respiratory distress leading to respiratory arrest

Immediate management

- ABC and initial survey for tension, as described previously
- ❶ If at this stage you suspect a tension pneumothorax, proceed directly to needle decompression. Insert a 16-G cannula in the second intercostal space (above third rib) in the midclavicular line on the affected side. On removing the needle, there should be a hiss of gas. Secure the cannula, and insert an intercostal chest drain (see *OHCM*, 7th edn, p. 754–5) on the affected side.
- CXR for measurement of air rim. This is now easily achieved by use of the mark-up tool on computerised radiology systems
- ABG (see p. 422–424) may be dictated by clinical condition. It is prudent to take a sample if the patient is overtly breathless or has significantly reduced SpO_2 on oximetry

Further management

Management from this point is dependent on the nature of the pneumo-thorax and clinical condition.

- A patient with primary pneumothorax, who is not breathless and is cardiovascularly stable, has uncompromised ABGs and a CXR showing a rim <2 cm can usually be discharged with advice to return if increasingly short of breath or uncomfortable. Recall to the chest clinic after 2 weeks allows the opportunity for radiological proof of resolution and reassurance for the patient
- Those with primary pneumothorax with either breathlessness or a rim >2 cm should be aspirated (see *OHCM*, p. 758). If unsuccessful, discuss with seniors; an intercostal chest drain is indicated. Remove chest drain 24 h after full re-expansion or cessation of air leak without clamping and consider discharge. If still unsuccessful, refer to chest team within 48 h
- In secondary spontaneous pneumothorax seen in patients who are breathless, >50 years of age or have a rim >2 cm, aspiration is most likely to fail. Proceed straight to intercostal chest drain insertion
- In patients with secondary spontaneous pneumothorax who are not breathless, are <50 years and have a rim <2 cm, aspiration should be attempted. If successful, admit for observation for 24 h, at which point discharge unless patient is still of clinical concern. If aspiration is unsuccessful, proceed to intercostal drain insertion as above
- Secondary traumatic/iatrogenic pneumothorax should be discussed with seniors. A chest drain is usually necessary owing the risk of progression to tension pneumothorax

A patient who is of any concern should not be discharged, even if intervention appears to have been successful. All presentations should be discussed with seniors before discharge, even if they are primary and not for any active intervention.

Investigations
- Posteroanterior CXR
  - Consider film in expiration or lateral decubitus film if high clinical suspicion for pneumothorax with negative PA chest radiograph
  - Look for visceral pleural line without distal lung markings—a visible lung edge parallel to chest wall, enlarged lateral costophrenic angle on supine film (deep sulcus sign)
  - Look also for signs of underlying lung disease
  - Any signs of trauma?
- As mentioned before, ABG sampling is definitely indicated in most types of pneumothorax; it would be prudent always to have at least one sample in all pneumothoraces
- Further investigations should be directed at suspected underlying cause, e.g. FBC and CRP for chest infection

Causes

Primary spontaneous
Caused by rupture of subpleural blebs/bullae. Smoking is a risk factor.

Secondary spontaneous
- Underlying lung disease predisposing to rupture of pleura
  - COPD
  - Asthma
  - Fibrotic lung disease
  - CF
  - Sarcoidosis
- Cavitating lung lesions
  - Lung carcinoma
  - Lung abscess
  - Cavitating pneumonia (*Staphylococcus/Klebsiella/Pseudomonas*)
  - TB
  - Pneumocystic pneumonia in immunocompromised patients
- Rarer causes
  - Ehlers–Danlos syndrome
  - Langerhan's cell histiocytosis
  - Pulmonary neurofibromatosis

Secondary iatrogenic
Invasive procedures such as internal jugular vein cannulation.

Secondary traumatic
Generally blunt or penetrating trauma resulting from RTAs, CPR or assault.

Further reading

- *OHCM*, 7th edn. Oxford: Oxford University Press, p. 174.
- Henry M, Arnold T, Harvey J. Pleural Diseases Group, Standards of Care Committee, British Thoracic Society. BTS guidelines for the management of spontaneous pneumothorax. *Thorax* 2003; **58** (Suppl 2):ii39–52.
- O'Connor AR, Morgan WE. Radiological review of pneumothorax. *BMJ* 2005; **330(7506)**:1493–7.

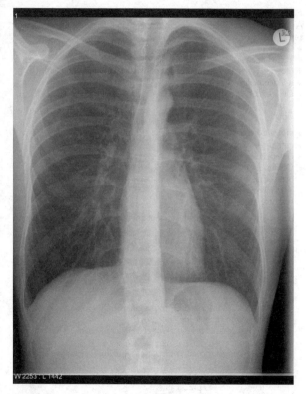

Fig. 4.4 CXR demonstrative a subtle pneumothorax

☼ Pneumonia

Definition

Symptoms and signs consistent with an acute lower respiratory tract infection, usually associated with new radiographic shadowing for which there is no other explanation. It can broadly be classified as either hospital or community-acquired in origin. Exacerbation of COPD is dealt with as a separate topic; see p. 212–215.

Presentation

A mixture of respiratory symptoms/signs and features of generalized sepsis.

- Cough (± purulent sputum)
- Tachypnoea
- Pleuritic chest pain (sometimes abdominal or shoulder tip pain)
- Reduced expansion
- Dull percussion
- Bronchial breathing
- Coarse crepitations

Symptoms associated with sepsis

- Lethargy/malaise
- Fever/rigors
- Confusion
- Nausea and vomiting
- Tachycardia
- Hypotension

It is also important to take a history of any foreign travel or exposure to birds, which may be a risk factor for atypical pathogens, in addition to checking immune status, the immunosuppressed being at substantially higher risk.

Immediate management

- ABC
  - Administer moisturized O_2 to maintain SpO_2 >95% (⚠ Caution in patients with chronic lung disease)
  - Good IV access is essential—pneumonia can cause severe fluid depletion
  - If hypotensive/shocked, resuscitate as per ABC technique (see p. 2–5)
- Quantitative assessment by ABG (see p. 422–424) should be performed as soon as practicable
- As soon as patient is stable, severity must be assessed using the CURB-65 scoring system (1 point for each criterion)
  - **C**onfusion (new onset)
  - **U**rea >7 mmol/l
  - **R**espiratory rate ≥30/min
  - **B**lood pressure <90 systolic and/or ≤60 diastolic

- **65**-years-old or over?
- Mild = 0–1; moderate = 2; severe ≥3
- Intravenous broad spectrum antibiotics at time of diagnosis are indicated for severe CAP
  - ⚠ Check for drug allergies
  - Cefuroxime, 1.5 g TDS IV
  - Clarithromycin, 500 mg BD IV
  - *and* Metronidazole, 500 mg IV should be given if aspiration is suspected
  - Penicillin-intolerant patients should be given fluoroquinolones in its place. Levofloxacin can be given IV (500 mg BD); moxifloxacin has yet to be licensed for either IV use or in severe CAP (community-acquired pneumothorax)
- Hospital-acquired pneumonia is treated according to local guidelines, which will take into account regional variation in likely pathogens

☎ Early decision about suitability for ITU admission is recommended if CURB-65 score is 4–5, or there is not a rapid response to initial therapy.

Investigations

- FBC, U&Es, LFT, CRP
  - ↑WCC indicates bacterial cause; ↑urea is a marker of severity; sepsis can affect renal or hepatic function; ↑CRP indicates infection and is useful for assessing response to treatment
- HIV serology in patients aged 15–54 with risk factors or an abnormal and unexplained WCC.
  - ⚠ **This test requires informed consent, which should be clearly documented in the patient's notes**
- ABG
  - PH <7.26 + pO_2 <8 + rising pCO_2 despite treatment are indications for ITU admission
- Routine microbiology
  - Blood culture (minimum 20 ml)
  - Sputum for Gram stain, culture and sensitivity—less commonly requested, but may still yield useful information
- Specific microbiology for at-risk populations
  - AFB/ZN stains for TB
  - Pleural fluid for Gram stain, culture and sensitivity, cell count and pH
  - Pneumococcal urine antigen test
  - Legionella tests—urine for antigen titre, sputum for culture and immunofluorescence, paired serum titres
  - Atypical pathogen tests—sputum for immunofluorescence, paired viral and atypical titres
- CXR
  - Lobar consolidation (indistinct heart/diaphragm border—see Figure); diffuse consolidation; lobar collapse; pleural effusion; may be normal

Further management
- Simple analgesia for pleuritic chest pain
- Nebulized bronchodilators if wheezing and saline to promote expectoration
- Close monitoring of vital signs
- Daily FBC/CRP to check response to antibiotics—WCC should be falling and CRP should decrease by 50% over 4 days if responding well

Antibiotic treatment

Table 4.1 Empirical antibiotic treatment in community-acquired pneumonia

Severity	Preferred treatment	Alternative treatment
Non-severe	Amoxicillin, 500 mg–1 g TDS PO +	Levofloxacin 500 mg OD PO or moxifloxacin 400 mg OD PO
7 days' treatment	Erythromycin 500 mg QDS PO or clarithromycin 500 mg BD PO	
Severe	Co-amoxiclav 1 g TDS IV or cefuroxime 1.5 g TDS IV or cefotaxime 1 g TDS IV or ceftriaxone 2 g OD IV +	Levofloxacin 500 mg BD IV or PO + benzylpenicillin 1.2 g QDS IV
10 days' treatment initially		
14–21 days for resistant or	erythromycin 500 mg QDS IV or clarithromycin 500 mg BD IV ±	
atypical infection	rifampicin 600 mg OD or BD IV	

Many hospitals will have local guidelines for treatment of chest infections. The above table is an empirical guideline, and should not override guidance from microbiologists.

Causes

Community-acquired
- Common: *Streptococcus pneumoniae*, *Haemophilus influenzae*, *Mycoplasma pneumoniae*, viral
- Rare: *Staphylococcus aureus*, *Legionella* spp, *Moraxella catarrhalis*, *Chlamydia* spp

Hospital-acquired
- Gram negative enterobacter, *Staph. aureus* (including MRSA), *Pseudomonas*, *Klebsiella*, *Bacteroides*, *Clostridia*

Aspiration
- Oropharyngeal anaerobes. A reactive chemical pneumonitis must also be considered here

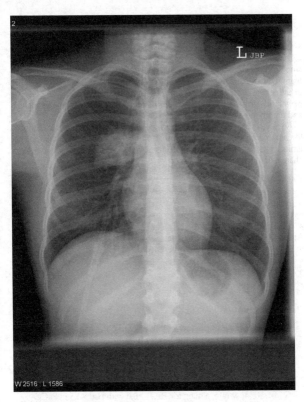

Fig. 4.5 Chest X-ray showing consolidation in the right middle zone

Immunocompromised patients
- *Strep. pneumoniae, H. influenzae, Staph. aureus, M. catarrhalis, M. pneumoniae, Gram negative bacilli, Pneumocystis carinii, fungi, viruses, Mycobacteria* spp

Further reading
- British Thoracic Society Guidelines (Pneumonia) 2001 + 2004 update www.brit-thoracic.org.uk
- *OHCM*, 7th edn. Oxford: Oxford University Press, p. 152–6.

⚠ **Acute exacerbation of COPD**

Definition

COPD is a progressive airway obstruction, usually related to tobacco smoking, at best only partially reversible. COPD is a spectrum of disease from mild exertional dyspnoea and chronic cough to a severe irreversible breathlessness at rest, requiring long-term oxygen therapy, and is the preferred term to encompass older diagnoses such as chronic bronchitis and emphysema.

An exacerbation is an acute worsening of symptoms which is prolonged and beyond any variation that the patient considers within normal limits. The worsening of symptoms should be sufficient to warrant a change in medication.

Presentation

- Increased dyspnoea, whether exertional or at rest
- Increased cough
- Increased sputum production
- Change in colour of sputum

Associated with this, there may be:

- Decreased level of exercise tolerance
- Increased leg oedema
- New or increased confusion
- Cachexia

Immediate management

- ABC—this is one of the few situations where the much over-quoted loss of hypoxic drive is at the forefront of management considerations
  - It is sensible to assume most patients in this population have a degree of Type II respiratory failure, so begin O_2 administration at 24–28% via Venturi mask
  - Titrate flow rate, aiming for PaO_2 >8.0 with rise <1.5 in $PaCO_2$
- Initial ABG (see p. 418–420), with frequent re-sampling during O_2 titration
- Nebulized salbutamol (2.5–5 mg PRN) and ipratropium (500 µg).
  - In severe Type II respiratory failure, these may need to be administered by air-driven nebulizer with supplemental O_2 via nasal cannulae
- IV access and bloods as detailed
- Commence corticosteroid therapy—prednisolone 30 mg orally if able to swallow or hydrocortisone 100–200 mg IV if not
- CXR may show any new infection, as well as give an idea of the extent of chest disease. Look for bullae, pneumothoraces, focal opacities, hyperinflation, oedema

Further management

- Optimum management involves frequent reassessment, both clinically and by ABG
- Increased sputum purulence or volume is an indication for antibiotic therapy. There is a wide range of suggested therapies, often guided by hospital microbiology departments. If information is unavailable, broad-spectrum cover (such as co-amoxiclav 1 g IV tds) should be prescribed
- Chest physiotherapy
- Prophylactic dose heparin is prudent, especially given increased risk of polycythaemia
- Look at fluid status carefully. If evidence of cor pulmonale, a controlled fluid balance regime may help prevent further decompensation
- Discuss aminophylline usage with senior. Load with 250 mg if not on theophylline, followed by 750–1500 mg over next 24 h
- Worsening or new CO_2 retention, acidosis or tiring after 1 h of optimum medical management is an indication for non-invasive ventilation (NIV)
  - Respiratory rate <12, pneumothorax, altered consciousness, agitation or inability to tolerate facepiece are all contraindications to NIV
  - Referral must not be made without discussion with senior medical on-call staff
  - ABGs should be sampled at least hourly
- Doxapram, a respiratory stimulant, is supported more by anecdote than evidence. If senior considers it suitable, 1 g in 500 ml 5% dextrose should be infused, starting at 1 ml/min. ABGs must be checked within the hour, with an infusion ceiling of 2 ml/min
- At this stage, a frank and focused discussion must be had with the patient and relatives. COPD is by its nature a terminal disease, but many patients may not have had this (or recall having it) explicitly explained to them. A detailed functional and social background is required from patient and family prior to discussion with ITU; they in turn need to be made aware that ventilation may not be considered appropriate, that the patient is now receiving maximum medical therapy and that this admission may not be survivable. If a decision is reached at this stage, ensure any appropriate DNAR is documented and initiated as per hospital protocol
- ☎ Contact ITU for further assessment.

Investigations

- Serial ABGs, ensuring FiO_2 at time of sampling is clearly documented
- FBC, U&Es and CRP—look for evidence of infection and its biochemical impact. Salbutamol causes cellular take-up of K^+, monitor serum level and correct if low, being especially aware that hypokalaemia potentiates the arrhythmogenic effects of β agonists and aminophylline
- Theophylline level if appropriate
- ECG—is there coexisting cardiac dysfunction?
- Sputum C&S
- Serial PEFR where possible

Causes

Non-infectious
- Air pollutants

Infectious
- Viral
  - Rhinovirus
  - Influenza species
  - Parainfluenza
  - Adenovirus
  - RSV
- Bacterial
  - *H. influenzae*
  - *Strep. pneumoniae*
  - *Moraxella catarrhalis*
  - *Pseudomonas aeruginosa* (less commonly)
  - *Chlamydia* and *Mycoplasma* spp. (rarely)

Non-respiratory causes
In patients known to have minimally problematic COPD normally, look for another cause of respiratory decompensation, such as head injury or opiate overdose.

Further reading
- Chronic obstructive pulmonary disease—management of chronic obstructive pulmonary disease in adults in primary and secondary care. NICE Guideline, February 2004.
- Rodriguez-Roisin R. COPD exacerbations 5: Management. *Thorax* 2006; **61**:535–44.
- *OHCM*, 7th edn. Oxford: Oxford University Press, p. 168–9.

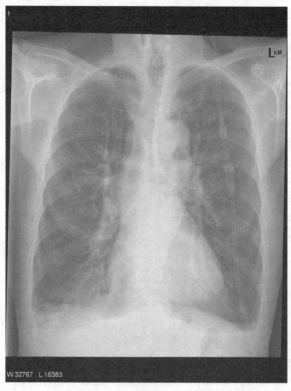

Fig. 4.6 CXR showing the Hallmark changes of COPD

① **Pleural effusion**

Definition

The accumulation of abnormal amounts of fluid in the pleural space. There is normally a small amount of fluid; 10 ml could be found in most of the population, but an accumulation implies an imbalance between formation and removal. Rarely a true emergency, patients often present when the progressive dyspnoea interferes too much with activities of daily living.

Presentation

- Dyspnoea
- Chest pain
- Syncope
- Cough
- Dull percussion note on affected side
- Reduced air entry on auscultation

Immediate management

- ABC
  - Caution with FiO_2 is required here—patients with existing chest disease (whether or not directly related to this effusion) may also have a degree of Type 2 respiratory failure. If any suggestion of this, controlled oxygen is indicated, otherwise high flow
  - Rapid assessment of chest. Look for trauma—is this definitely an effusion rather than haemothorax secondary to injury or massive infection?
  - If you have elicited history of chest disease, nebulized salbutamol may improve condition at this stage
- ABG
- CXR—this may need to be portable if hypoxia is profound. The image quality of this is poor, as there is a large positional distortion of the fluid levels. Be especially aware that in supine films, an effusion can appear as diffuse opacity rather than as a fluid level

Further management

- Aspiration ('tapping') of pleural fluid is essential as soon as stability permits. This will allow differentiation of exudate vs. transudate
  - Consider getting ultrasound guidance as to best site of aspiration— 'X' marks the spot!
  - See *OHCM*, p. 752 for procedure
  - Note macroscopic appearance of tap: clear, cloudy, bloody, purulent
  - Send specimen for Gram stain, C&S (to include AFB), cytology, protein, pH, glucose, amylase and LDH
  - If effusion is significant, a tap may be made therapeutic by taking further fluid. This is for symptomatic relief rather than formal drainage, however
  - Post-aspiration CXR to exclude pneumothorax should be considered mandatory

- A chest drain is likely to be appropriate; discuss with senior
- Take the time to elicit a detailed history for possible malignancy (e.g. weight loss, night sweats, postmenopausal bleeding, PR bleeding, altered bowel habit). Pleural effusion is not just a manifestation of intrathoracic disease

Investigations

- Light's criteria deem an effusion to be exudate if any of the following are met (otherwise it is a transudate):
    - Pleural fluid protein/serum protein >0.5
    - Pleural fluid LDH/serum LDH >0.6
    - Pleural fluid LDH >0.66 of normal serum LDH upper limit
- If transudate, consider:
    - Echo
    - USS abdomen
    - USS leg
    - CTPA or V/Q scan
    - 24-h urine protein collection
    - Thyroid function tests
    - CT thorax may be of benefit if above investigations reveal no other cause
- If exudate:
    - Discuss CT thorax with radiologist and chest physician
    - C&S sputum (include AFBs for TB)
    - Autoantibody screen
    - Amylase

Causes

Transudate

- Common
    - Left venticular failure
    - Hypoalbuminaemia
    - Cirrhosis
    - PE
- Uncommon
    - Mitral stenosis
    - Nephrotic syndrome
    - SVC obstruction
    - Constrictive pericarditis
    - Meig's syndrome

Exudate

- Common
    - Malignancy—pleural (mesothelioma), intrathoracic (e.g. small cell carcinoma lung) or extrathoracic (e.g. carcinoma of ovary)
    - Parapneumonic effusions
    - TB
    - Trauma

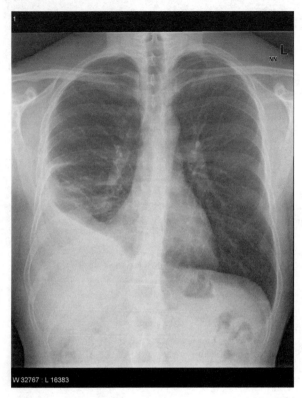

Fig. 4.7 CXR showing right-sided pleural effusion

- Uncommon
  - Pulmonary infarction
  - Asbestos-related effusion (benign)
  - Post-MI (Dressler's syndrome)
  - Pancreatitis
  - Rheumatoid arthritis, SLE or other connective tissue disorders
  - Fungal infection
  - Drugs—e.g. amiodarone, methotrexate, phenytoin, nitrofurantoin

Furhter reading
- *OHCM*, 7th edn. Oxford: Oxford University Press, p. 176–7.
- Maskell NA *et al*. BTS guidelines for the investigation of a unilateral pleural effusion in adults. *Thorax* 2003; **58**(Suppl. II):ii8–ii17.
- Chapman SJ, Davies RJO. Pleural effusions. *Clin Med* 2004; **4**:207–10.

Endocrine

☠ Diabetic ketoacidosis

Definition
- Capillary blood glucose >11.1 mmol/L
- pH <7.3
- Bicarbonate <15 mmol/L
- Base excess <−10

Metabolic acidosis secondary to uncontrolled catabolic state with insulin deficiency, resulting in hyperglycaemia and hyperketonaemia with severe fluid depletion. Free fatty acids are broken down into ketones in the liver causing acidaemia; dehydration is caused by the osmotic diuresis and vomiting secondary to acidosis.

DKA has an overall mortality rate of about 10% but can be as high as 50% in the elderly.

Presentation
DKA occurs almost always in Type I insulin-dependent diabetes and is a not infrequent mode of presentation. It rarely occurs in Type II diabetes with excessive counter-regulatory hormone secretion.
- Generally unwell
- Dehydration—can be severe
- Hyperventilation (Kussmaul breathing) with ketotic breath (pear drops)
- Nausea and vomiting—worrying signs, indicate significant acidosis
- Abdominal pain—can be severe, and be confused with an acute abdomen
- Confusion, stupor or even coma

Immediate management
- ABC (p. 422–424)—may be comatose, vomiting, etc
  - Large bore IV access required for fluid support
  - Monitoring where possible
- Bloods as detailed
- Cultures followed by broad spectrum antibiotics (use local protocol) if likely infective cause
- ABG
  - pH and base excess
  - K^+
- Fluid resuscitation
  - If hypotensive give 500 ml colloid stat and review
  - Otherwise give 1000 ml normal saline over 1 h

Further management

Fluid replacement

- 1000–2000 ml normal saline over first 2 h
- 1000 ml over next 4 h
- 4000 ml per 24 h thereafter
- Increase for other losses such as vomiting, remaining vigilant for signs of fluid overload
- Avoid half normal saline

Electrolyte and acid–base balance

- Plasma K^+ can be normal, low or high, but total body K^+ is low
  - K^+ 3.5–5.0 mmol/l, add 20 mmol KCl per litre of saline
  - K^+ <3.5 mmol/l, add 40 mmol KCl per litre of saline
  - K^+ >5.0 mmol/l, omit KCl (requires ECG +/– monitoring)
- pH is restored largely by fluid resuscitation and insulin treatment
  - Bicarbonate is no longer recommended as routine
- Check magnesium and phosphate

Insulin replacement

- Via intravenous infusion
  - Dilute 50 units of soluble insulin (e.g. Actrapid) in 50 ml normal saline
  - Initially 6 u/h (i.e. 6 ml/h) then reduce
  - Glucose >10 mmol/l—4 ml/h
  - Glucose 5–10 mmol/l—2 ml/h
  - Glucose <5 mmol/l—0.5 ml/h
- Investigate and treat any intercurrent illness, infection being the most common
- Consider LMWH—at risk of VTE
- Patients may require HDU, catheterization and central venous access, especially in severe DKA, the elderly or those with cardiac disease
- Hourly capillary blood glucose measurement
- 2-hourly ABGs will give indication both of acid–base balance and electrolytes
- When stable commence a standard sliding scale of insulin, 5% dextrose and potassium
- When able to eat and drink commence or review subcutaneous insulin regimen

Investigations

- Capillary blood glucose
- Blood cultures
- Venous blood glucose, HbA_{1C} for better indication of long-term control
- FBC, CRP, LFTs for infection
- U&Es for dehydration
- CXR—infection, fluid overload from initial resuscitation
- Urinalysis—monitor ketones
- ECG, cardiac enzymes if possible ischaemic event

Causes
- New presentation of Type I diabetes (common)
- Intercurrent illness—infection, trauma, surgery
- Omission or under dosing of insulin

Further reading
- *OHCM*, 7th edn Oxford: Oxford University Press, p. 814.
- Trachtenbarg DE. Diabetic ketoacidosis. *Am Fam Physician* 2005; **70(9)**:1705–14.

☢ **Hyperosmolar non-ketotic state (HONK)**

Definition
Uncontrolled hyperglycaemia in the absence of hyperketonaemia or acidosis, occurring largely in the Type II diabetes where sufficient circulating insulin prevents lipolysis and ketogenesis.

Presentation
Hyperglycaemia tends to be higher than in DKA (often over 50 mmol/l), with significant diuresis, dehydration and pre-renal renal failure. Plasma osmolality can be very high.
- Tends to be more insidious than DKA
- Frequently the mode of presentation of Type II diabetes
- 'Classical' hyperglycaemia symptoms
  - Thirst
  - Polydypsia
  - Polyuria
  - Tiredness
  - Weight loss
- Confusion, seizure, coma
- Signs of precipitating illness, e.g. pneumonia, UTI, etc.

Immediate management
- ABC
  - Large bore IV access, ideally to address significant dehydration
- Bloods as detailed
- ABG to exclude DKA
  - pH and base excess
  - K^+
- Fluid resuscitation
  - If hypotensive give 500 ml colloid stat and review
  - Otherwise give 1000 ml normal saline over 1 h

Subsequent management

Consider HDU care, catheterization, central venous access and monitoring, especially if elderly or significant co-morbidity.

Fluid replacement

- 1000–2000 ml normal saline over first 2 h
- 1000 ml over next 4 h
- 4000 ml per 24 h thereafter
- Increase for other losses such as vomiting, remaining vigilant for signs of fluid overload
- Beware of over-rapid correction of osmolality

Electrolyte and acid–base balance

- Hypernatraemia corrected by fluid resuscitation
- Avoid half normal saline
- Add 20 mmol/l KCl per litre initially
- Regular K^+ monitoring

Insulin replacement

- Via intravenous infusion 1 units/ml
    - Beware greater sensitivity to insulin than DKA patients
    - Initially 4 units/h
    - Glucose >17 mmol/l—4 ml/h
    - Glucose 11–17 mmol/l—3 ml/h
    - Glucose 7–11 mmol/l—2 ml/h
    - Glucose 4–7 mmol/l—1 ml/h
    - Glucose <4 mmol/l—0 ml/h

Anticoagulation

- Commence LMWH as prophylaxis for VTE
- Investigation and treatment of precipitating illness
- Most patients can be weaned off insulin
- Once stable eating and drinking, commence oral hypoglycaemics or insulin

Causes

- New presentation of Type II diabetes (common)
- Intercurrent illness—infection, MI
- Drugs, e.g. thiazide diuretics, glucocorticoids

Further reading

- *OCHM*, 7th edn. Oxford: Oxford University Press, p. 816.

:☉: Hypoglycaemia

Definition
Plasma glucose levels measured <3.0 mmol/l. Symptomatic patients require urgent correction of blood glucose levels. Further investigation is required if there is no obvious cause (e.g. DM).

Presentation
Presentation can be very variable, and does not necessary correspond to plasma glucose levels. Rate of fall, tolerance to hypoglycaemia and inter-current illness are all confounding factors.

- Routine capillary glucose measurement
  - Most common presentation. Clinical picture is much more important than measured level
- Adrenergic symptoms
  - Pallor, sweating, tremor
- Neuroglycopaenia
  - Confusion, altered behaviour, drowsiness
  - Seizure
  - Coma

Finger-prick capillary glucose tests are simple, quick and readily available, so should be used in all patients with the above presentations (even if cause appears to be obvious).

Immediate Management

Alert Patient
- Usually discovered on routine finger-prick capillary glucose testing
- Administer glucose
  - Oral route is preferential. Ideally give sugar and starch (short and long acting carbohydrates). Toast with jam is ideal.
  - If patient is NBM or unable to eat (e.g. vomiting) then give IV dextrose or IM glucagon (see below)
- Review oral hypoglycaemic agents or insulin regimen

Obtunded Patient
- ABC
  - Protect airway and give high flow O_2
  - Assess conscious level (AVPU/GCS)
- Stop any insulin infusions
- Gain IV access and send bloods (see below)
- Give IV dextrose
  - Use 50 ml boluses of 10% dextrose solution
  - Avoid 50% dextrose (causes phlebitis and increases risk of rebound hypoglycaemia following initial treatment)
- If IV access delayed/not available
  - Give glucagon 1 mg IM
- Expect a rapid and dramatic recovery
- If no recovery of conscious level in 10 mins

- - Recheck finger-prick capillary glucose level—consider other cause if it has normalised (see p. 72–75)
  - Repeat dextrose bolus if glucose level still low
  - Give hydrocortisone 100 mg IV
- Review the patient regularly with frequent blood sugar monitoring

Prolonged, refractory hypoglycaemia with coma
- ☎ Call for senior support
- Can be due to neurological insult (including cerebral oedema)
- May require mannitol & dexamethasone (under senior guidance)
  - Mannitol 20% solution 1 g/kg rapid IV infusion
  - Dexamethasone 10 mg IV bolus *then* 4 mg IV every 6 hours

Further management
- Once obtunded patients have become conscious again, encourage them to take some food—this will prevent relapse
- Frequent monitoring of glucose levels is important in the period following the hypoglycaemic episode
  - This may have to be over a prolonged period if the causative agent has a long half-life (e.g. some oral hypoglycaemic agents)
- ⚠ Patients with type 1 DM require insulin—do not withhold it
  - If an insulin infusion was stopped initially (see above), it will need to be recommenced once the blood glucose level is satisfactory—although the rate that the insulin/glucose needs to be infused may have to be altered
  - If unable to eat, they will need to be started on an IV insulin, glucose and potassium infusion
  - SC insulin doses may need to be adjusted according to the blood sugar profile from the previous 24 hrs (this will depend on the insulin regimen)—if unsure, seek senior advice

Investigation
Patients with diabetes
- Check laboratory plasma glucose
- Review management (insulin dose/regime, oral hypoglycaemic treatment & dietary habits)

Other investigations (where cause is not obvious)
- C-peptide
  - Raised if increased intrinsic production of insulin, e.g. insulinoma
  - Decreased if exogenous insulin has been administered (in patients not on insulin, this should raise the question of self-harm, poisoning or factitious illness)
- Insulin level
- Early morning cortisol/short synacthen test
- Plasma drug levels (paracetamol, salicylates, sulphonylureas)

Causes

Patients with diabetes

- Insulin
  - This is the most common complication of insulin therapy. It is due to over administration of insulin, reduced glucose intake or increased metabolic demands (e.g. exercise, illness). Patients can lose their adrenergic warning signs over time
- Some oral hypoglycaemic agents (sulphonylureas and meglitinides)

Non-diabetic patient

- Alcohol
  - Can occur 6-36 hrs post ingestion, usually in fasted, malnourished patients
  - Does not respond to glucagon administration
- Drugs
  - Paracetamol, salicylates, haloperidol, pentamidine, quinine and sulfonamides
- Organ Failure
  - Cardiac, renal or hepatic failure; sepsis with MOF
- Pancreatic causes
  - Pancreatitis, insulinoma (rare)
- Endocrine
  - Pituitary (↓ACTH, ↓GH, panhypopituitarism), adrenal (↓cortisol, ↓adrenaline)
- Infection
  - Bacterial, viral or parasite (especially malaria)
- Self harm, poisoning or factitious illness
  - Use of insulin or sulphonylureas
  - May require prolonged administration of large doses of glucose
- Reactive Hypoglycaemia
  - Chronic, transient episodes—often alcohol related

References

- Oxford textbook of Medicine. Vol 3. p. 1458.
- Moore C, Woollard M. Dextrose 10% or 50% in the treatment of hypoglycaemia out of hospital? A randomized Control Trial. *Emerg Med J* 2005; **22**: p. 512–515

☼ Lactic acidosis

Definition

A state of decreased systemic pH, acidosis results from either a primary increase in hydrogen ion or a reduction in bicarbonate (HCO_3^-) concentrations. The underlying aetiology of metabolic acidosis is classically categorised into those that cause an elevated anion gap (AG) and those that do not. Lactic acidosis, identified by a state of acidosis and a plasma lactate concentration significantly >2 mmol/l, is one type of elevated AG metabolic acidosis, with several potential causes.

Presentation

No single feature itself is indicative of the presence of lactic acidosis, as symptoms are dependent on the underlying aetiology. A careful history should pay particular attention to prescription drugs or toxins (including antiretroviral therapy). Lactic acidosis should be suspected in the presence of elevated AG metabolic acidosis; onset may be rapid (within minutes to hours) or progressive (over a period of several days).

Immediate management

- ABC + O₂
- IV access and bloods
  - FBC
  - U&Es
  - LFTs
  - Amylase
  - Lactate
- If volume replacement is required, avoid lactate-containing solutions; isotonic normal saline is a good starting point
- ABG
  - The base deficit gives an approximation of tissue acidosis, an indirect evaluation of tissue perfusion
  - Some blood gas analysers will also give a lactate value
- Catheterize and take specimen for urinalysis
- ECG
- Further treatment should be directed at underlying causes

Examination

- Respiratory
  - Shallow respiration with raised RR—Kussmaul hyperventilation (respiratory compensatory mechanism)
- Cardiac
  - Be watchful of cardiac monitor for onset of arrhythmia/fibrillation
  - Decreased myocardial contractility at low pH—reduced BP
- Neurological
  - Altered mental status and coma—check and regularly review AVPU/GCS
  - Increased sympathetic tone—pallor, sweating, nausea/vomiting, tachycardia, reduced CRT
- Abdominal
  - Check for tenderness—mesenteric ischaemia typically causes marked rise in lactate
- Other
  - Check peripheral pulses—could there be limb ischaemia?
  - Decreased renal perfusion—monitor UO
  - Increased metabolic rate and protein catabolism—is the patient cachexic?

Investigations

- Anion gap (AG) = [sodium + potassium] − [chloride + bicarbonate]
  - The normal anion gap generally ranges from 8 to 12 mmol/l
- Serum lactate
  - Neither the anion gap nor the arterial pH can be guaranteed to reflect the presence or severity of lactic acidosis reliably
  - The most accurate assessment is direct measurement of lactate level
  - Values above 4–5 mmol/l are indicative of lactic acidosis

Causes

Cohen and Woods' classification of lactic acidosis follows.

Type A

- Clinical evidence of decreased tissue perfusion
  - Left ventricular failure
  - Decreased cardiac output
- Or reduced oxygenation
  - Asphyxia
  - Hypoxaemia
  - Carbon monoxide poisoning
  - Life-threatening anaemia

Type B

No clinical evidence of poor tissue perfusion or oxygenation.
- B1—Underlying systemic diseases
  - Renal and hepatic failure
  - Diabetes mellitus
  - Pancreatitis
  - Malignancy
  - Vitamin B deficiency

- B2—Medication or intoxication
  - Metformin
  - Alcohols
  - Iron
  - Isoniazid
  - Salicylates
  - Statin therapy (very rare)
- B3—Inborn error of metabolism
  - Defects in gluconeogenesis
  - Defects in pyruvate dehydrogenase
  - Defects in the tricarboxylic acid cycle

Further management

This is directed at correction of the underlying disorder and may include:
- Administration of appropriate antibiotics
- Surgical drainage or debridement of a septic focus
- Discontinuation of potentially causative medications
- Dietary modification in inborn errors of metabolism
- Dialysis—may be useful when severe lactic acidosis exists in conjunction with renal failure or congestive heart failure. It also allows bicarbonate infusion without precipitating or worsening fluid overload
- Attempting to correct the arterial pH by lowering the $PaCO_2$ (indirectly by increasing the rate of ventilation)
- Sodium bicarbonate ($NaHCO_3$)—should be reserved for patients with severe metabolic acidosis to maintain the pH above 7.15 until the underlying process is corrected
  - The amount of $NaHCO_3$ required (mmol) is:

    $0.4 \times$ (body weight in kg) $\times$ (desired HCO_3^- – measured HCO_3^-)

    ⚠ Minute ventilation must be increased to expel CO_2 generated by bicarbonate administration, as it may precipitate ventilatory failure
- Thiamine deficiency may be associated with cardiovascular compromise and lactic acidosis. The response to thiamine repletion (initially 50–100 mg IV) may be dramatic and potentially life-saving

⚠ Avoid using vasoconstrictor drugs because of their potential to exacerbate ischaemia in critical tissue beds.

Further reading

- Bishop RL, Weisfeldt ML. Sodium bicarbonate administration during cardiac arrest. Effect on arterial pH PCO2, and osmolality. *JAMA* 1976; **235(5)**:506–9.
- Cohen RD, Woods HF. Lactic acidosis revisited. *Diabetes* 1983; **32(2)**:181–91.
- Cohen R, Woods H. *Clinical and Biochemical Aspects of Lactic Acidosis.* Oxford: Blackwell Scientific Publications, 1976.
- Cooper D, Walley K, Wiggs B. Bicarbonate does not improve hemodynamics in critically ill patients who have lactic acidosis. A prospective, controlled clinical study. *Ann Int Med* 1990; **112**:492–8.
- Fall PJ, Szerlip HM. Lactic acidosis: from sour milk to septic shock. *J Int Care Med* 2005; **20(5)**:255–71.
- Forsyth SM, Schmidt GA. Sodium bicarbonate for the treatment of lactic acidosis. *Chest* 2000; **117**:260–7.
- Frommer JP. Lactic acidosis. *Med Clin North Am* 1983; **67(4)**:815–29.
- Hindman BJ. Sodium bicarbonate in the treatment of subtypes of acute lactic acidosis: physiologic considerations. *Anesthesiol* 1990; **72(6)**:1064–76.
- Mizock BA, Falk JL. Lactic acidosis in critical illness. *Crit Care Med* 1992; **20(1)**:80–93.
- Oh M, Carroll H. The anion gap. *N Engl J Med* 1977; **297**:814–17.
- Stacpoole PW. Lactic acidosis: the case against bicarbonate therapy. *Ann Int Med* 1986; **105(2)**:276–9.
- Stacpoole P, Wright E et al. Natural history and course of acquired lactic acidosis in adults. *Am J Med* 1994; **97**:47–54.

☠ **Hyperthyroid crisis**

This uncommon medical emergency, also known as thyroid storm, is an acute life-threatening exacerbation of thyrotoxicosis that results in significant morbidity, disability or even death.

It occurs in patients with untreated or inadequately treated hyperthyroidism, and has an untreated mortality rate of 90%.

Presentation
- Tachycardia
- Atrial fibrillation
- Hypertension
- Nausea, vomiting and diarrhoea
- Jaundice
- Hyperpyrexia ± dehydration
- Delirium, seizure or coma
- Multisystem failure
  - Congestive heart failure with oedema
  - Congestive hepatomegaly
  - Respiratory distress
  - Hypotension and shock

Immediate management

Because thyroid storm is invariably fatal if left untreated, rapid diagnosis and aggressive treatment are critical; there should be no delay for lab results (which are often unremarkable). Treatment is directed at counteracting the effect of excess activity of TH.
- ABC as per p. 2–5
- ABG—acidosis?
- Capillary blood glucose—DKA?
- Antibiotics if infective cause suspected
- Control hyperthermia by applying ice packs and cooling blankets
- Establish thyroid control
  - Reduce hyperadrenergic effects of TH on peripheral tissues with use of β blocker (propranolol 20–200 mg orally, or 1–5 mg IV 6-hourly)
  - Decrease production of TH with antithyroid medications (propylthiouracil 150–250 mg or carbimazole 15 mg 6-hourly to reduce synthesis and sodium ipodate 500 mg IV to prevent secretion
  - Prevent further TH secretion and peripheral conversion of T4 to T3, using glucocorticoids (hydrocortisone 100–200 mg/day or dexamethasone 2 mg 6-hourly)

Further management
- Early and thorough investigation of primary cause (see later), as the condition cannot be controlled fully without treating this
- Fluid balance

Investigations
- FBC, CRP for infection
- Cultures
- fT3, fT4 (free thyroid hormones), TSH (should be suppressed)
- CXR ± echo if heart failure

Causes
- Thyroid surgery
- Radio-iodine
- Amiodarone
- Withdrawal of antithyroid drugs
- Iodinated contrast agents
- Toxaemia of pregnancy
- Anticholinergic and adrenergic drugs
- TH ingestion
- Hypoglycaemia or DKA
- Acute illness, e.g. infection, trauma
- Pulmonary thromboembolism
- Stroke

Further reading
- *OHCM*, 7th edn. Oxford: Oxford University Press, p. 816.
- Abraham P, Avenell A, Watson WA, Park CM, Bevan JS. Antithyroid drug regimen for treating Graves' hyperthyroidism. *Cochrane Database Syst Rev* 2005; **(4)**:CD003420.
- Allanic H, Fauchet R, Orgiazzi J et al. Antithyroid drugs and Graves' disease: a prospective randomized evaluation of the efficacy of treatment duration. *J Clin Endoc Metab* 1990; **70**:675.
- Cooper DS. Antithyroid drugs in the management of patients with Graves' disease: an evidence-based approach to therapeutic controversies. *J Clin Endocrinol Metab* 2003; **88**:3474–81.
- Cooper DS. Hyperthyroidism. *Lancet* 2003; **362**:459–68.
- Cooper DS. Antithyroid drugs. *N Engl J Med* 2005; **352**:905–17.
- Franklyn JA. The management of hyperthyroidism. *N Engl J Med* 1994; **330(24)**:1731–8.

☼ Myxoedema coma

Definition

Severe hypothyroidism associated with altered mental state and hypothermia. Associated with high mortality rates, it is now rare (11 admissions in England in 2004) owing to early diagnosis of hypothyroidism.

Presentation

This must be considered in patients with background of thyroid surgery or radio-iodine. It is rare for hypothyroid patients to present with true coma, but be alert for exaggerated symptoms of hypothyroidism.

- Altered mental state—due to cerebral oedema, hypoxia and hypercarbia
- Seizures—may precede coma in 25% of patients
- Hypothermia—usually <32.2°C
- Hypoventilation
- Hypotension
- Bradycardia
- Hypoglycaemia
- Dry skin and hair
- Goitre/scar from previous surgery
- Slow relaxing reflexes
- Non-pitting oedema—eyes, hands, eyelids
- Cerebellar ataxia

Immediate management

- ABC—very low threshold for anaesthetic assistance owing to airway risk from coma or seizures
- ABG—likely hypoxia, hypercarbia and lactic acidosis
- Bloods as detailed
- Initiate precise fluid balance
- Request close observations
- A reduced GCS at this stage with suspected thyroid primary cause should be referred to critical care outreach
- Initially, the precipitating illness needs to be identified and treated. Perform a thorough history and examination, looking for infections, especially UTIs and RTIs. Obtain an urgent CXR, urine dip, ECG and rectal core temperature
- Cautious correction of hypothermia by insulation rather than active rewarming, ensuring cardiac monitoring in place throughout
- Immediate thyroid replacement—thyroxine 300–500 µg IV, followed by daily maintenance of 50–100 µg. The dose must be considered in the context of the patient's age and clinical condition—a progressive regimen may well be most appropriate.

Further management

- Further elucidation and treatment of primary cause is the key to management
- Discuss broad spectrum antimicrobials with medical microbiology if suspected infective cause
- 50–100 mg hydrocortisone TDS, as temporary adrenal impairment is frequently seen

Investigations

- FBC—WCC suggestive of infection?
- U&Es—hyponatraemia common, owing to SIADH
- Serum glucose—hypoglycaemia common and should be treated early
- TFTs (f T4, TSH). Is the hypothyroidism primary or secondary?
- Blood cultures
- ABG—look for lactic acidosis
- Cortisol for Addison's disease
- Troponin S if suspected cardiac cause
- CXR for infection or effusions
- ECG—look for small complexes with prolonged QT interval, or generalized signs of ischaemia

Causes

- Infection
- Stroke
- Trauma
- MI
- Drugs, including phenothiazines, phenytoin, amiodarone, propranolol, lithium

Further reading

- *OHCM*, 7th edn. Oxford: Oxford University Press, p. 816.
- Burke CW. Adrenocortical insufficiency. *Clin Endocrinol Metab* 1985; **14**:947–76.
- Holvey JN, Goodner CJ, Nicoloff JT et al. Treatment of myxedema coma with intravenous thyroxine. *Arch Intern Med* 1964; **113**:89–96.
- Kearney D, Dang C. Diabetic and endocrine emergencies. *Postgrad Med J* 2007; **83**:79–86.
- Rodriguez I, Fluiters E, Perez-Mendez LF et al. Factors associated with mortality of patients with myxoedema coma: prospective study in 11 cases treated in a single institution. *J Endocrinol* 2004; **180**:347–50.

☼ **Acute adrenal insufficiency**

Definition

Acute adrenal insufficiency (also known as an Addisonian crisis) is caused by either primary adrenal failure (mostly due to autoimmune adrenalitis) or by hypothalamic–pituitary impairment of the corticotrophic axis (predominantly due to pituitary disease). It is a rare disease, but is life-threatening when overlooked.

Presentation

- Severe hypotension
- Acute abdominal pain
- Vomiting
- Fever

50% of patients will have had signs and symptoms of Addison's disease for more than 1 year prior to diagnosis being established, including:

- Fatigue
- Anorexia and weight loss
- Gastric pain, nausea, vomiting
- Fever
- Low BP, postural hypotension
- Myalgia, joint pain
- Dizziness
- Salt craving
- Dry and itchy skin, hyperpigmentation
- Loss of libido, loss of axillary/pubic hair

Immediate management

- ABC, remembering the potential speed of deterioration and requirement for inotropes. Involve critical care early
- ECG—cardiac monitoring to be requested if abnormal
- ABG—look for metabolic acidosis, respiratory failure
- Urgent bloods as detailed
- Correct any hypoglycaemia (remembering unreliability of capillary blood glucose in overwhelming systemic illness—may be best to wait for lab glucose)
- Do not withhold steroid replacement—give 10 mg dexamethasone IV (this will not interfere with cortisol assay)
- Assess for concurrent infections—CXR and urinalysis
- Discuss with medical microbiology—empirical broad antimicrobial coverage may be appropriate here
- Initiate strict fluid balance

Further management

- Request old notes, discuss with relatives or GP relevant past medical history. Previous use of steroid, general health, compliance with existing steroids
- If the patient is unstable, has ongoing hypotension or severe electrolyte abnormalities, management must be within the critical care environment
- If patient known to have Addison's disease and stable, definitive steroid therapy is commenced; otherwise a short Synacthen™ test is required
  - Baseline serum blood for cortisol assay
  - Tetracosactide (Synacthen™) 250 µg IV or IM administered
  - Further serum samples at 30 and 60 min
  - Normal results baseline >170 nmol/l, rising to >580 nmol/l after tetracosactide
  - May be equivocal, requiring long Synacthen™ test
- Follow up any suspected infection—focus antimicrobial therapy with culture results
- Fluid balance review

Investigations

- FBC—WCC suggestive of infection?
- U&Es—be alert to risk of hyponatraemia (p. 388–390) and hyperkalaemia (p. 394–395)
- Calcium—look for and correct hypercalcaemia (p. 404–406)
- Glucose—correct abnormalities (often caused by physiological stress, without pre-existing DM)
- Blood cultures prior to any antimicrobial therapy
- ABG
- TFT, remembering that Addison's and thyroid crises can coexist
- ACTH and cortisol
- Serum lactate if acidosis seen on ABG

Causes

The cause of the crisis is a physiologically stressful event, such as those listed, on a background of adrenal insufficiency, itself caused by several primary or secondary causes.

- Acute illness
- Rapid withdrawal of exogenous steroids
- Sudden stress
- Surgery
- Primary adrenal insufficiency
  - Autoimmune adrenalitis
  - Infectious adrenalitis—AIDS, TB
  - Genetic disorders
  - Bilateral adrenal haemorrhage—severe physiological stress, e.g. MI, complicated pregnancy, septic shock
  - Adrenal infiltration—metastases, sarcoid
  - Bilateral adrenalectomy
  - Drug induced—mitotane, etomidate

- Secondary adrenal insufficiency
  - Tumours—pituitary
  - Pituitary radiation
  - Sheehan's syndrome
  - Pituitary infiltration—TB, sarcoid
  - Trauma
  - Previous chronic glucocorticoid excess—exogenous >4 weeks, including long term widespread topical steroids

Further reading
- *OHCM*, 7th edn. Oxford: Oxford University Press, p. 818.
- Arlt W, Allolio B. Adrenal insufficiency. *Lancet* 2003; **361**:1881–93.
- Kearney T, Dang C. Diabetic and endocrine emergencies. *Postgrad Med J* 2007; **83**:79–86.

☼ **Phaeochromocytoma**

Definition
Tumours arising from the chromaffin cells of the adrenal medulla, phaeo-chromocytomas are associated with increased catecholamine production (usually adrenaline or noradrenaline). This section is predominantly to enable competent handling of a hypertensive crisis precipitated by phaeochromocytoma.

Presentation
May present as a hypertensive crisis or mimicking septic shock, but most are diagnosed during routine hypertensive screening. Other features include:
- Cardiac ischaemia
- Pulmonary oedema (may develop ARDS-like features)
- Headache, seizures or cerebrovascular events
- Palpitations
- Diaphoresis, pallor, cold extremities
- Anxiety
- Visual disturbance
- Abdominal pain
- Asymptomatic

Immediate management

- ABC, bearing in mind relative fluid depletion is likely at time of pres-entation
- Accurate fluid balance
- Urgent investigations as detailed
- Organize for continuous cardiac monitoring and a 12-lead ECG
- Contact senior help and/or critical care outreach team early—central access and invasive BP monitoring may be required

△ Treatment of a hypertensive crisis should be immediate—contact senior before taking these steps, as they can have a precipitous effect.
- Rehydration should be complete prior to initiation of alpha blockade, otherwise severe hypotension may occur
- Give phentolamine 2.5–5 mg IV bolus at 1 mg/min
- Repeat doses every 5 min until hypertension is adequately controlled
- Can also be given as infusion (100 mg phentolamine in 500 ml 5% dextrose) with continuous BP monitoring

---

Further management
- Patients with ongoing hypertension and electrolyte abnormalities need to be managed in a critical care bed
- Prevention of a hypertensive crisis
  - Especially important when marked catecholamine release is anticipated (during operation)

- Can be achieved by blocking adrenoreceptors, drug of choice being phenoxybenzamine 10 mg BD, gradually increased to 1 mg/kg/day in four divided doses
- Adequate alpha blockade is achieved within 10–14 days
- β blockade (atenolol 25 mg OD) is added afterwards to prevent reflex tachycardia
- Hypertensive crisis associated with undiagnosed phaeochromocytoma in pregnancy carries a high morbidity and mortality. Most frequently it is seen in the period surrounding delivery

Investigations

- U&Es—uraemia, hypokalaemia (p. 396–398)
- Glucose—hyperglycaemia
- Plasma metanephrines (Ix of choice)—raised
- Urinary vanillylmandelic acid (UVMA) level, although catecholamine metabolite, will be non-specific owing to dietary interference
- Urinary catecholamines (adrenaline, noradrenaline and dopamine) are more specific
- MRI (ideally) or CT to localize tumour. MRI has a high specificity for localizing both adrenal and extra-adrenal phaeochromocytoma
- MIGB (^{131}I-metaiodobenzylguanidine) is taken up selectively by adrenal tissues, localizing lesion
- CXR for pulmonary oedema
- Cardiac enzymes if index presentation with suspected cardiac ischaemia

Causes

Hypertensive crisis in association with phaeochromocytoma may be precipitated by emotion, voiding, postural change, direct manipulation during surgery or drugs. The lesions are referred to as the '10% tumour' because they are 10% inherited, are associated with a 10% risk of malignancy, 10% are bilateral and 10% are extra-adrenal.

- Idiopathic—commonest
- Inherited—occur as part of the following conditions:
  - Von Recklinghausen disease
  - Von Hippel–Lindau disease
  - Multiple endocrine neoplasia types 2a, 2b
  - Tuberous sclerosis
  - Sturge–Weber syndrome

Further reading

- *OHCM*, 7th edn. Oxford: Oxford University Press, p. 818.
- Brouwers FM, Lenders JWM, Eisenhofer GPK. Pheochromocytoma as an endocrine emergency. *Rev Endo Metab Dis* 2003; **4(2)**:121–8.
- Kearney, Dang C. Diabetic and endocrine emergencies. *Postgrad Med J* 2007; **83**:79–86.

Gastroenterology

⚙ **Liver failure**

Definition

Failure of hepatic function. The most common presentation will be of a patient with known chronic liver disease, who decompensates acutely. Another (rarer) presentation is acute liver failure, where there is evidence of hepatic failure in a patient with a previously healthy liver. The initial management of both of these presentations is similar, but the further management is much more complex. This topic will mainly cover that initial stabilisation.

Presentation

- Generally unwell
  - Nausea, vomiting, abdominal discomfort
- Jaundice
- Encephalopathy
  - Confusion, agitation, coma
- Coagulopathy
  - Bruising, epistaxis, PR bleed, etc.
- Abnormal LFTs
- 2–3 days following a paracetamol overdose
  - Accidental, deliberate or serial
- Ascites (usually in chronic liver failure)
- Decompensation of chronic liver failure may be precipitated by:
  - Progressive loss of liver function
  - Dehydration
  - Constipation
  - Additional liver insult (e.g. alcohol consumption, accidental or deliberate paracetamol overdose, hepatitis A infection)
  - Drugs (e.g. opioids)
  - Acute upper GI bleed
  - Infection (e.g. spontaneous bacterial peritonitis)
  - Non-compliance with treatment
  - ↑Portosystemic shunt (e.g. TIPSS insertion)
  - Renal failure
  - Hepatocellular carcinoma
  - Vascular impairment (e.g. acute portal vein thrombosis).

Immediate management

- ABC assessment
  - Patients with grade 3–4 encephalopathy (see below) are likely to be obtunded, so may require airway support ± ventilation
  - Patients with grade 2 encephalopathy can rapidly progress to grade 3–4—monitor closely
  - Nurse with a 20° head-up tilt
- DEFG—don't ever forget the glucose
  - Give IV dextrose bolus if hypoglycaemic (see p. 226–228)
  - Monitor BMs 4-hourly—there is a high risk of hypoglycaemia in liver failure

- Keep NBM initially, and start maintenance IVT
  - Consider using fluid containing 10% dextrose for maintenance, as this will help to avoid hypoglycaemia
  - If chronic liver failure is suspected, avoid using fluids with large amounts of NaCl, as it may precipitate/worsen ascites
- If there are clinical signs of bleeding
  - Give vitamin K, 10 mg IV OD for 3 days
  - Consider FFP ± platelet transfusion. ☎ Discuss with haematologist
- Treat the underlying cause, if known
  - e.g. paracetamol overdose (see p. 408–411).

Further management
Encephalopathy

Grading system for encephalopathy

Clinical grade of hepatic encephalopathy	Clinical signs	Flapping tremor
Grade 1 (prodrome)	Alert, euphoric, occasionally depression. Poor concentration, slow mentation and affect, reversed sleep rhythm	Infrequent at this stage
Grade 2 (impending coma)	Drowsiness, lethargic, inappropriate behaviour, disorientation	Easily elicited
Grade 3 (early coma)	Stuporous but easily rousable, marked confusion, incoherent speech	Usually present
Grade 4 (deep coma)	Coma, unresponsive but may respond to painful stimulus	Usually absent

- Avoid sedatives, opioids and diuretics
- The input of a specialist dietician may be of use
- Decrease intestinal transit time
  - Lactulose, 15–30 ml PO BD (then adjust dose to produce two soft stools daily)
- Consider gut decontamination (under specialist guidance)
  - Neomycin, 1 g PO QDS
  - *and* Metronidazole, 250 mg PO TDS
- Consider (under specialist guidance)
  - Sodium benzoate, 10 g/day PO
  - Ornithine aspartate, 9 g/day PO
  - Zinc acetate, 600 mg/day PO.

Ascites
- Sodium restriction
  - Aim for <90 mmol/day (in practice, is likely to be <110 mmol/day)

- NB. One litre of 0.9% NaCl contains 150 mmol!
- Fluid restriction
  - Limit to 1.5 l/day—will only work if sodium restricted as well
- Diuretics
  - Spironolactone, 100 mg OD
  - Furosemide, 40 mg OD
  - ⚠ Consult expert before prescribing if there is any evidence of encephalopathy
- Consider therapeutic large volume paracentesis if there is respiratory embarrassment
  - ⚠ This must be done aseptically, as there is a high risk of introducing fatal infection.

Other considerations
- Be sure to check for and treat alcohol withdrawal (see p. 258–260)
- Owing to the alteration of drug metabolism, always consult the BNF appendix on prescribing in liver failure when prescribing medication
- N-acetylcysteine treatment
  - Can be of benefit in acute liver failure, even if not caused by paracetamol overdose
- Consider PPI to reduce the risk of gastric stress ulcers
  - e.g. lansoprazole, 30 mg PO OD
- Carefully look for, and treat, any of the precipitating factors, e.g. dehydration, constipation
- Low threshold for antibiotic treatment if any sign of infection
  - Tailor to suspected site of infection (discuss with microbiologist)
  - If unsure of site, commence 'blind' treatment, e.g. cefotaxime, 2 g IV BD
- Take thorough drug history, and consider changing or stopping any medication which may be responsible or aggravating the situation
- Many patients (especially those with acute liver failure) should be discussed with the regional liver unit
  - Centres will have criteria for referral, often based around the suitability for transplantation.

Complications
- Spontaneous bacterial peritonitis
  - Occurs in 10–30% of hospitalised patients with cirrhosis and ascites
  - Suspect in this group if any signs of sepsis (especially fever)
  - ❶ Often, there will be no abdominal symptoms/signs, and 10% can be asymptomatic
  - Diagnosis made on ascitic tap (WCC >500 × 10⁹/L, neutrophils >250 × 10⁹/L, isolation of organism from Gram stain or culture)
  - Treat with broad spectrum antibiotic, e.g. cefotaxime, 2 g IV BD (clinically stable patients can be treated with ciprofloxacin, 750 mg PO BD)
  - Will require long-term antibiotic prophylaxis following resolution of acute episode
- Hepatorenal syndrome
  - This occurs in ~18% of patients, due to hypoalbuminaemia causing ↓GFR (renal histology is normal)

- ☎ Discuss with a nephrologist and the regional liver unit
- Patient may require IV albumin and glypressin/vasopressin ± haemodialysis
- Cerebral oedema
  - This can occur with patients with liver failure
  - Look for features of ↑ICP (headache, nausea/vomiting, ↓GCS, papilloedema, ↓HR + ↑BP)
  - Can be difficult to distinguish from encephalopathy
  - Patient will likely need to be ventilated to achieve ↓$PaCO_2$
  - Consider mannitol 20% solution, 1 g/kg IV
  - ☎ Discuss with regional liver unit.

Investigations

- FBC and CRP
  - Monitor inflammatory markers for indication of infection
  - Patients with chronic liver disease are prone to thrombocytopenia
- Coagulation screen
  - PT is probably the most useful marker for liver synthetic function, and is a very useful prognostic indicator
- Glucose
  - Can be lowered because of impaired glycogen storage and reduction of gluconeogenesis owing to poor liver synthetic function
- LFTs
  - Liver enzyme levels are likely to be grossly elevated, supporting the diagnosis of liver failure, although not always and not in alcoholic hepatitis
  - Normal levels can occur in chronic liver failure, if there are insufficient hepatocytes to produce the enzymes in large amounts
  - Serum albumin and bilirubin levels are also good indicators of liver synthetic function
- U&Es
  - Should be monitored to check for the development of hepatorenal syndrome (↑creatinine and ↑urea)
- Paracetamol level
  - May be normal if overdose was taken a significant amount of time ago (so is no substitute for careful history-taking)
- USS liver
  - Can check for structural liver problems, vascular problems (e.g. Budd–Chiari syndrome), and to check for ascites
- CT abdomen
  - Can provide more information about structural disease than USS, especially in obese patients, or those with significant ascites
  - Consider performing a scan with no contrast, to avoid precipitating renal failure
- Liver biopsy
  - Can be useful in establishing underlying diagnosis
  - Contraindicated in the presence of coagulopathy, thrombocytopenia and more than minimal ascites
- Tests to screen for underlying causes
  - Hepatitis A, B and C, EBV and CMV serology

- Ferritin (haemochromatosis)
- Serum free copper/caeruloplasmin levels (Wilson's disease)—if <40 years old
- Autoantibodies and immunoglobulin levels, especially ANA and ASMA (autoimmune hepatitis)
- α_1 anti-trypsin level.

Causes

- Alcoholic liver disease
  - Most common cause of chronic liver disease
- Acute alcoholic hepatitis
  - Most common cause of acute liver failure
- Paracetamol overdose
- Viral infection
  - Hepatitis A, B or C
- Drug reaction
  - Either to prescription, herbal or illicit drugs
- Toxins
  - *Amanita phalloides* mushroom
  - Organic solvents
  - Yellow phosphorus
- Vascular causes
  - Ischaemic hepatitis (possibly following severe blood loss, sepsis, etc.)
  - Budd–Chiari syndrome (hepatic vein thrombosis)
  - Portal vein thrombosis
- Haemochromatosis
- Cryptogenic
- Autoimmune hepatitis
- Primary biliary cirrhosis
- Primary sclerosing cholangitis
- Non-alcoholic fatty liver disease
- Malignancy
  - Primary or secondary
- Metabolic
  - Acute fatty liver of pregnancy
  - α_1 anti-trypsin deficiency
  - Fructose intolerance
  - Galactosaemia
  - Lecithin-cholesterol acyltransferase deficiency
  - Reye syndrome
  - Tyrosinaemia
  - Wilson's disease.

Further reading
- *OHCM*, 7th edn. Oxford: Oxford University Press, p. 250.
- *Oxford Textbook of Medicine*, 4th edn, vol. 2. Oxford: Oxford University Press, p. 741.
- *Oxford Handbook of Gastroenterology and Hepatology*, 1st edn. Oxford: Oxford University Press, p. 42.
- Moore KP, Aithal GP. Guidelines on the management of ascites in cirrhosis. *Gut* 2006; **55**:1–12.

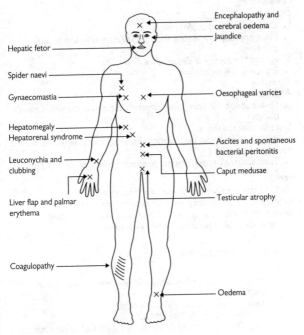

Fig. 6.1 Features of liver failure

⚠ **Exacerbation of inflammatory bowel disease**

Definition

Inflammatory bowel disease encompasses ulcerative colitis and Crohn's disease. These illnesses tend to run a relapsing/remitting course, and will occasionally require hospital admission for severe exacerbations.

Presentation

- Diarrhoea
  - Often with blood and/or mucus
  - More predominant in ulcerative colitis (especially with bloody diarrhoea
- ↑Urgency/↑frequency of defaecation
  - Especially waking at night
- Tenesmus
- Abdominal cramps
  - Severe abdominal pain is less common, but can occur with Crohn's disease
- Systemic manifestations
  - Pyrexia, nausea/vomiting, tachycardia, weight loss, dehydration
- Severe complications
  - Toxic megacolon, perforation, peritonitis, intestinal obstruction.

Severity

- Mild: <4 stools daily, no systemic manifestations
- Moderate: 4–6 stools daily, minimal systemic manifestations
- Severe: >6 stools daily, systemic disturbance (fever, tachycardia, anaemia, ESR >30, ↑platelets, ↑CRP, ↓albumin).

Immediate management

- ABC
  - Some patients will be hypovolaemic, and will require fluid resuscitation
- Commence steroid therapy (IV and topical)
  - e.g. hydrocortisone, 100 mg IV QDS
  - *and* e.g. Predfoam® (prednisolone), 20 mg PR ON (if proctitis is present)
- Stop drugs which may cause colonic dilatation
  - e.g. NSAIDS, opioids, anticholinergics, antidiarrhoeals
- Send urgent blood tests (see below)
- Get an urgent AXR to check for toxic megacolon (see below)
  - If any suspicion of this, also order an erect CXR to check for perforation
- Start DVT prophylaxis
  - e.g. tinzaparin, 3500 units S/C OD
  - *and* TED™ stockings

- ☎ Discuss management with gastroenterologist/colorectal surgeon
  - Call urgently if there is any evidence of toxic megacolon or perforation
- Examine patient BD to check for dilatation, bowel sounds and abdominal tenderness
  - ❶ Steroid therapy may mask these signs, so also keep a close eye on other indicators (e.g. pulse and BP)
- Ensure an accurate stool chart is kept, as this will guide further management.

Further management
- Start or increase aminosalicylates
  - e.g. Asacol® MR (mesalazine), 800 mg PO TDS
  - NB. Different preparations have different pharmacodynamics, so are not interchangeable (if patient is already on aminosalicylates, use the same preparation as their maintenance)
- Nutritional support
  - Patients with IBD are often malnourished when first admitted, and will have increased nutritional demands
  - There appears to be no benefit in stopping PO nutrition, so this route is preferable, but NG nutrition may be required if patient cannot tolerate PO diet
  - In certain patients with Crohn's disease, an elemental or polymeric diet may be of use (usually via NG tube as it is highly unpalatable)
  - Involvement of a specialist dietician can be extremely helpful
- Blood transfusion
  - May be indicated to keep Hb >10 g/dl
- Antibiotics
  - Consider if there is severe perianal disease
  - e.g. metronidazole, 400 mg PO TDS
- Immunosuppressant therapy
  - These should only be considered under the guidance of a specialist
  - Used if patient fails to respond to intensive steroid therapy
  - Agents used include ciclosporin, azathioprine, methotrexate and mercaptopurine
  - All have significant side-effects, and require close monitoring
- Infliximab
  - Can be of use in treatment-resistant Crohn's disease, but only under specialist guidance
- Surgery
  - Can be indicated acutely if there are complications (e.g. toxic megacolon, perforation)
  - Patients with IBD have a high chance of requiring surgery in the future (25–30% of patients with ulcerative colitis will require a colectomy, and 75% of patients with Crohn's disease will require surgery).

Investigations

- Stool tests
  - Send for *Clostridium difficile* toxin, to rule out pseudomembranous colitis (especially if patient has been on antibiotics)
  - Also send for virology and C&S to rule out infective colitis
- FBC and CRP
  - ↑CRP will indicate inflammation, and is useful in monitoring response to treatment
  - ↑WCC is also common, but can reflect chronic steroid use
  - ↓Hb with ↔/↓MCV
- ESR
  - Will usually be raised
  - Level >30 can indicate severe disease
- U&Es
  - Diarrhoea can cause significant hypokalaemia, which will require replacement
- LFTs
  - Most common is ↓albumin, due to malnutrition ± protein-losing enteropathy, and being in a catabolic state
  - Sclerosing cholangitis can occur with Crohn's disease, and will show an obstructive picture
- Haematinics, vitamin B_{12} and folate levels
  - A combination of GI blood loss, and malabsorption of iron, vitamin B_{12} and folate can cause anaemia
- AXR and erect CXR
  - Check for toxic megacolon (transverse colon ≥5.5 cm)
  - Look for signs of perforation (extraluminal gas, free air under diaphragm)
  - Dilated loops of bowel may indicate obstruction in Crohn's disease
- Contrast studies
  - These should only be performed under expert guidance
  - Barium enema can be diagnostic of IBD, and can allow differentiation between ulcerative colitis and Crohn's disease
  - Small bowel contrast studies can show changes consistent with Crohn's disease
- CT abdomen
  - Can demonstrate intra-abdominal abscesses or fistulae
- Colonoscopy
  - ❶ In severe flare-ups, there is a significant risk of perforation, so should only be performed by an expert operator, without bowel prep
  - Gold standard for diagnosis, as it allows for biopsy and histological analysis.

Complications

- Toxic megacolon
- Perforation
- Peritonitis
- Intestinal obstruction (Crohn's disease)
- High risk of thromboembolism

- Lower GI haemorrhage
- Increased risk of colorectal cancer.

Further reading
- *OHCM*, 7th edn. Oxford: Oxford University Press, p. 264.
- *Oxford Textbook of Medicine*, 4th edn, vol. 2. Oxford: Oxford University Press, p. 604.
- *Oxford Handbook of Gastroenterology and Hepatology*, 1st edn. Oxford: Oxford University Press, p. 244–9, 618.
- Carter MJ, Lobo AJ, Travis SPL. Guidelines for the management of inflammatory bowel disease in adults. *Gut* 2004; **53**:(Suppl. V):v1–v16.

☼ **Cholangitis**

Definition
Inflammation of the biliary system, usually caused by biliary stasis with superadded bacterial infection (often Gram negative). This can rapidly lead to septic shock and carries a high mortality rate (7–40%). Rapid recognition and treatment can significantly improve outcome.

Presentation
Charcot's triad
- Fever (>90%)
- Jaundice (65%)
- Right upper quadrant pain (>40%).

The presence of all three symptoms strongly suggests cholangitis, but will only occur in 20% of cases. There should be a high index of suspicion in any patient who may have biliary obstruction, and has a high temperature or any other signs of SIRS/sepsis (see p. 304–306).

It is also a common cause of sepsis in the elderly, who can often present without features of Charcot's triad.

Immediate management
- ABC assessment
  - Give patient high flow O$_2$ via a non-rebreath mask
  - Gain large bore IV access
  - Fluid resuscitation is likely to be necessary if patient is in septic shock (see p. 6–8)
- Give broad spectrum antibiotics
  - e.g. cefuroxime, 1.5 g IV TDS
  - *and* metronidazole, 500 mg IV TDS
  - *or, if patient is clinically well,* ciprofloxacin, 750 mg PO BD
- Keep patient nil by mouth
- Get an urgent abdominal USS
- ☎ Call gastroenterologist
  - Patient is likely to require urgent intervention (e.g. ERCP).

Further management
- Definitive intervention to alleviate the biliary obstruction will be required
  - ERCP with removal of stone/stenting is first choice
  - Percutaneous transhepatic cholangiogram (PTC) with drainage can be used, but has an increased risk of causing bacteraemia.

Investigations
- Urine dipstick
  - ↑Bilirubin and ↓urobilinogen indicates biliary obstruction
- FBC and CRP
  - Typically will show ↑WCC (with a neutrophilia) and ↑CRP

- U&Es
  - Sepsis may precipitate acute renal failure, especially if the patient is jaundiced (see p. 270–275)
- LFTs
  - Likely to show ↑bilirubin with a predominantly obstructive picture (i.e. ALP and GGT raised out of proportion to ALT/AST)
- Blood cultures
  - Positive in up to 50% of cases
- USS/CT abdomen
  - Will demonstrate a dilated biliary tree proximal to the obstruction, and strongly supports the diagnosis
  - Will also show if there is a hepatic abscess.

Causes

- Gallstone disease
- Post-ERCP
- Pancreatic cancer (especially in the head of the pancreas)
- Primary sclerosing cholangitis
- Hepatocellular carcinoma
- Biliary-enteric fistula
- Infestation (e.g. *Clonorchis, Ascaris, Fasciola*)
- Congenital intrahepatic biliary dilatation (Caroli's disease).

Further reading

- *OHCM*, 7th edn. Oxford: Oxford University Press, p. 590.
- *Oxford Textbook of Medicine*, 4th edn, vol. 2. Oxford: Oxford University Press, p. 706.
- *Oxford Handbook of Gastroenterology and Hepatology*, 1st edn. Oxford: Oxford University Press, p. 212.

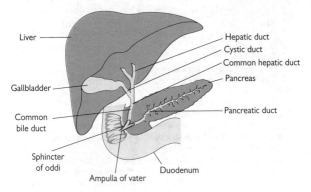

Fig. 6.2 Anatomy of the Biliary Tree

☼ Alcohol withdrawal

Definition
Sudden withdrawal from chronic alcohol use can be extremely dangerous, which is why it is important to take an alcohol history from every patient who is admitted to hospital. Prescribing adequate prophylactic treatment after identifying at–risk patients can often prevent this problem.

Some patients will, however, develop withdrawal symptoms, the extreme presentation of which is delirium tremens (DTs). This has a 5–35% mortality rate, so should be treated as a medical emergency.

Presentation
Alcohol withdrawal symptoms can start as early as 8 h after cessation or reduction in intake, but tend to be worst after 24–72 h. It is a clinical diagnosis, so be sure to rule out other causes for the symptoms (e.g. head injury or sepsis).

- Neuropsychiatric symptoms
  - Intention tremor, confusion, agitation, insomnia, hallucinations (of any modality), generalized seizures
- Autonomic instability
  - Tachycardia, hypertension, diaphoresis, tremor, pyrexia, mydriasis
- Delirium tremens
  - More severe manifestation of the above, particularly of the neuropsychiatric symptoms
  - This has a >20% mortality rate if left untreated.

Immediate management
- ABC assessment
  - If patient is fitting, see p. 76–79
  - Attach patient to cardiac monitor (risk of arrhythmia)
  - If patient is conscious, they are likely to be uncooperative. If this is the case, additional help may be required from security guards etc.
- DEFG—don't ever forget the glucose
  - Check the patient's BM, to rule out hypoglycaemia (see p. 226–228)
  - This can be a problem in chronic alcohol users, owing to depletion of glycogen stores
  - Start IV dextrose infusion whilst patient is not feeding well
- If the patient is showing severe signs of withdrawal, start on IV benzodiazepines
  - These patients should be managed in an HDU environment, as they will be at the most severe end of the spectrum. Most patients can be managed on PO treatment (see below, or local guidelines)
  - e.g. lorazepam, 1–4 mg IV 1–3-hourly (max 240 mg/day)
  - The frequency and dose should be titrated to response, and can vary significantly

- This should be slowly reduced over a 3–5-day period, or switched to PO regimen
- With a very agitated patient, gaining IV access may be impractical, so give IM drugs initially, then switch to IV once settled
  - e.g. lorazepam, 0.5–2 mg IM—repeat until settled
  - ± haloperidol, 3–5 mg IM—repeat until settled
- Patients with milder symptoms can be managed on a reducing PO regimen (see below)
- Start on thiamine
  - e.g. thiamine, 100 mg IV (to avoid precipitating Wernicke's encephalopathy), then 100 mg PO OD
- The patient will require close nursing supervision, and adequate PRN benzodiazepines
  - Aim to keep the patient calm, but still awake
  - Patients on high doses of benzodiazepines should be closely monitored for signs of respiratory depression.

Further management
- Perform a thorough history and examination to exclude any other cause for this presentation (see differential diagnosis)
- Reducing dose of chlordiazepoxide:

Table 6.1 Reducing dose of chlordiazepoxide (all doses are mg)

Day	0800	1200	1800	2200	Total dose
1	20	20	20	20	80
2	20	15	15	20	70
3	15	15	15	15	60
4	15	10	10	15	50
5	10	10	10	10	40
6	10	5	5	10	30
7	5	5	5	5	20
8	5	—	—	5	10
9	—	—	—	5	5
10	—	—	—	—	Stop

  - PRN dose: chlordiazepoxide, 5–20 mg PO, 2° PRN
  - Higher doses may be required initially in more severe cases
- Nutrition
  - Start patient on PO multivitamins and folic acid supplements
  - If patient is hypomagnesaemic, consider IV replacement
  - Monitor PO_4^{2-} very carefully over the first few days of admission, due to the risk of refeeding syndrome; if levels are low, give phosphate, 30 mmol IV over 24 h
  - Also check magnesium, calcium and zinc levels, and moitor regularly.

Investigations

Alcohol withdrawal is a clinical diagnosis, so investigations should be undertaken to rule out other causes which may need treatment.
- ABGs
  - Is the patient acidotic? (e.g. respiratory acidosis with COPD, metabolic acidosis with alcoholic or diabetic ketoacidosis)
  - Is the patient hypoxic?
- FBC and CRP
  - ↑WCC and ↑CRP may indicate underlying infection—could this be delirium?
  - ↑Hb, ↑MCV, and ↓platelets all suggest chronic alcohol overuse
- LFTs and coagulation screen
  - Liver enzymes are likely to be raised if patient has been drinking recently, although markers of synthetic function (e.g. albumin and clotting) tell most about underlying liver function
- Blood alcohol level
  - Severe withdrawal symptoms are rare if blood alcohol levels are high this should raise suspicion of another cause
- U&Es and bone profile (with Mg level)
  - Screen for any electrolyte disturbance which may be causing the symptoms
  - Low urea is common if patient is undernourished
  - Monitor PO_4^{2-} to check for refeeding syndrome (see above)
  - Hypomagnesaemia is common with chronic alcohol overuse
- CXR
  - Have low threshold if patient has any chest signs
  - Pneumonias are quite common, owing to patients becoming intoxicated and failing to protect their airway
- ECG
  - Check for underlying arrhythmia if tachycardic (e.g. AF)
- CT head
  - If there is any suspicion of head injury or intracranial bleed.

Differential diagnosis
- Hypoglycaemia
- Head injury/intracranial bleed
- Sepsis
- Hepatic encephalopathy
- Alcoholic ketoacidosis
- Drug intoxication
- Meningitis/encephalitis
- Electrolyte disturbance (e.g. hyponatraemia, hypercalcaemia)
- Wernicke/Korsakoff syndrome.

Further reading
- *OHCM*, 7th edn. Oxford: Oxford University Press, p. 274.
- *Oxford Textbook of Medicine*, 4th edn. vol. 3. Oxford: Oxford University Press, p. 1338.
- *Oxford Handbook of Gastroenterology and Hepatology*, 1st edn. Oxford: Oxford University Press, p. 146.

Renal and urology

☼ Pyelonephritis

Definition
Pyelonephritis is an infection of the kidney parenchyma, which may extend to involve the ureter, glomeruli and blood vessels. It is usually caused by infection ascending from lower down in the urinary tract.

Presentation
- Loin pain and tenderness
- Fever
- Nausea and vomiting
- Features of lower UTI
  - Urinary frequency, urgency, suprapubic pain, painful micturition

Immediate management
- ABC assessment
  - The patient may potentially be in septic shock (see p. 304–306)
  - Give high flow O_2 via a non-rebreath mask
  - Consider fluid boluses if patient appears poorly perfused—↑HR, ↓BP, ↑CRT, ↓UO (see p. 6–8)
- Gain IV access
- Give IV antibiotics (after taking blood and urine cultures)
  - e.g. cefuroxime, 1.5 g IV TDS
- Give adequate analgesia (see p. 10–11)

Investigations
- Urine dipstick
  - May show nitrites, leucocytes, blood, protein
- Urine microscopy + C&S (send before antibiotics are administered if possible)
  - Phase contrast microscopy can show bacteria, strengthening your diagnosis, although there may be less than in a typical lower UTI
  - C&S will guide further antibiotic treatment
- FBC and CRP
  - WCC is often significantly raised in pyelonephritis, as is CRP
- U&Es
  - Raised urea and creatinine may suggest renal failure
- Blood culture
  - Is the patient septicaemic?
- Renal USS
  - Should be performed to check for renal abscesses, hydronephrosis or other renal tract abnormalities
- KUB X-ray
  - May reveal renal calculi
- Further investigations may be required, under the direction of a renal physician or urologist

Further management

- If the patient's symptoms persist despite 3 days of culture-sensitive antibiotics, further investigation will be required to determine if there is a pyonephritis, perinephric abscess or emphysematous pyelonephritis
  - Discuss management with a urologist
  - You may want to consider this earlier in patients with DM, or with previous urological history
- Repeat urine C&S following course of antibiotics to ensure eradication
- A first episode in a sexually active female will probably not require any further follow-up
- Male patients or patients with recurrent infections should be referred to a urologist for follow-up
- Advice for women
  - Ensure good fluid intake, genital hygiene (wiping from front to back), urinate immediately following sex

Causes

- Gram-negative aerobic bacteria (e.g. *E. coli*)
  - 95% caused by ascending infection, remaining 5% by haematogenous spread
- Urinary catheterization
- Renal calculi
- Dehydration
- Vesicoureteric reflux/incompetent ureterovesical valve
- Pregnancy
- Diabetes
- Faecal incontinence (especially women)
- Prostatic disease
- Unprotected anal intercourse (men)
- Structural abnormality
- Post-cystoscopy or other urinary tract surgical procedures
- Neurogenic dysfunction
- Immunocompromise
- TB (rare)
- Fungal infections (rare)

Complications

- Renal scarring
  - Recurrent pyelonephritis can cause chronic renal failure
- Pyonephritis (pus in the kidney)
  - Will require surgical drainage
- Perinephric abscess
  - Will require surgical drainage
- Septicaemia/septic shock
- Acute renal failure

Further reading

- *OHCM*, 7th edn. Oxford: Oxford University Press, p. 282.
- *Oxford Textbook of Medicine*, 4th edn, vol. 3. Oxford: Oxford University Press, p. 423.
- *Oxford Textbook of Clinical Nephrology*, 3rd edn. Oxford: Oxford University Press, Chapter 7.1.

! Obstructive uropathy

Definition

Structural or functional changes in the urinary tract that hinder normal urine flow. It may lead to permanent renal dysfunction, i.e. obstructive nephropathy. The obstruction can be at any level from the renal tubules (casts, crystals) to the external urethral meatus. Obstructive uropathy is an emergency because of the potential for permanent kidney damage, renal failure, septicaemia or death. This can be prevented or limited by early intervention to relieve the obstruction.

Presentation

Symptoms and signs can vary with the site of obstruction, degree of obstruction, and rapidity of onset.

Upper tract obstruction
- Flank pain, often with loin/renal angle tenderness
  - Can be intermittent or persistent
  - Dull, sharp or colicky, usually of varying intensity
  - Often radiates to iliac fossa, inguinal area and groin
  - Can be provoked by alcohol, diuretics or ↑fluid intake
- Symptoms of UTI or renal calculi
  - Dysuria, frequency, frank/microscopic haematuria
- Sepsis
- Complete anuria suggests bilateral (or unilateral if patient only has one kidney) complete obstruction

Lower tract obstruction
- Often follows a history of symptoms of chronic obstruction of bladder outflow
  - Urinary hesitancy, poor stream, terminal dribbling, feeling of incompletely voided bladder
- Severe suprapubic pain (unless superimposed on chronic retention or underlying neuropathy)
- Suprapubic mass, which is dull to percussion

Chronic obstruction
- Pain is often less of a feature
- Patients can present with features of renal failure
  - Lethargy, nausea, anorexia, uraemia
- Some patients may become polyuric if the obstruction is relieved
- Hypertension
- Oedema

Immediate management

- ABC assessment
  - If there is an underlying infective cause, the patient may be septic (see p. 304–306)
  - Fluid management can be problematic, as polyuric patients may be significantly hypovolaemic and patients with renal failure may be overloaded. ☎ Discuss with seniors if unsure

- Give adequate analgesia (see p. 10–11)
- Consider antibiotics if infective cause is suspected
  - e.g. cefuroxime, 1.5 g IV TDS
- Consider urinary catheterization
  - If a large volume of urine is drained, this indicates bladder outflow obstruction
  - The urine should be drained rapidly and completely from an obstructed bladder—studies have shown minimal problems with rapid bladder decompression (frank haematuria can occur following this, but is always self-limiting—inform urologists non-urgently)
  - If little or no urine is drained, the catheter position should be checked by instilling water—if the water returns freely, this indicates that the catheter is in the bladder and that the obstruction is in the upper renal tract
- Ensure that strict fluid balance recording (including hourly urine output) is performed
- If there is proximal obstruction, or you are unable to pass a catheter, ☎ call urologists early
- ☎ Call nephrologists if there is any indication of renal failure

Investigations
- Urine
  - Leucocytes and nitrites indicate infection
  - Haematuria can be caused by infection, calculi, neoplasm
- FBC and CRP
  - ↑WCC and ↑CRP point towards an infective cause
  - Polycythaemia can be caused by chronic obstruction and ↓Hb can be caused by chronic renal failure
- U&Es and blood gas
  - A hyperkalaemic normal anion gap metabolic acidosis often occurs with urinary obstruction
  - ↑Urea and ↑creatinine occur in renal failure, although may not occur until there is a 50% decrease in GFR
- Imaging studies
  - Usually done under the guidance of a urologist/nephrologist
  - e.g. renal tract USS, KUB X-ray, IVU and CT

Further management
- The initial goal is to relieve the obstruction. If this cannot be done with simple interventions (e.g. catheterization), then urgent urological intervention will be required
  - This includes expert catheterization, nephrostomy, lithotripsy, stenting and open surgery
- If the patient is in renal failure, they will require nephrology involvement

Causes

Urethral obstruction
- Benign prostatic hypertrophy
- Neoplasia
  - Prostate, bladder, cervical or colorectal cancer
- Phimosis
- Urethral stricture
- Trauma
- Blood clot
- Inflammation from sexually transmitted diseases
- Calculi
- Neuropathic bladder
  - DM, MS, spinal cord lesions, Parkinson's disease, anticholinergic medications, alpha blockers

Obstruction of the ureter
- Calculi
- Trauma
  - e.g. Postoperative
- Blood clot
- Vesicoureteric reflux
- Papillary necrosis
  - Pyelonephritis, DM, sickle cell disease
- Pregnancy
- AAA
- Neoplasm impinging on ureter
- Retroperitoneal fibrosis
- Inflammatory bowel disease
- TB
- Sarcoidosis
- Post-radiotherapy

Intrarenal obstruction
- Calculi—e.g. staghorn calculus
- Protein casts—myeloma, amyloidosis

Further reading
- *OHCM*, 7th edn. Oxford: Oxford University Press, p. 286.
- *Oxford Textbook of Medicine*, 4th edn, vol. 3. Oxford: Oxford University Press, p. 447.
- Vaughan ED Jr, Gillenwater JY. Recovery following complete chronic unilateral ureteral occlusion: functional, radiographic and pathologic alterations. *J Urol* 1971; **106(1)**:27–35.

⚙ Acute renal failure

Definition

Acute renal failure (ARF) is defined as a significant reduction in the excretory function of the kidney, occurring over hours or days. It is a frequently occurring problem for unwell patients, particularly those with pre-existing renal impairment (e.g. the elderly). Prompt diagnosis and treatment is essential to preserve remaining kidney function.

ARF is often divided up into three types, based on the underlying pathological process, to simplify investigation and management. It should be noted that certain disease processes can cause damage through more than one mechanism.

- Pre-renal failure
  - Reduction in renal blood flow, leading to ↓GFR
  - The most common cause of ARF in the hospital setting
- Intrinsic renal failure
  - Disease process causing damage to the nephrons, reducing the number of functioning glomeruli, hence causing ↓GFR
- Post-renal failure
  - Caused by obstruction to urine flow away from the kidney, resulting in increased pressure in the renal tubule, causing ↓GFR
  - It is very important to identify this cause, as prompt intervention can preserve renal function (see p. 266–268)

Presentation

As it can be asymptomatic, ARF is often only picked up when routine U&Es are taken. For this reason, all unwell patients who are admitted to hospital should have baseline U&Es taken. The presenting features are often caused by the underlying disease process.

Clinical features of ARF

- ❶ Arrhythmia/cardiac arrest
  - Due to hyperkalaemia
- Uraemia
  - Anorexia, nausea, vomiting, diarrhoea, bruising, muscle cramps, encephalopathy

Pre-renal failure

- Symptoms of hypovolaemia (see p. 96–100)
  - Tachycardia, hypotension, ↑CRT, ↓urine output (<0.5 ml/kg/h, <400 ml/day), thirst, postural hypotension
- History of excessive fluid loss
  - e.g. Vomiting, diarrhoea, bleeding, polyuria
  - Daily fluid balance charts and daily weights can demonstrate fluid loss
- Severe cardiac failure
- Sepsis

Intrinsic renal failure

- History consistent with nephritic syndrome
  - Haematuria, oedema and hypertension

- History of severe hypotension
  - e.g. cardiac arrest, haemorrhage, sepsis, surgery
  - Can cause acute tubular necrosis (ATN)
- Nephrotoxic drugs
  - See below
- Any history of rhabdomyolysis or severe haemolysis
  - Muscle tenderness, limb ischaemia, precipitating drugs, prolonged fitting, recent blood transfusion, 'haematuria' on dipstick (myoglobinuria will cause dipstick to be positive for blood)
- Severe allergic reactions

Post-renal failure (see p. 266–268)
- Loin/flank pain
- History of bladder outflow obstruction
  - Lower urinary tract symptoms (e.g. hesitancy, frequency, poor flow, terminal dribbling)
- Recent abdominal surgery
- History of renal calculi
- Intra-abdominal tumours

Immediate management

- ABC assessment
  - The initial priority is to treat any life-threatening complications (see below)
  - If patient is unwell, give high flow O_2 via a non-rebreath mask
  - Use caution when giving fluid-resuscitation, as some patients are at high risk of becoming fluid-overloaded, but patients with pre-renal failure will urgently need IV fluid
- Management of ARF is complicated. ☎ Call seniors or nephrologists early

Life-threatening complications
- Hyperkalaemia (see p. 394–395)
  - Put patient on cardiac monitor until serum K^+ is known
  - Perform 12-lead ECG
  - Treat as a priority
  - Severe, refractory hyperkalaemia is an indication for haemodialysis
- Pulmonary oedema
  - Suspect this if the patient is SOB, hypoxic, oedematous and has widespread crepitations in their chest
  - Sit upright
  - Give high flow O_2 via a non-rebreath mask
  - Furosemide is unlikely to be helpful
  - Give small doses of morphine, e.g. morphine, 2.5–5 mg IV, titrated to effect (ensure that naloxone is available, as the impaired renal function may cause accumulation)
  - Consider IV venodilators, e.g. glyceryl trinitrate—initially 10 µg/min IV infusion, titrate to response
  - Definitive treatment is haemodialysis

- Hypovolaemia
  - Patients with pre-renal failure are likely to be volume-depleted, so will require fluid resuscitation
  - This should be corrected carefully, as patients with inadequate renal function will be susceptible to volume overload
  - Give 5 ml/kg boluses of 0.9% NaCl, and assess response (e.g. pulse, BP, CRT, postural BP drop), repeating if necessary
  - Ensure strict fluid balance charts are kept, and that the patient is weighed daily

Investigations
- Urine output
  - Can provide a clue as to underlying aetiology
  - Anuria (<100 ml/day)—urinary tract obstruction, renal artery occlusion, rapidly progressive glomerulonephritis, bilateral diffuse renal cortical necrosis
  - Oliguria (100–400 ml/day)—pre-renal failure, hepatorenal syndrome
  - Non-oliguric (>400 ml/day)—acute interstitial nephritis, acute glomerulonephritis, partial obstructive nephropathy, ATN, radiological contrast-induced ARF, rhabdomyolysis
- Urine microscopy
  - Normal—pre-renal, post-renal, haemolytic uraemic syndrome (HUS), thrombotic thrombocytopenic purpura (TCP), vasculitis, renal emboli
  - Granular casts—ATN, glomerulonephritis, interstitial nephritis
  - Red cell casts—glomerulonephritis, malignant hypertension
  - White cell casts—acute interstitial nephritis, pyelonephritis
  - Eosinophiluria—acute allergic nephritis, renal emboli
  - Crystalluria—aciclovir, sulphonamides, methotrexate, ethylene glycol poisoning, radiological contrast
- U&Es
  - Monitor for hyperkalaemia
  - ↑Urea and ↑creatinine indicates renal failure, and levels can be used to monitor progress
  - eGFR can be calculated using the MDRD equation:

  $$\text{eGFR (ml/min/1.73m}^2) = 186.3 \times (\text{creatinine}^{-1.154} \times \text{age}^{-0.203} \times$$
  $$(0.742 \text{ if female}) \times (1.21 \text{ if Afro-Caribbean}))$$

  (Normal value = >70 ml/min/1.73m^2)

  - Try to obtain any previous results as they will provide clues as to previous renal impairment
  - A urea: creatinine ratio of >20 favours a diagnosis of pre-renal failure
- Urine biochemistry
  - Calculation of the fractional excretion of sodium (FENa) can help to differentiate pre-renal failure from ATN

  $$\text{FENa (\%)} = (\text{urine Na} \times \text{plasma creatinine})/(\text{plasma Na} \times \text{urine creatinine}) \times 100$$

- Make sure that urine and plasma creatinine levels are both given in the same units (e.g. mmol/l)
  - FENa <1% indicates pre-renal failure
  - FENa >1% indicates ATN
- FBC
  - Leucocytosis is common in ARF
  - Leucopenia and thrombocytopenia may suggest SLE
  - Anaemia may indicate myeloma, or could suggest chronic renal failure
- LFTs and coagulation screen
  - Abnormal LFTs and coagulopathy may indicate underlying liver disease—?hepatorenal syndrome
- Blood gas
  - ARF can cause renal tubular acidosis—a normal anion gap metabolic acidosis
  - Patient may require PO bicarbonate replacement
- Bone profile
  - ↓Ca^{2+} & ↓PO_4^{2-} are common in ARF, and should be treated (see p. 400–402)
- Creatine kinase (CK)
  - Elevated levels could indicate rhabdomyolysis
- 12-lead ECG
  - Check for changes consistent with hyperkalaemia or heart failure
- CXR
  - Can aid the diagnosis of pulmonary oedema
- Renal USS
  - Bilaterally small kidneys may indicate chronic renal failure/impairment
  - This can demonstrate collecting system dilatation if there is an obstruction
- Other imaging studies
  - Should be done under the guidance of the nephrologists (e.g. DMSA, MAG3, etc.)
- Renal biopsy
  - Under the guidance of the renal team

Further management

- Close involvement with the renal team is vital
- Fluid intake
  - Following the correction of any fluid depletion, careful consideration should be given to the patient's fluid intake
  - Generally, the patient should be given the previous day's total fluid loss, plus 500 ml either IV or PO
  - If patient is polyuric, just give the previous day's urine output
  - The fluid status of the patient should be reviewed daily, and fluid intake adjusted accordingly
- Sodium
  - Monitor sodium intake very carefully, and adjust according to the plasma sodium level

- Potassium
  - Patients should initially have their potassium level checked daily when diagnosed with ARF
  - They will require a low potassium diet—the importance of this should be explained to the patient, as it is often very restrictive and difficult to comply with
  - The involvement of a renal dietician is invaluable
- Nutrition
  - Patients with ARF will be catabolic, and weight loss has been shown to be an indicator of poor prognosis—this is another area in which a renal dietician can help
- Drug doses
  - Many drugs are excreted by the kidneys, so caution should be used when prescribing for patients with ARF
  - The BNF has an appendix dealing with prescribing for patients with renal impairment
- Dialysis
  - Will be instigated by the renal physicians, but it is useful to know the indications:
    —Refractory hyperkalaemia
    —Intractable fluid overload
    —Acidosis producing circulatory compromise
    —Overt uraemia, with encephalopathy, pericarditis or uraemic bleeding

Causes
Pre-renal failure
- Reduced effective arterial blood volume
  - Hypovolaemia
  - Sepsis
  - Cardiac failure
  - Liver failure
- Reduced renal artery flow
  - Renal artery stenosis
  - Renal emboli
  - AAA

Intrinsic renal failure
- ATN
  - Often secondary to hypoperfusion/ischaemia from pre-renal failure
- Toxins
  - Antibiotics: aminoglycosides, tetracyclines, cephaloridine, amphotericin B, sulphonamides, polymyxin/colistin, bacitracin, pentamidine, vancomycin
  - Radiological contrast media
  - Anaesthetic agents: methoxyfluranea, enflurane
  - Chemotherapy/immunosuppressive drugs: ciclosporin A, cis-platinum, methotrexate
  - Organic solvents: glycols (e.g. ethylene glycol), hydrocarbons (e.g. carbon tetrachloride, toluene)

- Poisons: venoms, stings, insecticides/herbicides, mushrooms, herbal medicines
- Most illegal drugs
- Heavy metals
- Endogenous toxins: myoglobin, haemoglobin, urate, phosphate (tumour lysis syndrome), immunoglobulin light chains
- Interstitial disease
  - Acute interstitial nephritis, drug reactions, autoimmune diseases (e.g. SLE), infiltrative disease (sarcoidosis, lymphoma), infectious agents (Legionnaire disease, hantavirus)
- Acute glomerulonephritis
- Vascular diseases
  - Vasculitis, malignancy hypertension, polyarteritis nodosa

Post-renal

- See p. 266–268

Further reading

- *OHCM*, 7th edn. Oxford: Oxford University Press, p. 292, 820.
- *Oxford Textbook of Medicine*, 4th edn, vol. 3. Oxford: Oxford University Press, p. 248.

⚠ **Nephrotic syndrome**

Definition

Nephrotic syndrome is a condition that is caused by excessive loss of protein into the urine. It has a number of different causes, involving all damage to the glomerulus. It can cause serious complications, including pulmonary oedema, hypovolaemia, thrombophilia and increased risk of infection.

It can be defined as a triad of:
- Heavy proteinuria—usually >3.5 g/24h or urinary albumin: creatinine ratio of >400 mg/mmol
  - If patient is profoundly hypoalbuminaemic, then the level of proteinurea can be less than this
- Hypoalbuminaemia—<30 g/dl
  - Oedema often does not occur until albumin is <25 g/dl
- Oedema

Presentation

- Oedema
  - Increasing oedema over days or weeks
  - Usually dependent oedema, which can extend up to the abdomen
  - Ascites can occur
  - Facial swelling (often around the eyes), particularly in the mornings
- Non-specific symptoms
  - Lethargy, weakness, reduced appetite, abdominal pain
- SOB
  - Occurs with pulmonary oedema or a pleural effusion
  - Can cause exacerbation of existing cardiac failure
- Polyuria
- Frothy urine
- Thrombotic complications (e.g. DVT)
- Infections—particularly pneumococcal
- Renal failure

Immediate management

- ABC assessment
  - The patient may be SOB due to pulmonary oedema
  - Give high flow O_2 via a non-rebreath mask
  - ⚠ Be very careful with fluid resuscitation—although patient may be oedematous, they can have intravascular fluid depletion (i.e. hypovolaemia). Equally, they may be in cardiac failure and additional fluid could be harmful. ☎ Discuss with seniors if in any doubt
  - Avoid using fluids with high concentrations of sodium (i.e. use colloids for fluid resuscitation)
- ☎ Contact nephrologists early for advice
- Consider diuretics if patient very oedematous
  - e.g. furosemide—initially 40–80 mg/day PO

- ± spironolactone, 100–200 mg/day PO (monitor serum K$^+$ carefully)
- Be careful not to precipitate intravascular fluid depletion, which can in turn worsen renal impairment—aim for weight reduction of 0.5–1 kg/day
- Consider IV albumin if very hypoalbuminaemic—consult seniors
  - Only use if absolutely necessary—albumin is a blood product
  - Use sodium-depleted albumin solutions
  - e.g. 20% albumin solution, 100 ml/day by slow IV infusion
- Consider high dose steroids—under the guidance of the nephrologists
  - This is generally only useful for patients with minimal change nephropathy
- Give antibiotics if any indication of sepsis
  - e.g. Cefuroxime, 1.5 g IV TDS
  - If suspicious of spontaneous bacterial peritonitis, add metronidazole, 500 mg IV TDS
- Check Wells' score to assess for DVT risk
- Ensure strict input/output records are kept, along with daily weights

Investigations
- Urine analysis
  - Dipstick testing is a very quick, useful way of monitoring proteinurea
  - 24-h protein collection will more accurately measure proteinurea
  - Albumin:creatinine ratio is also useful for diagnosis (usually >400 mg/mmol)—use an early morning sample
  - 24-h creatinine clearance can help to estimate renal function
- FBC and film, coagulation
  - Useful screening test for haematological malignancy
  - Check platelets and coagulation if patient will be undergoing renal biopsy
- U&Es
  - Check for ↓Na$^+$
  - Monitor K$^+$ if on diuretics
  - Urea and creatinine are helpful in estimating renal function (calculate eGFR)
- Autoantibody screen
  - Particularly looking for SLE (anti-nuclear antibody, anti-double-stranded DNA antibody)
- Serum complement level
  - Patients are likely to be complement-deficient
- Hepatitis B and C serology
- Serum immunoglobulins
  - Patients are likely to have reduced immunoglobulin levels
- Plasma protein electrophoresis
  - Look for evidence of myeloma
- Varicella serology
  - Check if immune

- ASOT
  - Has there been a recent streptococcal infection?
- Lipid profile
  - Patients are likely to be hypercholesterolaemic
- Renal USS
  - Check for any obvious abnormalities
- Renal biopsy is usually indicated unless there is an obvious clinical cause (e.g. DM with chronic proteinuria)

Further management
- Dietary modification
  - It is advisable to limit fluid intake to 1.5 l per day, or 1 l per day if severely oedematous or hyponatraemic
  - It is also advisable to reduce sodium intake, by avoiding high sodium foods, and not adding any extra salt to meals
  - Patients should have a full calorie diet, with ~1 g/kg/day of protein
  - It is useful to involve a dietician
- Treatment of infection
  - Patients with nephrotic syndrome are particularly susceptible to bacterial (particularly pneumococcal) infection
  - Good skin care is essential, as the combination of oedema and reduced immunity predisposes to cellulitis
  - Pneumococcal vaccination should be considered for patients who are recovering
  - Prophylactic penicillin can be considered
  - Monitor patients with ascites very carefully, as they are at high risk of developing spontaneous bacterial peritonitis—perform an ascitic tap if suspicious
  - If patient is Varicella non-immune, they may warrant Zoster immune globulin (ZIG) if they come into contact with chicken pox. Patients who develop chicken pox should receive aciclovir
- Thromboembolism
  - Owing to the increased risk of thromboembolism, it would seem sensible to supply TED stockings to patients, and to give prophylactic low molecular weight heparin to patients who are immobile, e.g. tinzaparin, 3500 units S/C OD
  - Have a low threshold for investigating for PE if there are any clinical indications (e.g. persistent tachycardia, chest pain, SOB—see p. 200–202)
  - Loin pain, worsening renal function or increasing proteinuria may indicate renal vein thrombosis—arrange an USS if this is suspected, and liaise with nephrologists
- Hyperlipidaemia
  - There is debate as to whether this should be treated with statins or not, as it does tend to be transient whilst the patient is hypo-albuminaemic—seek advice from a nephrologist
- Treatment of underlying condition
  - There are many different causes for nephrotic syndrome, some of which are amenable to immunosuppression (e.g. minimal change nephropathy)

- Immunosuppression should be considered under the guidance of the renal team

Complications

- Infection
  - Particularly pneumococcal disease, cellulitis and spontaneous bacterial peritonitis
- Renal vein thrombosis
- Arterial thrombosis
- Hypovolaemia
- Acute/chronic renal failure
- Iron deficiency anaemia secondary to loss of transferrin and iron
- Muscle wasting
- Accelerated atherosclerosis
- DVT/PE

Causes

Glomerulonephritides

- Minimal change nephropathy
- Membranoproliferative glomerulonephritis
- Membranous glomerulonephritis
- Focal segmental glomerulosclerosis
- Mesangial proliferative glomerulonephritis
- IgA nephropathy (Berger's disease)

Other causes

- Connective tissue disease
  - SLE, rheumatoid arthritis, polyarteritis nodosa
- Diabetic nephropathy
- Post-infection
  - e.g. Streptococcal infection, malaria, TB, hepatitis B and C
- Henoch–Schönlein purpura
- Amyloidosis
- Malignancy
  - Leukaemia, myeloma, Wilm's tumour
- Allergic reactions
- Drugs and metals
  - Gold, lithium, mercury, cadmium, captopril, penicillamine, analgesics and NSAIDs, including phenacetin, aspirin and paracetamol
- Congenital nephrotic syndrome
- Sickle cell disease
- Pre-eclampsia (rare, more often associated with heavy proteinuria)

Further reading

- *OHCM*, 7th edn. Oxford: Oxford University Press, p. 290.
- *Oxford Textbook of Medicine*, 4th edn, vol. 3. Oxford: Oxford University Press, p. 227.

① **Testicular torsion**

Definition

Testicular torsion occurs as a consequence of a testis and the spermatic cord twisting around in the tunica vaginalis of the scrotum. This causes venous occlusion and raised venous pressure, eventually causing failure of the arterial supply and infarction of the testis. Prompt diagnosis and surgery is necessary to prevent loss of the testis.

Presentation

There should be a high degree of suspicion of torsion in a patient with testicular pain, and all male patients presenting with abdominal pain should have their scrotums examined. The presentation of epididymitis and orchiditis can be very similar, but be very sure of the diagnosis before ruling out torsion.

- Sudden onset lower abdominal pain ± testicular pain and tenderness
  - Pain will ease later, as testis becomes necrotic
  - Transient testicular pain can occur with intermittent torsion
  - Pain is usually severe, but can be mild
- Testicular swelling with horizontal lie of the testis
- Mass in scrotum
- Scrotal erythema
- Nausea and vomiting
- Fever (uncommon)

Risk factors

- Age
  - Most common in first year of life and between 12–18 years, although it can occur at any age
- Can present following trauma to groin
- Previous testicular torsion

Immediate management

- ABC assessment
  - It is very unlikely for the patient to be severely unwell, although they may be in severe pain and vomiting
- Give adequate analgesia (see p. 10–11)
- ☎ Call urologist urgently
  - ⚠ This is a urological emergency which requires urgent surgery if torsion is suspected

Further management

- The patient is likely to require surgery, so ensure that all preoperative preparations are completed
  - e.g. Keep nil by mouth, check when last fed, check if any previous adverse reaction to anaesthetics, ask about cardiovascular risk factors, bloods and ECG if indicated

- Surgery is required for definitive treatment
  - Untwisting of the testis, removal of dead tissue and fixation of the testis in the scrotum (orchidoplexy)—necrotic testes are removed (orchidectomy)
  - An orchidoplexy is always performed on the contralateral testis at the same time, to prevent torsion in the future

Investigations

There is no test that can accurately rule out a testicular torsion, so a clinical judgement is required as to whether a patient will require surgical exploration. Investigations can be used as a guide in the more equivocal cases, but don't waste time organizing scans if there is high clinical suspicion.

- Urine dipstick
  - Usually normal, but up to 30% will have leucocytes
- FBC
  - Up to 60% of cases will have ↑WCC
- Colour Doppler
  - Very specific for torsion (100%), but not very sensitive (86%)— therefore there will be some false-negative results
- Radionucleotide scans
  - Reduced uptake in one testis indicates reduced blood flow (i.e. torsion), and is quite accurate (will pick up 90–100%)
  - Often not available at short notice, and involves a dose of ionizing radiation

Causes

- Idiopathic
- Trauma
- Vigorous exercise
- Sexual arousal/activity
- Active cremasteric reflex

Further reading

- *OHCM*, 7th edn. Oxford: Oxford University Press, p. 600.

⑦ Paraphimosis

Definition

Paraphimosis is a urological emergency occurring in uncircumcised or partially circumcised males in which the prepuce of the foreskin is retracted behind the corona of the glans penis and becomes trapped. This can cause lymphatic engorgement, compromising blood flow to the glans, eventually leading to ischaemia and necrosis.

Presentation

- Pain, swelling, erythema and tenderness of the prepuce and inability to pull the foreskin forward
- Blackened tissue around the tip of the penis indicates necrosis
- Urinary retention
- This can often happen following examination of the penis, or procedures such as catheterization or cystoscopy, when the foreskin has been left retracted
  - ⚠ Always remember to replace the foreskin after examination, catheterization, etc
  - This is particularly important in confused or unconscious patients, as they may not alert you to the problem until permanent damage has been done

Immediate management

- ABC assessment
  - The patient is unlikely to be severely unwell with this problem
- Analgesia (see p. 10–11)
  - This will be required before any attempt is made to manipulate the foreskin
  - Topical analgesia may be required in addition to oral pain relief— e.g. lidocaine gel, or a penile nerve block
- Consider removing a urinary catheter if you are confident you can replace it
- Attempt to replace the foreskin
  - Facing the glans, gently grasp the penis and push the glans penis away from you with your thumbs whilst pulling the foreskin forwards between the index and middle fingers
- If unsuccessful, ☎ contact urologists urgently

Further management

- If attempts to return the foreskin are unsuccessful, there are other techniques to reduce the oedema. These should be undertaken by a urologist
  - Puncture technique—a 21-G needle is used to create several punctures in the oedematous foreskin, to allow interstitial fluid to drain out
  - Dorsal slit—an incision is made into the preputial ring, to relieve constriction, and allow replacement of the foreskin

- Occasionally, an emergency circumcision is required
- Always examine the penis following the reduction
  - Is there a discharge indicating infection?
  - Are there any skin lesions which may be neoplastic? (e.g. squamous cell carcinoma)
- An elective circumcision may be indicated to prevent recurrence

Causes

- Iatrogenic
  - Not returning the foreskin after penile examination, urinary catheterization, cystoscopy or similar procedures
- Chronic infection
  - Often secondary to poor hygiene
- Chronic balanoposthitis
  - Especially in patients with DM
- Post-circumcision
  - Sclerosis of excessive skin
- Vigorous sexual intercourse
- Trauma
  - e.g. following piercing

Further reading

- *OHCM*, 7th edn. Oxford: Oxford University Press, p. 66.

Haematology, oncology and infectious diseases

☠ Neutropenic sepsis

Definition
- Pyrexia of more than 38°C at a single reading or 37.5°C on two occasions over 1–2 h
- *and* Neutrophil count of <1.0×10^9/l

Neutropenia is common in patients receiving chemotherapy, usually occurring 10–12 days after the first day of a new treatment cycle. It is not uncommon for some agents, such as the taxanes, to cause neutropenia more quickly.

Immediate management

Any infection in a neutropenic patient should be considered an emergency, requiring rapid clinical review and action.
- Follow ABC approach as described on p. 2–5. It must be borne in mind that speed of decompensation in this patient group is much more rapid, so early senior and/or critical care review is vital
- Take multiple sets of blood cultures from different sites—consult local guidelines as approaches vary. Bear in mind difficulty of access, risk of introduction of further infection and potential coagulation defects when doing so

⚠ Start IV antibiotics as soon as possible, even if infective site not known. The first dose should be given within 1 h of presentation. Follow your own hospital protocol; if unsure contact local microbiologist. Recommended combinations are:
- Piperacillin–tazobactam and gentamicin
- Ciprofloxacin/ceftazidime *and* teicoplanin/vancomycin
- ☎ Contact haematologist
- Instruct regular observation and set next review time.

History
- Chemotherapy regimen, agents and current day of cycle
- Respiratory system
  - Shortness of breath
  - Purulent sputum
  - Cough
- ENT
  - Sinusitis
  - Sore throat
  - Coryzal symptoms
- Gastrointestinal
  - Diarrhoea
  - Abdominal pain
  - Vomiting
- Skin lesions
  - Rash (do not forget immunosuppression may cause re-activation of Herpes and Varicella)

- Infected ulcers
- Surgical incisions
- Vascular access sites
  - Are rigors associated with use of central venous access?
- Any blood products in the past 24 h?
- Genitourinary
  - Discharge
  - Rashes
  - Dysuria
  - Loin pain
  - Frequency
  - Haematuria
- Neurological
  - Altered level of consciousness
  - Odd behaviour
  - Confusion
  - Visual disturbance
  - Weakness
  - Paraesthesia

Investigations

- Minimum of two new venepunctures for blood cultures
- Cultures from venous access if *in situ*; do not remove central lines or Hickman lines without advice from haematologist
- CXR—consolidation or effusion suggestive of infection
- FBC—what is the patient's current haematological status?
- CRP—initial value may not be indicative of severity but can be used to track progress
- U&Es—renal function may deteriorate and is important for antibiotic choice and dose
- LFTs—any sign of biliary sepsis?
- Coagulation screen—be extremely alert to risk of DIC in these patients
- Swab any rashes or sites of infection
- Stool samples for microscopy, culture and *C. difficile* toxin
- Urine dipstick and MSU
- Sputum sample
- Throat swab
- Viral serology

Causes
- Bacterial—most commonly Gram-positive cocci or Gram-negative bacilli. Consider *Mycobacterium* and PCP if additional risk factors present
- Fungal—*Aspergillus*, *Candida*
- Viral—Varicella zoster, Herpes, CMV if following bone marrow transplant, HIV

Further management
- Daily progress bloods
  - FBC
  - CRP
  - U&Es
  - LFTs
  - Coagulation
  - Repeat blood cultures if no improvement
- Daily review by medical microbiologist, haematologist or infectious diseases consultant is desirable

Further reading
- *OHCM*, 7th edn. Oxford: Oxford University Press, p. 336.
- Northern Cancer Network NHS. Guidelines on the inpatient management of infection in neutropenic patients. July 2001. www.cancernorth.nhs.uk
- Vidal L, Paul M, Ben-Dor, Pokroy E, Soares-Weiser K, Leibovici L. Oral versus intravenous antibiotic treatment for febrile neutropenia in cancer patients. *The Cochrane Database of Systematic Reviews* 2007, Issue 3. www.library.nhs.uk

☠ Disseminated intravascular coagulation

Background

In essence, disseminated intravascular coagulation (DIC) is intravascular activation of fibrin, causing consumption of clotting factors and platelets and leading in the acute scenario to features of either bleeding or thrombosis, which may be localized or generalized. The activation may arise from damage to endothelium or tissue and, in practice, often results in further damage to it.

Presentation

- Spontaneous bleeding suggestive of reduced coagulability
    - e.g. bleeding gums, petechial rash, oozing from venepuncture sites, epistaxis
- Cardiovascular compromise consistent with distributive shock (see p. 96–100)
    - tachycardia, hypotension, shortness of breath
- Focal neurological deficit is rare, but clouding of sensorium may occur
- Oliguria or other signs of renal compromise
- Pleural rub or other features of ARDS
- Localised thrombosis
- Skin infarction and gangrene
- Haematoma or surgical wound oozing

Immediate management

- The ABC resuscitation approach (p. 2–5) must be used to address the actual or potential compromise caused by DIC. Fluid balance becomes complex, but in the first instance there must be secure means by which to administer IVT
- First line investigations should be requested immediately, as detailed
- An ABG will give an indication of the respiratory and metabolic effects of the syndrome and help direct immediate management

❶ If this seems a likely clinical diagnosis, a senior colleague should be made aware. Even if in control of the situation currently, a critical care review will both offer additional support and make the ITU team aware that this patient is in the hospital, and thus that a bed may be required in due course.

- The emphasis of management is correction of the primary cause whilst monitoring and supporting clotting and fluid balance, so timely further investigations are key.

Investigations

- Blood tests
  - FBC will give an absolute value to confirm thrombocytopenia ($<100 \times 10^9$). Check Hb to assess extent of blood loss. Is WCC raised? (suggestive of toxic granulation)
  - U&Es—is there any renal compromise?
  - D-dimer will confirm the presence of fibrin degradation
  - A coagulation screen is likely to indicate lengthened PT and APTT
  - Note that diagnosis is not absolute from any one of the above tests. The overall combination of thrombocytopenia, lengthened PT/APTT and positive D-dimer in the presence of the clinical picture described is the most reliable diagnostic approach
- CXR—the altered capillary permeability associated with the condition has the potential to cause pulmonary problems lying within the spectrum of ARDS
- Further coagulation investigations offer confirmation—prothrombin fragment I and II are abnormal in 90% of patients with DIC, for example. Liaise with haematology to establish what is available locally and recommended by them
- Investigate local effects—haematomas, for example, can be better assessed by USS
- Further exploration of any likely causes, e.g. serum βhCG if suspicious of intrauterine causes
- Baseline investigations must be frequently repeated to monitor progress. Involve haematology and critical care—decide what the monitoring tool is going to be, and when to escalate care

Further management

- As previously mentioned, management consists of three main elements
  - Correct primary cause, which should in turn see a correction of coagulability
  - Continuing physiological support during this time
  - Close monitoring
- Continued involvement of critical care team is advisable, both for another clinician's input and the physiological support available for the patient by escalating care.

Causes

- Infection
  - Bacterial—Gram-negative sepsis, Gram-positive infections, *Rickettsia*
  - Viral—HIV, CMV, hepatitis
  - Fungal—*Histoplasma*
  - Parasitic—malaria
- Malignancies, either haematological or metastatic
- Trauma
- Transfusion reaction
- Acute liver failure
- Placental abruption, retained products of conception, amniotic fluid embolism
- Haemolytic reactions
- Vasculitic disorders
- Inflammatory bowel diseases

❶ One form of endothelial damage is aortic aneurysm. Be very suspicious of a DIC (especially subacute) picture with no evident rashes or bleeding—is this local DIC due to an aneurysm?

Further reading

- *OHCM*, 7th edn. Oxford: Oxford University Press, p. 332–3.
- *Oxford Textbook of Medicine*, 4th edn. Oxford: Oxford University Press, p. 770–1.
- Levi M, Opal SM. Coagulation abnormalities in critically ill patients. *Crit Care* 2006; **10**:222.

ⓘ **Thrombocytopenia**

Definition

Platelet count less than 150×10^9/l.

Presentation

Bleeding is uncommon with a platelet count greater than 30. Common presentations include:

- Easy or excessive bruising
- Petechial rashes
- Spontaneous nosebleeds or bleeding from gums
- Prolonged bleeding time from cuts or venesection
- Malaena or haematemesis
- Haematuria
- Abnormally heavy menstrual flow
- Preceding bloody diarrhoea (HUS)

Immediate management

- Thrombocytopenia is an emergency if it is associated with significant bleeding or circulatory compromise. In these circumstances, aggressive resuscitation by ABC is required

❶ An actively bleeding and compromised patient will almost definitely need platelets, which will take time to procure. Call a senior, an on-call haematologist, or both, now.

- Rapid history, discussion with nurses and assessment of drug chart. Is the patient receiving chemotherapy?
- Nearly all further management is based on correction of the primary cause, so timely investigations result in timely treatment. Initiate investigations as detailed.

Further management

Management will depend on the cause of the thrombocytopenia; if no cause can be found then it may be classified as idiopathic thrombocytopenic purpura (ITP). Before diagnosing ITP:

- Exclude any causative illness
- Stop any possible culprit drugs
- Ensure the patient is stable
- Involve a haematologist

Thrombocytopenia due to aplasia or chemotherapy

- The mainstay of treatment here is platelet transfusion, to be discussed with the haematology team
- Liaise with the oncology team if chemotherapy is implicated

Idiopathic thrombocytopenic purpura

- In non-emergency situations, patients with platelet counts of more than 30 do not usually require treatment and should be referred to a haematologist for monitoring
- First line treatments
  - Methylprednisolone ± cyclophosphamide (discuss with haematologist)
  - Prednisolone 1 mg/kg body weight daily for 2–4 weeks will improve platelet counts in two-thirds of patients and is the usual first choice of agent
  - Current evidence suggests that IV Ig has comparable response rates and long term need for second line treatments, but it may be more useful for short term elevation of platelets, e.g. before surgery
- Second line treatments
  - Splenectomy—two-thirds of of patients who receive a splenectomy will achieve a normal platelet count
  - IV Ig, vinca alkaloids, danazol and anti-D are considered in less acute cases

Thrombotic thrombocytopenic purpura

- Patients with TTP require specialist care, potentially necessitating transfer to a regional centre. It carries a 90% mortality rate if incorrectly treated
- First line treatment is plasma exchange ± corticosteroids
- Second line includes aspirin (prevents relapse), vincristine, immunosuppression

Haemolytic uraemic syndrome

- Requires specialist treatment as 50% of those affected will require dialysis
- Blood transfusion, platelet replacement, and sometimes plasma exchange are necessary

Investigations

- Establish thrombocytopenia
  - Platelet count and blood film to ensure an automated count is correct

- Establish cause
  - Elevated white cell counts suggestive of leukaemia or sepsis
  - Excessive alcohol ingestion is suggested by a macrocytosis
  - Cancerous bone marrow invasion or aplastic anaemia may be demonstrated by pancytopenia
  - Bone marrow biopsy is often required to make a firm diagnosis
- Consider complications
  - U&Es (consider HUS)
  - CRP (look for signs of sepsis)
  - CXR
  - Pregnancy test
  - Urine

Causes

- Low production of platelets in bone marrow
  - Myelosuppression by drugs, especially chemotherapeutic agents
  - Aplastic anaemia
  - Cancerous invasion of the marrow, e.g. leukaemia, lymphoma, breast, lung or GI malignancy
  - Viral infection, e.g. HIV, EBV, hepatitis C
  - Heavy alcohol ingestion
- Intravascular destruction of platelets
  - Immunologically-mediated drug destruction—quinidines, heparin, cefalosporins
  - Idiopathic thrombocytopenic purpura
  - Thrombotic thrombocytopenic purpura
  - Systemic autoimmune disease, e.g. SLE
  - Haemolytic uraemic syndrome—the combination of thrombocytopenia, microangiopathic haemolytic anaemia and renal faliure
  - Pregnancy—causes a mild thrombocytopenia normally but can cause HELLP syndrome
  - DIC
  - Paroxysmal nocturnal haemoglobinuria
- Extravascular destruction of platelets
  - Hypersplenism

Further reading

- *OHCM*, 7th edn. Oxford: Oxford University Press, p. 330.
- ASCO Guidelines Compendium. Online at www.asco.org
- British committee for standards in Haematology: General haematology task force. Guidelines for the investigation and management of idiopathic thrombocytopenic purpura in adults, children and pregnancy. *Br J Haematol* 2003; **120**:574–96.
- Yang R, Zhong CH. Pathogenesis and management of chronic thrombocytopenic purpura: an update. *Int J Haematol* 2000; **71**:18–24.

⊙ **Superior vena cava obstruction**

Definition

Partial or complete blockage of the superior vena cava (SVC), most commonly due to lung cancer.

Presentation

- Swelling of the face, eyelids, neck and arms
- Headache or sensation of 'fullness' in the head
- Dyspnoea
- Engorged veins across shoulders, arms and upper torso
- Dizziness, often positional on leaning forwards
- Dysphagia
- Blurred vision
- Drowsiness

Immediate management

Treatment is directed at the primary cause; there is no justification for treatment without tissue diagnosis unless there is airway obstruction or cerebral oedema. Blind treatment carries no mortality benefit; simple measures which will benefit most patients include:

- Raising the head of the bed
- Supplemental oxygen

Once confident of basic airway security and any first line ABC measures (see p. 2–5), seek senior help. Little more can be done now without further investigations.

Further management

- Medical
    - Corticosteroids, e.g. dexamethasone 8–40 mg initially followed by 4–6 mg 6–8-hourly may offer symptomatic relief
    - Diuretics may relieve oedema but may cause dehydration
    - Antiemetics for relief of nausea
- Chemotherapy
    - For chemosensitive tumours, such as lymphoma, this is the treatment of choice
- Radiotherapy
    - Used for symptom relief in non-chemosensitive tumours
- Thrombolysis
    - Thrombolysis or thrombectomy is required when the obstruction is caused by a thrombus
- Stenting
    - Often used in non-malignant SVC obstruction or in non-responsive tumours
    - At risk of occluding if no anticoagulants are given
    - May be used in an emergency if no tissue diagnosis is possible
- Surgical bypass is mainly indicated in benign SVC obstruction

Causes

- Up to 75% of SVC obstruction is caused by lung cancer, either by direct invasion of the SVC by the primary tumour or by pressure from paratracheal lymph nodes
- Other tumours
  - Local, e.g. thyroid, lymphoma
  - Metastatic, e.g. testicular, breast
- Scarring and fibrosis
  - TB
  - Histoplasmosis
  - Post-radiotherapy
- Thrombosis
  - Primary
  - Secondary to central venous access
- Inflammatory lymphadenopathy

Investigations

- FBC
- U&Es
- LFTs (consider metastases)
- Tumour markers (do not request without discussion with senior colleagues)
- CXR for mediastinal mass
- CT thorax
- A tissue diagnosis is essential for management
  - Biopsy of lymph nodes (supraclavicular, cervical)
  - Needle biopsy of mediastinal mass
- If suspicious of lung cancer
  - Sputum for cytology
  - Bronchoscopy

Further reading

- *OHCM*, 7th edn. Oxford: Oxford University Press, p. 514.
- Abner A. Approach to the patient who presents with superior vena cava obstruction. *Chest* 1993; **103**(4 Suppl):394S–7S.
- Baker GL, Barnes HJ. Superior vena cava syndrome: etiology, diagnosis, and treatment. *Am J Crit Care* 1992; **1(1)**:54–64.
- Beckles MA, Spiro SG, Colice GL, Rudd RM. Initial evaluation of the patient with lung cancer: symptoms, signs, laboratory tests, and paraneoplastic syndromes. *Chest* 2003; **123**:97–104.
- Chen BC, Bongard F, Klein SR. A contemporary perspective on superior vena cava obstruction. *Am J Surg* 1990; **160(2)**:207–11.
- Rodrigues CL, Njo KH, Karim AB. Hypofractionated radiation therapy in the treatment of superior vena cava syndrome. *Lung Cancer* 1993; **10(3–4)**:221–8.
- Würschmidt F, Bünemann H, Heilmann HP. Small cell lung cancer with and without superior vena cava syndrome: a multivariate analysis of prognostic factors in 408 cases. *Int J Radiat Oncol Biol Phys* 1995; **33(1)**:77–82.

:⚙: **Tumour lysis syndrome**

Definition

The severe and life-threatening metabolic derangements which result from rapid tumour breakdown, comprising:

- Hyperuricaemia
- Hyperkalaemia
- Hyperphosphataemia
- Hypocalcaemia

Presentation

Typically, tumour lysis syndrome is precipitated by the onset of chemotherapy in patients with chemosensitive tumours, with a characteristic risk period lasting up to 3 days after onset of chemotherapy. It is also possible for TLS to occur spontaneously in tumours as a result of fulminant apoptosis. Symptoms occur less regularly than laboratory evidence of metabolic abnormalities, and include:

- Symptoms of the underlying malignancy
- Hyperkalaemia (see p. 394–395)
  - Cardiac arrhythmias
  - Muscle weakness
  - Paraesthesia
- Hypocalcaemia (see p. 400–402)
  - Anorexia
  - Confusion
  - Tetany
  - Carpopedal spasm
  - Cardiac arrest
- Hyperuricaemia
  - Renal colic
  - Lethargy
  - Nausea
  - Vomiting
- Hyperphosphataemia—this is usually asymptomatic
- The most concerning consequence of TLS is renal failure, which may present with weakness, fatigue, irritability, volume overload, drug toxicity, pericarditis

Immediate management

- Management is all corrective, starting with ABC (p. 2–5)
- Correct imbalances as per their individual guidelines (see above)
- Secondary prevention as detailed below

Prophylaxis with no metabolic derangement

- Good hydration as per fluid balance guidelines (see p. 6–8)
- Allopurinol in reducing dose
- Prophylactic sodium bicarbonate (consider starting then discontinuing if uric acid does not rise)

- 12–24 hourly U&Es, Ca^{2+}, uric acid and phosphate
- 4-hourly BP and urine output

  ⚠ Discuss transfer to HDU for CVP monitoring with seniors if there are any concerns over ability to manage fluid balance accurately.

Prophylaxis with pre-existing metabolic abnormalities
- Hydration; a thiazide diuretic may be used to ensure diuresis if confident of adequate input
- Allopurinol as above if normal renal function. Consider lower dose in renal failure. British Committee for Standards in Haematology guidelines currently recommend the use of allopurinol for reduction of uric acid; however, recent studies have shown that rasburicase may be superior for the prevention of hyperuricaemia-related complications. Ask your senior for advice regarding this
- Sodium bicarbonate to maintain urine pH >7.0
- Intravenous calcium and activated vitamin D if symptomatic hypocalcaemia
- Promptly treat hyperkalaemia.

Further management
- Close observations with particular attention to fluid balance
- Liaise with renal team—management may ultimately require haemodialysis

Investigations
- FBC—monitor WCC and platelet levels
- Coagulation screen—a coagulopathy may be associated with TLS; also consider DIC
- Serum magnesium—treat any coincidental hypomagnesaemia
- U&Es 12–24-hourly
- CRP to monitor any intercurrent infection

Causes
Prevention is, without doubt, much better than cure. Know your patients and be aware of those at risk of TLS. Patients at high risk of TLS include those with:
- Tumours with high growth rate or those very sensitive to chemotherapy
- Bulky abdominal disease
- Elevated pre-treatment uric acid levels
- Elevated LDH levels
- Prior poor urine output or renal impairment

Common causes
- NHLs (high grade)
- Lymphoma—acute lymphoblastic leukaemia (ALL), acute myeloblastic leukaemia (AML), acute promyelocytic leukaemia (APML), chronic lymphoblastic leukaemia (CLL) and chronic myelocytic leukaemia (CML; blast crisis)
- Breast cancer
- Testicular/germ cell
- Soft tissue sarcomas
- Small cell lung cancer
- Merkel cell carcinoma
- Neuroblastoma
- Medulloblastoma

Less common causes
- Corticosteroids
- Interferon
- Hyperthermia
- Radiotherapy
- Spontaneous

Further reading
- *OHCM*, 7th edn. Oxford: Oxford University Press, p. 514.
- British Committee for Standards in Haematology Guidelines in diagnosis and treatment and therapy: nodal non-Hodgkins lymphoma. 2005: www.bcshguidelines.com
- Lorrigan PC, Woodings PL, Morgenstern GR, Scarffe JH. Tumour lysis syndrome, case report and review of the literature. *Ann Oncol* 1996; **7**:631–6.

☠ SIRS and sepsis

Background

SIRS

A clinical response, provoked by a variety of physiological insults, both infective and non-infective. This definition was reached by consensus opinion, and includes clinical and laboratory findings, as detailed below.

Presence of two or more of:
- Temperature >38°C or <36°C
- Heart rate >90 beats/min
- Respiratory rate >20 breaths/min or $PaCO_2$ <4.3 kPa
- White cell count >12 × 10⁹/l or <4 × 10⁹/l or >10% immature forms

Non-infective causes of SIRS include pancreatitis, severe trauma, burns, hepatic failure and immunological disorders, amongst others.

SEPSIS

Sepsis is the systemic inflammatory response which results from infection (proven or suspected). Criteria for diagnosis are as for SIRS, with the addition of a proven or strongly suspected source of infection. Further subcategories exist:

- **Severe sepsis**: sepsis with evidence of resultant organ dysfunction, hypotension or hypoperfusion (e.g. oliguria, altered mentation, lactic acidosis)
- **Septic shock**: sepsis with hypotension despite adequate fluid resuscitation, plus evidence of hypoperfusion

Presentation

The mortality rate of septic shock remains high, despite advances in intensive care management. Although notoriously difficult to study with unbiased clinical trials, current evidence suggests that early recognition of the most unwell patients, with aggressive and meticulous supportive management, is the key to improving outcomes. To this end, many hospitals have introduced 'Early Warning Systems', which trigger urgent medical or critical care team review when a variety of 'scored' physiological variables deviate sufficiently from baseline 'normal' values. Presentation may, therefore, simply be a request to review a patient with deranged physiological parameters.

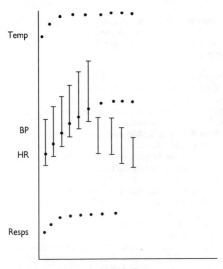

Fig. 8.1 Example observation chart showing SIRS with decompensation developing later

Immediate management

The initial management of this presentation hinges on thorough, systematic ABC approach, with good planning and awareness of potential pitfalls.

- Restore adequate tissue perfusion and thereby oxygenation with fluid, e.g. 500–1000 ml crystalloid or 250–500 ml colloid, repeated according to response
- Aim for urine output of ≥0.5 ml/kg/h
- Aim for blood pressure within normal range for patient or mean arterial pressure ≥65 mmHg
- Central venous pressure monitoring may help in assessing response to fluid, and requirement for further fluid boluses. Trend and response to fluid boluses is more important than absolute value, but a target of 8–12 mmHg is a reasonable starting point for many patients
- A central line also allows blood sampling for estimation of central venous oxygen saturation. $ScvO_2$ ≥70% may indicate adequate tissue perfusion with normal oxygen extraction; values below this level suggest supranormal oxygen extraction owing to impaired tissue blood flow (assuming arterial oxygen saturation is adequate)
- Serum lactate (often estimated by newer blood gas analysers) offers an indication of global tissue perfusion, but is non-specific.

❶ No or poor response to initial resuscitation is an indication for immediate referral to ITU. To resuscitate beyond this, central venous and arterial access is required, and vasopressor therapy likely. Do not allow administrative steps to delay this.

- Diagnosis
  - May be obvious from clinical history, but where due to infection, accurate identification of causative organisms is crucial
  - Send appropriate specimens, e.g. repeated blood cultures (including samples from longstanding vascular access devices), urine, sputum, CSF, pus, wound swabs
  - Ultrasound-guided drainage of collections may be useful, both diagnostically and therapeutically
  - If a discrete collection is identified, early consideration of surgical or radiologically-guided drainage should be made
- Antibiotic therapy
  - Where indicated, early administration (within first 3 h of admission or assessment) of appropriate antibiotic therapy should be a priority
  - Ideally, culture specimens should be obtained prior to administration of antibiotic
  - Choice of specific drug should be dictated by presumed source of infection and hence likely pathogens. Use local prescribing policies and seek advice from microbiologist.

Further management

Should be undertaken in an appropriate clinical environment. Transfer to a critical care unit should be organized early where indicated.

- Invasive monitoring (central venous if not in place already; arterial; invasive haemodynamic assessment if appropriate)
- Inotropic and vasopressor therapy guided by haemodynamic response
- Respiratory support with non-invasive or invasive ventilation where indicated, utilizing 'lung-protective' strategies
- Close control of blood glucose level (e.g. <8.3 mmol/l with sliding scale insulin has shown benefit in certain subgroups of ICU patients
- Consider low-dose 'physiological' steroid therapy
- Establish early enteral nutrition where possible
- Consider recombinant activated protein C (drotrecogin alfa) therapy
- DVT prophylaxis
- Renal replacement therapy where required
- Stress ulcer prophylaxis

Further reading

Dellinger *et al.* Surviving sepsis campaign guidelines for management of severe sepsis and septic shock. *Crit Care Med* 2004; **32(3)**:858–73.
🖳 http://www.survivingsepsis.org/documents/SSCGuidelines.pdf

Blood transfusion reactions

Definition

An immediate or delayed response to transfusion of blood products, infective or immunological in origin.

Presentation

- Bronchospasm
- Hypotension
- ↓SpO$_2$
- Angioedema
- Agitation, flushing
- Fever
- Pain at venepuncture site; abdominal/flank pain
- Oozing from puncture sites
- Urticarial rash
- Abdominal pain

Immediate management

- Stop transfusion immediately
- Inform transfusion department/haematologist and return intact blood pack with giving set to transfusion department
- Check patient identity and labelling of blood packs
- Keep IV access open with 0.9% saline infusion
- If suspected anaphylaxis, administer 0.5 mg adrenaline 1:1000 IM, chlorphenamine 10 mg slow IV and 200 mg hydrocortisone slow IV
- Monitor vital signs, including urine output (catheterize)
- Treat hypotension with rapid infusion of crystalloid (20–30 ml/kg)
- If persistent hypotension despite this, discuss with HDU/ICU—consider invasive haemodynamic monitoring, inotrope/vasopressor therapy
- Take blood samples for ABG, FBC, U+Es, coagulation studies, culture, repeat crossmatching, direct antiglobulin test, plasma haemoglobin (discuss with haematologist)
- If bacterial contamination is suspected from clinical condition, discuss with microbiologist and haematologist on call. Full cover of Gram and aerobic spectrum is essential.

Further management

- Maintain urine output of at least 1.5 ml/kg/h: consider furosemide/mannitol
- Watch for hyperkalaemia owing to acute renal failure and treat as necesssary
- If evidence of DIC, transfuse blood components as indicated (rematched blood does not carry an increased risk of a second haemolytic reaction)

- Discuss with senior whether re-transfusion for original indication is necessary—the original need for haemoglobin, although masked by this situation, is not cured!
- If TRALI is suspected, the transfusion department must be informed so that the donor of the implicated unit is removed from the donor panel
- Continual monitoring of respiratory function is essential in TRALI—if there is evidence of deterioration (e.g. from serial ABG), discuss with ITU on call—ventilation may be required

❶ Immediate reactions

1. Acute haemolytic reaction
- Most commonly due to ABO incompatibility, as a result of clerical errors
- Signs and symptoms can occur after as little as 5–10 ml blood transfused

2. Severe allergy/anaphylaxis
- Rare; may be associated with anti-IgA antibodies in an IgA-deficient patient
- If a patient is known to be IgA-deficient, seek expert advice before any transfusion

3. Transfusion-related acute lung injury (TRALI)
- Rapid onset of dyspnoea and non-productive cough
- Diffuse bilateral infiltrates on CXR
- Features identical to those of ARDS
- Due to donor plasma antibodies reacting to recipient leucocytes

4. Bacterial contamination
- Rapid onset hypotension and collapse
- Fever and rigors
- Otherwise, has a similar clinical picture to acute haemolytic reaction
- Bacterial contamination is rare but carries a high mortality rate

5. Circulatory overload
- Treat as for acute heart failure (p. 144–146)

6. Non-haemolytic febrile transfusion reaction
- Fever and shivering within 30–60 min of beginning transfusion
- Slow or stop transfusion
- Give paracetamol (1 g PO)
- Restart transfusion at controlled rate with close observations
- Reassurance to patient and nursing staff that this is not uncommon
- Recurrent problems may necessitate discussion with haematology—is leucodepleted or filtered blood indicated here?

Delayed reactions

1. Delayed haemolytic transfusion reaction

- Occurs in patients who have developed red cell antibodies as a result of previous exposure, either due to a previous blood transfusion or following pregnancy
- Haemoglobin does not rise as much as expected following transfusion, or falls more rapidly than expected
- Haemoglobinuria
- Elevated serum bilirubin 4–14 days post-transfusion
- Positive direct antiglobulin test
- The severity of presentation relates to the volume of blood transfused, but is rarely clinically significant

2. Transfusion-associated graft-vs.-host disease

- Rare complication, caused by T lymphocytes. Usually fatal
- Skin rashes
- Diarrhoea
- Altered liver function
- Bone marrow failure
- There is no effective treatment for the condition
- Those at risk of transfusion-associated graft-vs.-host disease include recipients of allogeneic bone marrow transplant, fetuses receiving intrauterine transfusion or an immunocompetent recipient of products from a near relative. Graft-vs.-host disease is prevented by gamma irradiation of cellular blood components prior to transfusion

Further reading

- *Handbook of Transfusion Medicine*, 3rd edn. London: **HMSO**, 2001.
- *OHCM*, 7th edn. Oxford: Oxford University Press, p. 571.

Neurology and neurosurgery

ⓘ **Stroke**

Definition

The acute loss of circulation to an area of the brain, resulting in ischaemia and loss of neurological function.

Presentation

Clinically it is very difficult to distinguish stroke due to infarction from that due to haemorrhage. Both present with a sudden onset focal neurological deficit and may additionally exhibit:

* Confusion
* Reduction in conscious level
* Seizures
* Coma

Patients with intracerebral haemorrhage often appear generally more unwell. More specifically, intracerebral haemorrhage may also include:

* Headache
* Neck stiffness
* Vomiting
* Dramatically reducing consciousness

Immediate management

* ABC, noting that supplemental oxygen is proven to be of no benefit in stroke unless hypoxaemia is demonstrated on ABG analysis
* ECG—arrhythmias, especially AF. If seen, a potential thrombotic cause of stroke has already been identified and the patient should therefore not be cardioverted (this risks further thromboembolic events)
* ABG—hypoxaemia. Is this due to aspiration?
* Bloods as detailed
* Urinalysis
* Detailed history and examination (explore risk factors detailed later, exclude mimicking conditions such as infections and establish co-morbidities, important for later management)
* Assess and classify deficit by Bamford classification (see later). This correlates well with subsequent neuro-imaging findings
* Unenhanced CT brain will exclude haemorrhage immediately. An infarct may not yet be evident, however, so this scan may only offer essentially binary information to exclude haemorrhage
* Notify a senior clinician, preferably involving a stroke unit. Rehabilitation starts at admission, with earlier appropriate management demonstrating better outcomes
* Swallow assessment is important and patients should be kept nil by mouth until they have been deemed safe. Any evidence of compromise from this, such as chest crackles on auscultation or reduced SpO_2, should be investigated by CXR and treated accordingly
* Treat any seizures as for seizures of any other aetiology

Further management

Ischaemic stroke

- Once proven, stat dose aspirin 300 mg
- Consider thrombolysis with TPA (alteplase). There are strict inclusion criteria (National Institute of Neurological Disorders and Stroke Protocol)
  - Age ≥18 years old
  - Clinical diagnosis of acute ischaemic stroke
  - Assessed by experienced team
  - Measurable neurological deficit
  - Well established time of symptom onset
  - CT/MRI and blood test results available
  - CT/MRI consistent with diagnosis
  - Treatment could begin within 3 h of symptom onset
- Exclusion by
  - Symptoms minor or rapidly improving
  - Haemorrhage on pre-treatment CT/MRI
  - Suspected SAH
  - Active bleeding from any site
  - GI or GU tract bleed in last 21 days
  - Platelet count <100 × 10^9/l
  - Recent treatment with heparin and raised APTR
  - Recent treatment with warfarin and INR raised
  - Major surgery or trauma within last 14 days
  - Recent post-MI pericarditis
  - Neurosurgery, serious head trauma or stroke in last 3 months
  - History of any intracranial haemorrhage
  - Known AV malformation or aneurysms
  - Recent arterial puncture at a non-compressible site
  - Recent lumbar puncture
  - BP consistently >185 systolic or >110 diastolic
  - Abnormal blood glucose (<3 mmol/l or >20 mmol/l)
  - Suspected or known pregnancy
  - Active pancreatitis
  - Epileptic seizure at stroke onset
- Admission to a stroke unit
- Carotid duplex if carotid artery stenosis/obstruction is suspected—possible need for carotid endarterectomy
- Echocardiogram if cardiogenic embolism is suspected—is anticoagulation needed?
- Regular antiplatelet therapy
- Management of hypertension, heart disease, DM, hyperlipidaemia and any other modifiable risk factors
- Speech therapy, dysphagia care, physiotherapy, occupational therapy
- Address specific neurological issues such as epilepsy, pain, incontinence

Haemorrhagic stroke
* Urgent neurosurgical opinion
* Evacuation of the haematoma may be necessary, especially if the patient is comatose or has signs of coning; the outcome is usually poor in this case
* Admission to ITU should be considered, dependent on neurosurgical opinion
* Rehabilitation principles are the same as in non-haemorrhagic stroke, remembering that antiplatelet therapies and anticoagulation are, of course, contraindicated

General
* If neurological symptoms last for less than 24 h, and after proper investigation are attributed to thrombosis or embolism, a diagnosis of transient ischaemic attack (TIA) is made. This may be a precursor to a full-blown stroke and is an ideal time to implement secondary prevention measures
* Treat risk factors such as cholesterol (aim for <3.5 mmol/l) and blood pressure (>140/85 for >2 weeks should be treated with combination of thiazide diuretic and ACE inhibitors, such as indapamide and perindopril)

Complications and sequelae
* Acute
  * Cerebral oedema
  * Raised intracranial pressure and herniation
  * Haemorrhagic transformation of ischaemic stroke (spontaneous or following thrombolysis)
  * Aspiration pneumonia
  * Seizures
* Within 72 h
  * Pneumonia
  * Thromboembolic
  * UTI
  * Pressure sores
  * Contractures
  * Spasticity
* Longer term—depression. Royal College of Physician guidelines recommend screening and early treatment for depression within 1 month of stroke, with good surveillance for mood alteration subsequently

Investigations
* FBC—thrombocytopenia?
* ESR—vasculitic disorders? (so risk of cerebral vascular pathology)
* U&Es—hypertension and renal damage?
* Coagulation—hypocoagulable state causing haemorrhage?
* Glucose—risk factor and plan secondary prevention
* Cholesterol—risk factor and plan secondary prevention
* CXR for aspiration
* CT head, MRI subsequently if inadequate information from CT

Causes
- Ischaemic stroke thrombosis or embolism (82%)
- Haemorrhagic stroke
  - PICH (15%)
  - Subarachnoid haemorrhage (3%)

Risk factors
- General
  - Increasing age
  - Hypertension
  - Diabetes mellitus
  - Positive family history
  - Hyperlipidaemia
  - Homocysteinaemia
- Lifestyle
  - Drug abuse
  - Smoking
  - Excess alcohol consumption
  - Oral contraceptive pill
  - Hormone replacement therapy
- Cerebral
  - Cerebrovascular disease
  - Berry aneurysm
  - Cerebral AV malformation
- Cardiac
  - Atrial fibrillation
  - Myocardial infarction
  - Left ventricular aneurysm
  - Ischaemic heart disease
  - Cyanotic heart disease
  - Patent foramen ovale
  - Endocarditis
- Peripheral vascular
  - Carotid stenosis
  - Ehlers–Danlos
  - Carotid dissection
  - Vasculitis
- Haematological
  - Hypercoagulable states
  - Polycythaemia
  - Sickle cell disease
  - Warfarin (haemorrhage)
  - Thrombolysis

Further reading
- *OHCM*, 7th edn. Oxford: Oxford University Press, p. 462.
- *Oxford Handbook of Neurology*, Oxford: Oxford University Press, p. 104.
- Bamford J et al. Classification and natural history of clinically identifiable subtypes of cerebral infarction. *Lancet* 1991; **337**:1521–6.

- Becker JU, Wira CR, Arnold JL. emedicine: Stroke, ischemic. Online: http://www.emedicine.com/EMERG/topic558.htm. 5 September 2006.
- Clarke CRA. Neurological disease. In: Kumar P, Clark M(eds). *Clinical Medicine*, 6th edn. London: Elsevier Saunders, 2005:1173–1271.
- Jaunch EC, Kissela B, Stettler BA. emedicine: acute stroke management. Online: http://www.emedicine.com/neuro/topic9.htm. 5 October 2005.
- Nassisi D. emedicine: Stroke, hemorrhagic. Online: http://www.emedicine.com/EMERG/topic557.htm. 18 November 2005.
- Neurological emergencies. In: Ramrakha P, Moore K(eds). *Oxford Handbook of Acute Medicine*, 2nd edn. New York: Oxford University Press, 2004:405–532.
- van Gijn J. Stroke: cerebrovascular disease. In: Warrell DA, Cox TM, Firth JD, Benz EJ (eds). *Oxford Textbook of Medicine*, 4th edn, vol. 3. New York: Oxford University Press. 2003; 1022–34.

☠ Subarachnoid haemorrhage

Subarachnoid haemorrhage (SAH) is arterial bleeding into the subarachnoid space and accounts for 3–5% of all strokes, with an annual incidence of around 6 per 100 000. Although technically a subclass of stroke, its high mortality rates, wide age range of patients and clinically distinct presentation merits individual discussion.

Presentation

- Key feature: sudden, severe 'thunderclap' headache that is maximal immediately or in first few minutes, and lasts for more than 1 h
- Meningism—nausea and vomiting, photophobia, neck stiffness
- Loss of consciousness, either transient or persistent, is present in around 50% of cases
- Seizures occur in around 6% of cases
- Focal neurology such as dysphasia, hemisensory or motor symptoms

Immediate management

- ABC as per p. 2–5
- Bloods as detailed (see Investigations)
- Diagnosis cannot be made from clinical picture alone—unenhanced CT brain is required
  - 95% sensitivity at 24 h from onset of pain
  - Reduces to 50% sensitivity at 3 days
- CXR—pulmonary oedema, aspiration
- 12-lead ECG
- Grade on World Federation of Neurological Surgeons (WFNS) scale

WFNS	Glasgow Coma Scale (sum score)
I	15
II	14 or 13 without focal deficit*
III	14 or 13 with focal deficit
IV	12–7
V	6–3

* Cranial nerve palsies are not considered a focal deficit.

- Discuss with senior clinician and neurosurgeons
- Airway management and sedation decisions need to be made. Involve on-call anaesthetist now, allowing time for ITU logistics to be addressed if admission likely to be required. In general, a patient with GCS <8 will require endotracheal intubation and sedation

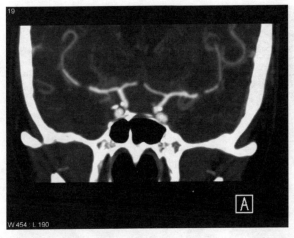

Fig. 9.1 CT cranial angiogram showing SAH

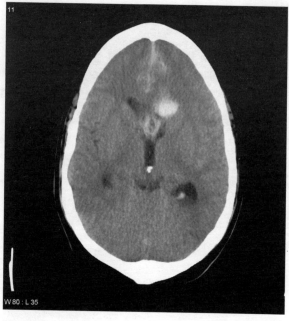

Fig. 9.2 CT brain showing SAH and associated features of raised ICP

Further management

- Lumbar puncture if CT is negative
  - Needs to be >6 h and preferably >12 h after onset of symptoms
  - Examine CSF for pressure, protein, cells, glucose, xanthochromia
  - Bacterial meningitis may clinically mimic SAH, so C&S CSF should also be requested
- Cerebral angiography is required in CT-positive patients, allowing identification of the source and an operative plan to be formed. Some CT-positive bleeds may still have negative angiography due to thrombosis or spasm; repeat angiography may need to be performed before further intervention is planned
- A major complication is cerebral vasospasm (>50% of patients), usually controlled by oral nimodipine (60 mg/4 h). When discussing a scan-positive patient with neurosurgeons, specifically check if this should be prescribed (if interhospital transfer is planned, significant delay to therapy may ensue if not initiated by diagnosing clinician)
- Radial artery cannulation offers invasive beat-on-beat monitoring and a portal for serial ABG sampling. Lowering pCO_2 is a further means by which vasospasm can be reduced, achievable by adjusting ventilation parameters in ITU
- Blood pressure should be maintained, and hypertension left untreated unless persisting >220 mmHg systolic. This is of further benefit in reducing vasospasm
- Surgical treatment may be either open by craniotomy or endovascular with platinum coils. Choice is largely by location and therefore ease of surgical approach; posterior fossa bleeds are particularly suited to endovascular access
  - A body of debate exists over whether evacuation of haematoma at the time of initial surgery is optimum management. Evacuation of clot is associated with reduced vasospasm; cases have been reported, however, of the mechanical trauma of excessive evacuation causing significant swelling and even intracerebral haemorrhage
- Vigilance is required for rebleeding (30% probability with 40% mortality rate) by close neurological observations. of those surviving 1 month, 90% will be alive at 1 year

Investigations

- FBC
- U&Es
- Coagulation
- Glucose
- Magnesium—hypomagnesaemia is a common finding and is associated with poor outcome)
- CXR for aspiration or associated injuries in traumatic causes
- CT brain without contrast
- Angiography—MR/CT angiography is yet to demonstrate equal quality of imaging due to resolution

Causes
- Spontaneous
  - Berry aneurysm in patients over 40 years
  - Arteriovenous malformations (AVMs) in those under 40 years
- Trauma

Further reading
- *OHCM*, 7th edn. Oxford: Oxford University Press, p. 470.
- *Oxford Handbook of Neurology*, 1st edn. Oxford: Oxford University Press, p. 316.

☺ **Extradural haematoma**

Definition

Accumulation of blood in the extradural space, often following tearing of a meningeal artery; or rarely, from a dural venous sinus.

Presentation

- Characteristic picture is head injury and short period of unconsciousness, followed by a period of regained consciousness (lucid interval). Subsequent reduction in GCS is seen
- Headache
- Vomiting
- Seizures
- In severe cases
  - Progressive hemiparesis and stupor
  - Rapid transtentorial coning with ipsilateral dilated pupil
  - Progression to bilateral fixed and dilated pupils
  - Tetraplegia
  - Respiratory arrest

Immediate management

- ABC as per p. 2–5, bearing in mind all other possible injuries from the mechanism
- Treat seizures
- Early decisions about airway and sedation are required. Anaesthetic on-call staff should be contacted if any impairment in GCS is seen; mild impairment may evolve, leading to airway compromise
- Bloods as detailed (see Investigations)
- Inform senior clinician
- Urgent CT head
- Contact neurosurgical team whilst scan in progress if good clinical history of EDH
- Ensure neuro obs documented at least every 15 min
- Check local policy on mannitol for raised ICP

Further management

- Early surgical evacuation of haematoma is linked to good outcome
  - Burr holes for haematoma evacuation are indicated if access to neurosurgery is unavailable or delayed
  - Site of drainage over the pterion, natural weak point
- Preoperative resuscitation should be addressed in transit
- Recovery is dependent on preoperative GCS
  - GCS >8 90–100% recovery
  - GCS <8 30% mortality, 50–60% good outcome

Causes

- Most common is tearing of a meningeal artery, usually the middle or one of its branches
- More rarely:
  - Tearing of a dural venous sinus
  - Intracranial infection
  - Anticoagulant therapy

Investigations

- FBC, U&Es, coagulation for preoperative assessment
- CT head
  - Biconvex lesion (bleeding constrained by skull and dura)
  - Careful review of whole scan—50% of EDHs are associated with other injuries, e.g. contrecoup, SDH, etc
  - Timing—20% will still be evolving at 36 h post-injury

Further reading

- *OHCM*, 7th edn. Oxford: Oxford University Press, p. 474.
- *Oxford Handbook of Neurology*, 1st edn. Oxford: Oxford University Press, p. 380.
- Clarke CRA. Neurological disease. In: Kumar P, Clark M(eds). *Clinical Medicine*, 6th edn. London: Elsevier Saunders, 2005:1173–271.
- Neurological emergencies. In: Ramrakha P, Moore K(eds). *Oxford Handbook of Acute Medicine*, 2nd edn. New York: Oxford University Press, 2004:405–532.
- Price DD, Wilson SR. emedicine: Epidural Hematoma. Online: http://emedicine.com/EMERG/topic167.htm. 8 March 2006.

⚙ Subdural haematoma

Definition

A subdural haematoma (SDH) is an accumulation of blood in the subdural space following rupture of a vein or artery in contused brain matter.

Presentation

Acute SDH usually follows head injuries and can present very similarly to EDH, with presentation up to several days following head injury. Chronic SDH is usually preceded by head injury, but this is often very slight and patients are therefore unable to recall it. Onset may be several weeks following head injury.

A high index of suspicion is required in patients who have a tendency to fall, e.g. alcoholics.

Acute and chronic SDH can present as:
- Head injury ± skull fracture
- Headache
- Vomiting
- Drowsiness
- Confusion
- Focal neurological deficit
- Seizures
- Papilloedema

Immediate management

- ABC as per p. 2–5. The mechanism must also be considered when considering primary survey and management—trauma sufficient to cause acute subdural haematoma (ASDH) also risks C-spine damage. Ensure head injury does not distract from any other injury by thorough survey
- Bloods as detailed
- Seizure termination as detailed previously
- CT head, urgency dictated by timeframe of symptoms. Suspected ASDH must be investigated as a matter of priority
- Close neurological observation, ensuring documentation of serial GCS and pupil status
- ASDH must be referred to neurosurgical on-call team, as definitive management is craniotomy and evacuation
- Mannitol is often advocated—this should be discussed with either the neurosurgical team or the anaesthetist who will be dealing with the patient

Further management

- Transfer to neurological centre if intervention required
- Dexamethasone is often prescribed in chronic cases (4 mg QDS)— discuss with senior before commencing

- SDH has a tendency to resolve spontaneously. More severe cases, such as those resulting in hydrocephalus, may still benefit from burr holes, sometimes with drainage left in situ
- An acute SDH may turn into a chronic SDH
- Complications of chronic SDH include:
  - Recurrent haematomas
  - Infection (subdural empyema)
  - Seizures

Causes

- Head injury
- Old age—bridging veins stretched by cortical atrophy
- Chronic alcohol abuse
- Anticoagulant therapy

Further reading

- *OHCM*, 7th edn. Oxford: Oxford University Press, p. 474.
- *Oxford Handbook of Neurology*, 1st edn. Oxford: Oxford University Press, p. 381.
- Clarke CRA. Neurological disease. In: Kumar P, Clark M(eds). *Clinical Medicine*, 6th edn. London: Elsevier Saunders, 2005:1173–271.
- Meagher RJ, Young WF. emedicine: Subdural hematoma. Online: http://emedicine.com/NEURO/topic575.htm. 2 November 2006.
- Neurological emergencies. In: Ramrakha P, Moore K(eds). *Oxford Handbook of Acute Medicine*, 2nd edn. New York: Oxford University Press, 2004:405–532.
- Scaletta T. emedicine: Subdural hematoma. Online: http://medscape.com/files/emedicine/topic560.htm. 11 May 2006.

:☹: **Meningitis**

Definition

Acute inflammation of the meninges, usually from an infective cause. Bacterial meningitis can kill very quickly, but early recognition and treatment will give your patient the best outcome.

Presentation

- Meningism
  - Headache
  - Neck stiffness
  - Photophobia
  - Kernig's sign (extension of the knee with the hip flexed causes hamstring spasm)
  - Brudzinski's sign (passive flexion of the neck causes flexion at the hips)
- Raised intracranial pressure (↑ICP)
  - Nausea/vomiting
  - Confusion/irritability
  - Papilloedema
  - ↓GCS
  - ↓HR and ↑BP (late sign)
- Sepsis
  - Pyrexia
  - Hypoperfusion (↑HR, ↑CRT, ↓BP)
  - A non-blanching petechial or purperic rash indicates meningococcal septicaemia (this can occur without meningitis as well)

Immediate management

- ABC assessment
  - Patient is likely to require airway support if GCS <8
  - Give high flow O_2 via a non-rebreath mask
  - If patient has septic shock, they are likely to require fluid resuscitation (see p. 6–8, 304–306)
  - Consider early referral to ITU if patient is unstable
- If patient has signs of septic shock or ↑ICP, give IV antibiotics immediately
  - e.g. Cefotaxime, 2 g IV QDS
  - *and* Ampicillin 2 g IV QDS (if patient is over 55 years old)
- Give steroids with or after first dose of antibiotics
  - e.g. Dexamethasone 10 mg IV QDS (for 4 days)
- If there is evidence of ↑ICP
  - Patient should be managed in ITU/HDU
  - Keep head elevated
  - Be cautious with fluid resuscitation
  - There should be a low threshold of intubation/ventilation
  - Consider mannitol 20% solution 1 g/kg IV, if severely compromised

Investigations

- FBC and CRP
  - Will often show ↑WCC and ↑CRP
  - ↓Platelets may indicate the development of DIC
  - Sepsis can develop rapidly, so inflammatory markers may be normal initially
- Coagulation screen
  - Coagulopathy may indicate DIC
- U&Es
  - ↓Na$^+$ can be caused by SIADH
  - Sepsis can precipitate acute renal failure (↑urea and ↑creatinine)
- LFTs
  - Elevated liver enzymes may indicate organ disturbance due to sepsis
- Blood cultures
  - Preferably before antibiotics are administered
  - Can reveal causative organism
- Nasopharyngeal swabs
  - Check for nasal carriage of likely organisms
- Serum meningococcal PCR
  - Can identify *Neisseria meningitides,* especially if antibiotics are administered prior to LP
- CT head
  - Indicated if there is ↑ICP, to exclude mass lesions and hydrocephalus, prior to LP
  - NB. It cannot exclude ↑ICP
  - CT can also be useful if symptoms have not diminished with adequate doses of IV antibiotics, as it can reveal collections/abscesses
- LP
  - Is diagnostic of meningitis, and can often identify causative organism
  - Is contraindicated if the patient is severely unwell, has ↑ICP or has a coagulopathy
  - Collect three samples (three plain tubes and one fluoride oxalate sample)
  - Send first (or most bloody) plain sample for C&S
  - Send second plain sample for protein level
  - Send third (or least bloody) plain sample for Gram stain, microscopy and cell count
  - Send fluoride oxalate sample for glucose level
  - If suspicious of viral meningitis or encephalitis, a further sample can be sent for PCR
  - Take a blood glucose sample at the same time, for comparison of blood/CSF glucose levels

Table 9.1

	Normal	Bacterial meningitis	Viral meningitis	TB meningitis
Appearance	Clear	Cloudy	Normal	Cloudy/normal
Pressure	5–18cmH$_2$O	Normal/raised	Normal	Normal/raised
WCC	0–4 mm^{-3}	1000–5000 (polymorphs)	10–2000 (lymphocytes)	50–5000 (lymphocytes)
Microbiology	Sterile	Organisms (may not be present if partially treated)	Viruses may be detected by PCR	TB may be detected by ZN stain or TB culture
Protein	<0.45 g/l	Raised	Normal/raised	Raised
Glucose	>60% blood glucose level	Low	Normal	Low

Further management

- Following identification of a causative organism, the antibiotic regimen should be altered accordingly
  - This is best done in consultation with your local microbiology team
- Inform the Health Protection Agency (HPA)
  - Both meningitis and meningococcal sepsis are notifiable diseases
  - Contact tracing and prophylactic antibiotic treatment of exposed people is often required
- Arrange hearing tests after discharge, to identify any sensorineural deafness which may have developed
- Following recovery, ensure that the patient has received the meningococcal C vaccine

Complications

- Cerebral oedema
- Cranial nerve deficits (particularly VI, III, VII, VIII and II)
- Central venous sinus thrombosis
- Intracranial collection

Causes

- Bacterial
  - *Neisseria meningitides*
  - *Streptococcus pneumoniae*
  - *Listeria monocytogenes*
  - *TB*
  - *Staphylococcus aureus* (following trauma)
  - *Haemophilus influenzae*
- Viral
  - Enteroviruses (echovirus, Coxsackie, polio)
  - Mumps
  - Influenza

- Herpes simplex
- Varicella zoster
- EBV
- HIV
- Other infectious causes
  - *Cryptococcus neoformans*
  - *Candida*
  - *Histoplasma*
  - *Toxoplasma*
  - Amoeba
- Non-infective causes
  - Malignant disease (usually metastatic)
  - Sarcoidosis
  - SLE
  - Behçet's disease
  - Mollaret's meningitis

Further reading

- *OHCM*, 7th edn. Oxford: Oxford University Press, p. 806.
- *Oxford Handbook of Neurology*, 1st edn. Oxford: Oxford University Press, p. 288.
- *Oxford Textbook of Medicine*, 4th edn, Section 24.14.1. vol. 3. Oxford: Oxford University Press, p. 1115–29.
- Early management of suspected bacterial meningitis and meningococcal septicaemia in immunocompetent adults (2nd edn). Meningitis research foundation (www.meningitis.org).

☼ Encephalitis

Definition

Inflammation of the brain parenchyma resulting in impairment of cerebral function, usually of viral origin. Untreated, mortality is in the region of 70%.

Presentation

- Headache
- Vomiting
- Fever
- Altered conscious level
- Convulsions
- Focal neurological signs
- Psychiatric/behavioural symptoms

Patients with viral encephalitis may have undergone a prodrome lasting several hours or days, including fever, lethargy, myalgias and meningism.

Immediate management

- ABC as per p. 2–5
- A senior clinician from the on-call medical or neurology team should be contacted
- Bloods as detailed, ensuring cultures are taken before any antibiotic administration
- If meningitis is suspected, start antibiotic therapy. In practical terms, prior to LP and CT the two are harder to distinguish and it is prudent to cover both meningitis and encephalitis initially
- Aciclovir is associated with a decrease in mortality rate (to around 20%) and morbidity in encephalitis; given that viruses are the most common causative pathogen, aciclovir is given empirically. 10 mg/kg should be infused over 60 min every 8 h
- Seizure termination as with seizures of any other aetiology
  - Lorazepam, up to 4 mg as a slow bolus into a large vein
  - Phenytoin infusion 18 mg/kg at a rate of 50 mg/min
- Treat fevers with antipyretics

Further management

- CT scan is urgent in patients with focal neurological symptoms. There may be areas of low attenuation surrounded by cerebral oedema, particularly in the temporal lobes in patients with HSV encephalitis. MRI scan is more sensitive to these changes
- If ICP is raised secondary to cerebral oedema then dexamethasone or mannitol should be considered. The use of dexamethasone should be discussed with a senior clinician as there is some evidence that steroids may cause spread of herpes virus
- Lumbar puncture
  - CSF pressure may be raised, especially in HSV—monitor patient closely
  - CSF analysis: lymphocytes predominate, red cell count is usually raised, protein is increased (↑proportion IgG) and glucose is normal. CSF may be normal
  - Serology for viral titres (IgM and IgG) and specific viral tests
- EEG, even if patient is not having seizures. In HSV there may be periodic high-voltage slow wave complexes over the temporal cortex
- Screen for mimicking conditions, such as diffuse encephalopathy resulting from liver failure, drug toxicity, etc.

Causes

Britain has a different pattern of causation from central Europe and North America.

- Viral
  - Mumps
  - Echoviruses
  - Coxsackie viruses
  - Measles
  - Herpes zoster and simplex
  - Epstein–Barr viruses
  - Adenoviruses
- Non-viral
  - *Mycobacterium tuberculosis*
  - *Mycoplasm pneumoniae*
  - *Legionella*
  - *Brucella*
  - Toxoplasmosis
  - Schistosomiasis
  - Cryptococcus
  - Aspergillosis
  - Candidiasis
- Tick-borne encephalitis (TBEs)
  - Louping ill is the only TBE native to Britain
  - Central Europe, the Far East, Russia and North America are all travel destinations with their own associated TBEs, hence travel history is important

- Acute disseminated encephalomyelitis (ADEM)—a post-viral condition that may follow one of many viral infections, rarely also following immunization against rabies, influenza or pertussis. Similar to acute viral encephalitis, characterized by focal lesions in brainstem and/or spinal cord due to demyelination

Further reading

- *OHCM*, 7th edn. Oxford: Oxford University Press, p. 807.
- *Oxford Handbook of Neurology*, 1st edn. Oxford: Oxford University Press, p. 292.
- Clarke CRA. Neurological disease. In: Kumar P, Clark M(eds). *Clinical Medicine*, 6th Edn. London: Elsevier Saunders, 2005;1173–271.
- Kennedy PG. Viral encephalitis. *J Neurol* 2005; **255(3)**:268–72.
- Neurological emergencies. In: Ramrakha P, Moore K(eds). *Oxford Handbook of Acute Medicine*, 2nd edn. New York: Oxford University Press, 2004;405–532.
- Tyler KL. Update on Herpes simplex encephalitis. *Rev Neurolog Dis* 2004; **1(4)**:169–78.
- Warrell DA, Farrar JJ. Viral infections in the central nervous system. In: Warrell DA, Cox TM, Firth JD, Benz EJ(eds). *Oxford Textbook of Medicine*, 4th edn, vol. 3. New York: Oxford University Press, 2003; 1129–40.

! **Spinal epidural abscess**

Definition

Infection of the epidural space.

Presentation

- Severe back pain, usually localisable
  - 50% Thoracic
  - Lumbar
  - Cervical least frequent
- Fever
- Systemically unwell
- Concurrent meningism (13%)
- If history is longer, may already have developed:
  - More specific radicular pain
  - Focal sensorimotor deficit at the infected level

Immediate management

- ABC (p. 2–5), remembering that this infection often carries a severe septic burden (see also sepsis, p. 304–306)
- Bloods as detailed, ensuring minimum two sets of cultures taken before antibiotic administration (S. aureus most common pathogen)
- Full neurological examination
- Plain X-rays unlikely to offer any information unless infection is of contiguous spread from osteomyelitis
- Any clinical history with supporting examination should be discussed with neurosurgery on-call at this stage; gold standard imaging is MRI with gadolinium, generally only available to neurosciences clinicians
- Establish from neurosurgeons and microbiologist what initial antibiotics should be prescribed (note that the selection has to be highly mobile across the blood–brain barrier)

Further management

- This is a surgical emergency, the definitive management of which is decompression and debridement of the abscess (via laminectomy or discectomy dependent on position of lesion)
- Antibiotics are indicated for several weeks after surgery, ideally with daily microbiology review
- Significant compromise from sepsis may indicate ITU admission for invasive monitoring and aggressive fluid control
- Mortality rate stands at <20%, with highly variable recovery from neurological deficits. Prognostic factors include speed of onset, degree of paralysis and persistence beyond 36 h
- Liaison with nursing staff over wound care, mobility and rehabilitation is important. The immobility induced by the condition and communicating wound site make bedsores a serious risk
- Immobility also indicates anticoagulation, to be discussed with seniors and neurosurgical team

Investigations
- FBC, CRP and ESR for leucocytosis and inflammatory markers
- U&Es, G&S and coagulation for surgery
- ABG if systemically unwell from infection
- MRI with gadolinium, to be arranged by neurosurgical team
- CT brain if concurrent meningism

Causes
- Haematogenous—cases have been described of abscess resulting from endocarditis and dental infection
- Contiguous—such as from vertebral osteomyelitis. Usually anterior when vertebral source
- Direct—from surgery or epidural anaesthesia site

Further reading
- Reihsaus E, Waldbaur H, Seeling W. Spinal epidural abscess: a meta-analysis of 915 patients. *Neurosurg Rev.* 2000 **23(4)**:175–205.

① **Central venous sinus thrombosis**

Definition

Thrombosis of one of the major sinuses in the brain, most commonly the superior sagittal sinus (72%).

Presentation

Evolution tends to be over days to weeks. Typically, three groups of presentations are seen:
- Focal neurological deficit and headache (up to 75%)
- Seizures and residual (Todd's) paresis (30–50%)
- Headache, papilloedema and visual disturbances, mimicking benign intracranial hypertension (18–38%)

Immediate management

- ABC (p. 2–5), bearing in mind the potential airway compromise in the patient with seizures
- Bloods as detailed
- Seizure termination
- Initiate fluid balance now if patient systemically unwell
- ABG if unwell
- CT head offers distinction between CVST and ICH, abscess or other structural lesion. Magnetic resonance venography (MRV), however, is the gold standard imaging for this condition
- LP offers no diagnostic value in CVST, but is an important means of exclusion of SAH and meningitis
- Any septic primary cause should be treated early, in liaison with medical microbiology. Severe sepsis should be discussed with ITU for appropriate goal-directed therapy
- There is a weight of evidence towards the heparinisation of CVST patients, even those with preceding bleeds. This step must, however, be discussed with the neurosurgical team

Further management

- Deterioration after heparinisation or poor clinical condition at presentation are indications for catheter-guided local thrombolysis where available. Discuss with local neurosurgery team or interventional radiologist
- Ensure underlying primary cause is addressed, as this has a direct effect on morbidity, especially when there is sepsis or malignancy
- Oral anticoagulation should be maintained for 3–6 months

Investigations
- FBC, U&Es, CRP for septic causes (8%)
- Coagulation both for cause of thrombosis and impact of any ongoing sepsis
- ABG if systemically unwell
- CXR if hypoxic
- CT brain MRV
- LP to exclude other causes

Causes
- Infective
  - Open head injury
  - Intracranial infection
  - Systemic infection and sepsis
- Head injury
- Surgery (local from neurosurgery, disseminated from immobility)
- Stroke and haemorrhage
- Intracranial masses
- Malignancies, paraneoplastic syndromes and endocrine
- Haematological
  - RBC disorders
  - Thrombocythaemia
  - Disordered coagulation
- Autoimmune and inflammatory (IBD, sarcoidosis, etc.)

Further reading
- *OHCM*, 7th edn. Oxford: Oxford University Press, p. 472.
- *Oxford Handbook of Neurology*, 1st edn. Oxford: Oxford University Press, p. 487.

:O: Status epilepticus

Definition

Seizures lasting >30 min or repeated seizures without improved consciousness between. Seizures may be generalized tonic–clonic or more subtle absence with constant tics.

Immediate management

- ABC, being wary of teeth in any attempted airway manoeuvres
- Cannulation should be of biggest veins accessible, i.e. antecubital fossa
- Bloods as detailed
- Lorazepam 4 mg IV or diazepam 10 mg IV (or PR if no IV access available)
- ABG—prolonged seizures result in marked acidosis
- BM—treat hypoglycaemia see p. 226–228
- Pabrinex if background alcohol abuse or malnutrition
- Repeat lorazepam or diazepam within 10 min if still fitting
- Give normal antiepileptic medication

Further management

- If second dose fails, call anaesthetist
- Antiepileptic infusion; one of below with cardiac monitoring
  - Fosphenytoin 18 mg/kg phenytoin equivalents (PE) up to 150 mg/min
  - Phenytoin 18 mg/kg up to 50 mg/min
  - Phenobarbital 10 mg/kg up to 100 mg/min
- Failure to terminate at this point is an indication for sedation and ITU admission

Investigations

- FBC, CRP for infection
- CXR if? aspiration
- Pregnancy test in women of child-bearing potential—eclampsia most likely cause of fits
- CT head if index presentation, for structural causes (see later)
- Urinalysis for UTI or hypertensive renal damage

Causes

- Mass lesion, present in >50% of patients presenting with status epilepticus as first seizure
- Eclampsia
- Hypertensive encephalopathy
- Infection
- Head injury
- Inadequate medication of known epilepsy
- Alcohol

Further reading

- *OHCM*, 7th edn. Oxford: Oxford University Press, p. 808.
- *Oxford Handbook of Neurology*, 1st edn. Oxford: Oxford University Press, p. 146.

Orthopaedics, rheumatology and dermatology

⚠ **Compartment syndrome**

Definition

The compromise of circulation and function of tissues within a closed musculoskeletal compartment. This occurs when an abnormally increased intracompartmental pressure rises above capillary perfusion pressure.

Presentation

Essentially a clinical diagnosis, compartment syndrome is suggested by:
- Pain
  - Out of all proportion to the associated injury
  - On passive stretching of involved compartment
  - On palpation of soft tissues of involved compartment
- Sensory deficit of any nerve traversing involved compartment
  - Dependent on location
  - May present as paraesthesia or numbness

⚠ Do not rely on peripheral pulses. Compromise in distal pulse pressure is a very late and unreliable sign, and worsening compartment syndrome may be seen with palpable pulses.

Immediate management

- ABC, paying particular attention to peripheral circulation. Request hourly observations from nursing staff
- Establish IV access and take bloods
  - FBC—is the bleeding secondary to haematological abnormality or postoperative blood loss?
  - Renal function—a baseline is important to assess for renal effects of rhabdomyolysis
  - LFTs/clotting profile—is there a coagulopathic bleed in the compartment?
  - G&S
- History and examination
  - Recent operations?
  - Has the patient got dressings on?
  - Has the patient got a cast on?
  - Has there been an injury in that location?
  - Could the patient have received iatrogenic intra-arterial drugs?
  - Has the patient undergone recent vigorous exercise?
- Send off a urine sample to the laboratory for analysis of muscle breakdown products
- Make nil by mouth, communicating this to patients, relatives and staff
- Administer analgesia with antiemetic as required

Further management

- Prompt senior review—delayed fasciotomy is associated with worse outcomes
- Review imaging. If no X-rays already available (unlikely in the trauma context), ensure limb is X-rayed
- Control limb pressure pending surgery
  - Aim for normotension
  - Gentle elevation, aiming to keep limb at level of heart
  - Split cast or take down constricting dressings
- Pay close attention to ongoing good fluid and pain management pre-operatively

Causes

The syndrome involves a downward spiral of decreasing tissue perfusion, leading to increased ischaemia and resultant altered vascular permeability, further compromising perfusion. Early action prevents catastrophic complications.

In order for compartment syndrome to occur there must be an insult to the bone or soft tissues that results in an increase in pressure within a defined fascial compartment. This must be enclosed by a resisting envelope such as deep fascia, skin, casts and dressings. Such insults may be due to:

- Decrease in compartment size
  - Seen as localized external pressure
  - Plaster cast, tight dressings, inadvertent compression during positioning in theatre
- Increase in intracompartmental contents
  - Bleeding
  - Increased capillary permeability—post-ischaemia swelling, post-exercise muscle swelling, trauma and burns
  - Increased capillary pressure—following exercise, muscle hypertrophy and venous obstruction

Further reading

- Finkelstein JA, Hunter GA, Hu RW. Lower limb compartment syndrome: course after delayed fasciotomy. *J Trauma* 1996; **40(3)**:342–44.
- Garfin SR, Tipton CM, Mubarak SJ, Woo SL, Hargens AR, Akeson WH. Role of fascia in maintenance of muscle tension and pressure. *J Appl Physiol* 1981; **51(2)**:317–20.
- Hargens AR, Schmidt DA, Evans KL et al. Quantitation of skeletal-muscle necrosis in a model compartment syndrome. *J Bone Joint Surg Am.* 1981; **63(4)**:631–6.
- Koval KJ, Zuckerman JD. *Handbook of Fractures*, 2nd edn. Philadelphia Lippincott Williams & Wilkins, 2002.
- Mars M, Hadley GP. Raised intracompartmental pressure and compartment syndromes. *Injury* 1998; **29(6)**:403–11.
- Miller MD. *Review of Orthopaedics*, 4th edn. Philadelphia: Saunders, 2004.

- Whitesides TE, Haney TC, Morimoto K, Harada H. Tissue pressure measurements as a determinant for the need of fasciotomy. *Clin Orthop Relat Res* 1975; **113**:43–51.
- Willis RB, Rorabeck CH. Treatment of compartment syndrome in children. *Orthop Clin North Am* 1990; **21(2)**:401–12.

! Septic arthritis

Definition

An inflammatory process within a joint, characterised by effusion, pain and decreased movement, as a result of the presence of an infective pathogen. Its potential for joint surface destruction means that rapid diagnosis and treatment is absolutely essential.

Presentation

Septic arthritis may present at all ages from neonate to the elderly, with features and causative organisms more specific to each group.

Children
- Limping
- Loss of appetite
- Generalized irritability
- Fever
- Limb held in fixed position (particularly the leg in flexion, abduction and external rotation—the obturator sign)
- Crying when limb is moved (such as when changing nappies)
- Intercurrent ear or local soft tissue infection

Adults
- Recent onset joint (commonly knee) pain
- Fever
- Associated inability to bear weight through or move the joint

There is much debate as to the reliability of symptom profiling and diagnostic tools in this condition. Overall, the following should raise a strong degree of suspicion:

- History of fever
- Non-weightbearing
- ESR higher than 40 mm/h
- WBC count higher than 12×10^9/l

Immediate management

- Establish intravenous access and request blood tests as detailed
- Note all observations and ask nursing staff to repeat these hourly
- Thorough systemic assessment—the source of sepsis is as important as the joint in management of this condition
- Urinalysis
  - Ward test for rapid exclusion of urinary source
  - CSU and microscopy
- Good analgesia is essential (see p. 10–11)
- Make the patient nil by mouth, communicating this to staff, the patient and the relatives
- Discuss with senior
- Early joint aspiration is important, but must be discussed with senior owing to potential for further complications
- Take blood cultures
- Antibiotics may now be considered—discuss with senior, input from medical microbiology also likely to be required

History

Points to consider within the context of age and activity are:

- Birth and developmental
  - Immunisations
  - Achievement of developmental milestones
  - Nutritional history
- Previous musculoskeletal or dermatological concerns— developmental problems, previous surgery, old open fractures or injuries
- Previous joint replacement surgery
- Concurrent coryzal or gastrointestinal illness, recent upper respiratory symptoms
- Mobility prior to discomfort
- Sexual history
- Foreign travel
- Intravenous drug use
- Genitourinary symptoms
- Recent trauma

Examination

* Joint
  * Effusion
  * Erythema and warmth
  * ↓ Range of motion actively and passively
* Systemic
  * Lymphadenopathy
  * Rashes
  * Inspect distant joints
  * Otoscopy

Further management

* If currently under medical care, patient to be discussed with orthopaedic on-call team
* A septic joint needs to be washed out or extensively aspirated, followed by close orthopaedic surveillance
* Further imaging may be beneficial to assess extent of joint damage after washout
  * CT ably demonstrates loss of articular structure
  * MRI will show soft tissue changes caused by the arthritis in addition to screening surrounding bone for concomitant osteomyelitis
* Further washouts are required if reaccumulation is suspected
* Daily FBC and inflammatory markers will help track progress
* Follow-up microbiology from aspirate and any other cultures—is the patient on the right antibiotics?

Investigations

* FBC—WCC and differential
* U&Es, to include serum uric acid for crystal arthropathy diagnosis
* Inflammatory markers—ESR and/or CRP (local availability and protocol dictating)
* LFTs and coagulation profile—could this be a haemarthrosis?
* Blood cultures—can a pathogen be isolated?
* Joint aspiration
  * Before antibiotic administration
  * Send for Gram stain, culture and sensitivities, leucocyte count and analysis for crystals and glucose
  * Gram stain around 45% specific—organisms less numerous in synovial fluid than in membranes in early infection
* X-rays
  * Request plain film radiographs (AP and lateral) of the affected joint), although findings are often normal
  * Look for soft tissue swelling around the joint, widening of the joint space, and displacement of tissue planes. Pseudogout may be represented by extensive soft tissue calcification
* Ultrasound
  * Highly sensitive for demonstration of effusion
  * Cannot determine if the fluid is infective in nature
* Genitourinary screening, if suspicious of associated infection

Causes

- Organisms include *Staphylococcus aureus*, *Haemophilus influenzae*, *E. coli* and group B streptococci
- In the sexually active population Neisseria gonorrhoeae should be suspected as well as *S. aureus* and the Gram-negative anaerobes
- With gonococcal infections, there may be multiple joint involvement with associated rash (up to two-thirds of patients), and a quarter of patients will describe associated genitourinary symptoms. Other routes of infection must be considered, including that resulting from intravenous drug abuse which may predispose to *Pseudomonas* infection

Further reading

- Faraj AA, Omonbude OD, Godwin P. Gram staining in the diagnosis of acute septic arthritis. *Acta Orthop Belg* 2002; **68(4)**:388–91.
- Frick SL. Evaluation of the child who has hip pain. *Orthop Clin North Am* 2006; **37(2)**:133–40.
- Harrington L, Schneider JI. Atraumatic joint and limb pain in the elderly. *Emerg Med Clin North Am* 2006; **24(2)**:389–412.
- Jung ST, Rowe SM, Moon ES, Song EK, Yoon TR, Seo HY. Significance of laboratory and radiologic findings for differentiating between septic arthritis and transient synovitis of the hip. *J Pediatr Orthop* 2003; **23(3)**:368–72.
- Levine MJ, McGuire KJ, McGowan KL, Flynn JM. Assessment of the test characteristics of C-reactive protein for septic arthritis in children. *J Pediatr Orthop* 2003; **23(3)**:373–7.
- Miller MD. *Review of Orthopaedics*, 4th edn. Philadelphia: Saunders, 2004.

⚙ Proximal femoral fracture

Background

Although often thought of as a problem solely dealt with by orthopaedic surgeons, 'broken hips' are without exception injuries requiring in-depth assessment. Equally, their inclusion here is partly due to the number caused by in-hospital accidents, almost always the domain of the medical house officer initially.

Presentation

- Typically, there will be a history of trauma with subsequent pain in and around the hip, and immobility
- As this group of fractures is the end stage of a disease process of the bone, lack of trauma does not exclude fracture
- In patients with cognitive impairment or communication difficulties, physical signs may be the only indication of the injury
- The affected limb will generally be shortened and externally rotated

Immediate management

- ABC (p. 2–5). Remember the potential blood loss in this injury is high (around 1 l)—gain access and prescribe fluids accordingly
- Analgesia
- Full examination, paying particular attention to neurovascular integrity of the distal limb, any open skin lesions or skin pressure areas
- Mark the limb with an indelible marker
- Request hourly observations pending senior review and operative decision
- Initiate accurate fluid balance (p. 6–8) and assess Waterlow score for skin integrity
- Make nil by mouth, communicating this to patient, relatives and staff
- It is imperative that an accurate picture of events leading up to the fracture is gained. Although mechanical falls are often implicated, the cause may just as well be cardiovascular, cerebrovascular or systemic illness
- An idea of premorbid mobility, domestic arrangements and cognitive ability is required
- If in doubt of cognition, recorded assessment of mental state is necessary—has this patient the capacity to consent? (see p. 14–16)
- Initiate investigations now—a full profile of blood tests, X-rays and occasionally cardiac physiology is required before surgery can progress

Further management

- Fracture management
  - Conservative management possible in those not fit for anaesthesia, with concomitant burden of lengthy inpatient convalescence
  - Reduction and fixation of the fracture carries lower recovery burden but higher risk at and around operation

- Choice of fixation depends on site and nature of the fracture. Any fracture appearing to risk avascular necrosis of the femoral head will require hemiarthroplasty
  - Other factors in operative decision include age, mobility, bone quality, co-morbidity and acetabular condition
- Postoperative care
  - Postoperative FBC and U&Es should be checked at 48 h
  - A check X-ray should also be performed at 48 h
- Thromboprophylaxis
  - High risk of developing DVT/PE
  - Prescribe aspirin 150 mg daily for 35 days after surgery, or use local protocol if available
  - LMWHs should be reserved for those with multiple risk factors or those in whom aspirin is contraindicated
  - Compression stockings do not decrease the risk of DVT in this patient group
- Involvement of geriatric medicine team if patient is elderly
  - Physicians specialising in the care of the elderly should ideally be involved in admission and subsequent care of these patients
  - Physiotherapy, occupational therapy and social work input are all required and need careful coordination

Investigations

Imaging

- AP pelvis and lateral X-ray of affected hip. These must be adequate views to classify fracture, important in blood supply to femoral head and therefore operative plan
  - Intracapsular (subcapital, transcervical and basicervical) fractures occur within the area of the femur surrounded by the hip joint capsule, lying proximal to the intertrochanteric line
  - Extracapsular (trochanteric, intertrochanteric and subtrochanteric) fractures occur between the intertrochanteric line proximally and 5 cm from the distal part of the lesser trochanter distally
- Most units using a fast-track system (direct admission from Accident and Emergency to trauma ward) require CXR
- For cases where the diagnosis is in doubt, MRI offers confirmation
- Consider long leg views of the femur if a pathological fracture is suspected from the initial views

Blood tests

- FBC
  - Is there an anaemia that may complicate surgery?
  - Platelet count is essential if considering regional anaesthesia
- U&Es
  - To assess renal function and hydration status
  - Hyponatraemia is a common finding in this population
- Calcium
  - Low energy fractures may be caused by underlying malignancy such as metastatic disease or myeloma

- LFTs
  - A useful guide to nutritional status
  - Synthetic dysfunction may highlight underlying coagulation abnormalities
- Coagulation screen
- G&S
  - Perioperative transfusion is a common requirement
- ECG
  - Close scrutiny for ischaemia and arrhythmia
- Echocardiogram
  - Aortic stemosis (AS), a common cause of falls, is a contraindication to spinal anaesthesia

Further reading

- Aitken E, Yu G. Orthogeriatric rehabilitation: which patients benefit most? *Hosp Med* 1998; 59:274–6.
- Boyce WJ, Vessey MP. Rising incidence of fracture of the proximal femur. *Lancet* 1985; 8421:150–1.
- Parker MJ, Handoll HHG. Intramedullary nails for extracapsular hip fractures in adults. *The Cochrane Database of Systematic Reviews*, Issue 2. Art. No. CD004961. DOI: 10.1002/14651858.CD004961.pub2, 2005.
- Parker MJ, Handoll HHG. Replacement arthroplasty versus internal fixation for extracapsular hip fractures in adults. *The Cochrane Database of Systematic Reviews*, Issue 2. Art. No. CD000086. DOI: 10.1002/14651858.CD000086.pub2, 2006.
- Parker MJ, Handoll HHG, Bhargava A. Conservative versus operative treatment for hip fractures in adults. *The Cochrane Database of Systematic Reviews*, Issue 4. Art. No. CD000337. DOI: 10.1002/14651858.CD000337, 2004.
- Parker MJ, Handoll HHG, Griffiths R. Anaesthesia for hip fracture surgery in adults. *The Cochrane Database of Systematic Reviews*, Issue 4. Art. No. CD000521. DOI: 10.1002/14651858.CD000521.pub2, 2004.
- Scottish Intercollegiate Guidelines Network. Prevention and Management of Hip Fracture in Older People. A national clinical guideline. SIGN publication no. 56, 2002.
- The National Confidential Enquiry into Peri-operative Deaths report. Extremes of Age. http://www.ncepod.org.uk/report/htm, 1999.

⊙ **Acute blistering disorders**

Erythema multiforme (EM) and Stevens—Johnson syndrome–toxic epidermal necrolysis (SJS–TEN) were formerly thought of as part of the same disease spectrum. However, these diseases are now considered as separate disorders with distinct causes.

Erythema multiforme

This is a relatively common condition which predominantly affects young individuals in the second to fourth decades. It is usually self-limiting but may be recurrent and occasionally persistent. There is a seasonal variation, with it being more common in spring and summer.

Aetiology
- The majority of cases of EM have an infective cause
- HSV is the most common and can cause recurrent cases. Adenovirus, Coxsackie, and EBV can also cause it, as can bacteria such as *Mycoplasma* spp
- Occasionally epidemics may occur (e.g. in military camps)

Presentation
- Sudden onset of progressive, symmetrically distributed round maculopapules 1–2 cm in diameter
- Most commonly involves soles and palms and the extensor surfaces of the limbs
- Some or all of the lesions have a bluish colour change centrally due to ischaemia. These are the classic *target lesions*
- Oral lesions may occur and usually present as multiple painful ulcers

Stevens-Johnson syndrome–toxic epidermal necrolysis

This is essentially a drug hypersensitivity reaction (although such a reaction has been reported in GVHD and *Mycoplasma* infection) affecting adults. SJS and TEN are different points on the spectrum of disease severity, and the classification is based on the extent of detached or detachable skin at the worst stage of the illness (<10% in SJS and >30% in TEN with a recognised intermediate category). Mortality in SJS is around 5%, whereas TEN is more extensive and carries a higher mortality rate, of up to 40% accordingly.

Presentation
- Non-specific prodromal illness
  - Pyrexia
  - Malaise
  - Myalgias
  - Arthralgias
  - Headache
  - Sore throat
  - Cough
  - Nausea, vomiting and diarrhoea
- Painful rash
  - Commonly starting on the face, neck and shoulders

- Subsequently becomes more generalized
- Irregular, erythematous (sometimes purpuric), flat, atypical target lesions (occasionally typical lesions overlapping with erythema multiforme may be a feature)
- SJS–TEN is a multisystem disease which can affect any epithelial tissue
  - Ocular—conjunctivitis, Sicca syndrome, trichiasis and keratitis (all can cause long-term morbidity)
  - Gastrointestinal—oesophageal stricture, hepatitis and pancreatitis are occasional manifestations
  - Respiratory—tracheobronchial involvement and ARDS
  - Haematological—anaemia and leucopenia

Immediate management

- ABC assessment
  - Early anaesthetic assistance if respiratory distress or evidence of tracheobronchial lesions and an impending threat to the airway
- Bear in mind the fluid management implications of severe skin disease
  - Patients may require fluid resuscitation initially
  - Management of ongoing fluid loss, electrolyte loss and increased metabolic demand should be done in consultation with seniors
  - Patients may not be able to manage PO fluid if there is severe mouth involvement
  - Urinary catheterization may aid fluid management
- Immediate withdrawal of any suspected causative drug
- Adequate analgesia
- Estimation of body surface involvement (see below)
- Investigations as detailed
- Urgent referral to dermatology team for possible
  - Steroid therapy
  - Immunoglobulins
  - Early plasmapheresis
  - Ciclosporin
  - Granulocyte colony stimulating factor (GCSF)
- Transfer to ITU or a burns unit

Further management

- As cause is frequently not immediately evident, thorough history and examination is required to identify the culprit
- Ensure urology team is involved in the management of phimoses
  - If a period of obstruction has preceded presentation, follow-up is by renal function checks and USS
- Involve ophthalmology team in management of eye symptoms
- Skin care
  - Meticulous wound care must be observed to avoid secondary infection of lesions
  - Patients are at high risk of pressure sores and should be put on a low-pressure mattress

- Rinsing with warm saline or local anaesthetic solutions may help to relieve oral lesions

Investigations

- FBC, CRP and ESR
  - ↑WCC, ↑CRP or ↑ESR can occur with infection, but are also raised owing to generalized inflammation
- U&Es
  - Monitor at least daily, as the patient's fluid and electrolyte balance will be severely deranged
  - ↑Urea out of proportion to creatinine should lead to consideration of upper GI bleed
- Swab lesions for bacterial, viral and fungal causes
- Infection screen
  - Blood culture
  - Sputum for C&S
  - MSU for C&S
- CXR
  - Look for evidence of infection, pulmonary oedema or ARDS

Complications

- Sepsis (typically *S. aureus* and *Pseudomonas* spp.)
- Cardiac failure
- PE
- DIC
- GI bleeding

Further reading

- Lamoreux M, Sternbach M, Teresa W. Erythema multiforme. *Am Fam Phys Kansas City* 2006; **74(11)**: 1883.
- Léauté-Labrèze C, Lamireau T, Chawki D, Maleville J, Taïeb A. Diagnosis, classification, and management of erythema multiforme and Stevens-Johnson syndrome. *Arch Dis Child* 2000; **83(4)**: 347–52.
- Schofield JK, Tatnall FM, Leigh IM. Recurrent erythema multiforme: clinical features and treatment in a large series of patients. *Br J Dermatol* 1993; **128(5)**:542–5.

① Giant cell arteritis

Definition

An inflammatory granulomatous arteritis of large arteries, often occurring in association with polymyalgia rheumatica. It is the involvement of the ophthalmic and/or posterior ciliary arteries, potentially leading to ischaemic optic neuropathy, that makes this condition an acute medical emergency.

Presentation

Onset tends to be gradual, with systemic symptoms in about half of patients.

- Headache
  - Present in over two-thirds of patients
  - Pain felt over inflamed superficial, temporal or occipital arteries
- Temporal artery tenderness (e.g. on combing hair). It may be thickened, nodular, tender or erythematous
- Jaw claudication—muscles of mastication, tongue or swallowing

❶ Visual symptoms—one-fifth of patients present with partial or complete loss of vision in one or both eyes. If untreated, the other eye becomes affected within 2 weeks. Once established, visual impairment is usually permanent.

- Neuropathies
- Dry cough
- Polymyalgia symptoms are present in 40%
- Arm claudication—owing to narrowing of subclavian/axillary arteries

Immediate management

- ABC (p. 2–5)
- Immediate ophthalmological assessment
- Bloods as detailed
- Immediate high dose steroid therapy
  - Prednisolone 40 mg (60–80 mg if visual loss)
  - 50% of those with visual loss given steroids within 24 h of onset demonstrate some recovery

Further management

- Ensure regular reviews by rheumatology and ophthalmology team
- Temporal artery biopsy required for formal diagnosis (three of the five criteria required for diagnosis)

Criterion	Definition
Onset ≥50 years	
New headache	Localised pain
Temporal artery abnormality	Tenderness or decreased pulsation
ESR	≥50 mm/h
Abnormal biopsy of temporal artery	Demonstrates vasculitis

Investigations

- FBC—anaemia of chronic disease
- LFTs—raised ALP
- CRP and ESR will both be significantly raised

Further reading

- Calvo-Romero J. Giant cell arteritis. *Postgrad Med J* 2003; **79(935)**:511–15.
- Chan C, Paine M, O'Day J. Steroid management in giant cell arteritis. *Br J Ophthalmol* 2001; **85(9)**:1061–4.
- Danesh-Meyer H. Giant cell arteritis: managing the ophthalmic medical emergency. *Clin Exp Ophthalmol* 2003; **31(3)**:173–5.
- Nordborg E, Nordborg C. Giant cell arteritis: epidemiological clues to its pathogenesis and an update on its treatment. *Rheumatol*, 2003; **42**:413–21.
- Salvarani C, Cantini F, Boiardi L, Hunder GG. Polymyalgia rheumatica and giant-cell arteritis. *New Engl J Med* 2002; **347(4)**:261–71.

☼ Erythroderma

Definition

Inflammation of the skin affecting >90% of the body surface. This is usually associated with a significant breakdown of skin function and is a dermatological emergency.

Presentation

- Erythematous skin
- Scaling or desquamation
- Itch
- Underlying skin disorder present, e.g. psoriasis, lichen planus
- Ectropion (out-turning of eyelids)—resulting from oedema (NB. mucous membranes themselves are normally spared)
- Hair loss
- Lymphadenopathy—underlying lymphoma?
- Peripheral oedema (increased capillary permeability)
- Tachycardia (this is a hypovolaemic state, may also be septic)
- Pyrexia or hypothermia, resulting from cutaneous vasodilation and loss of temperature control mechanism

Immediate management

- ABC, maintaining close watch on physiological parameters
- Is warmed fluid indicated by patient's clinical condition and core temperature?
- Bloods as detailed
- The potential precipitating illness needs to be identified and treated—detailed history required
- Commence empirical prophylactic antibiotics particularly to cover *S. aureus*

Further management

- Treat existing infections
- All non-essential drugs should be stopped
- Patients should be nursed in a warm room with regular monitoring
- Encourage oral fluids, high calorific food and protein. Discuss with dietician. Nasogastric feeding may be required
- Remove any unnecessary cannulae which may act as a source of infection
- Frequent and large quantities of simple, bland emollients should be applied
- Oral antihistamines such as hydroxyzine 25 mg QDS may have some effect on pruritus but is more useful as a sedative
- Involve dermatology early for management advice and further investigation into underlying cause

Investigations

- FBC—infection, haematological malignancies
- U&Es—hydration status, effects of sepsis
- LFTs—does albumin reflect chronic disease?
- Calcium—erythroderma has been described in association with hypoparathyroidism and consequent hypocalcaemia
- Blood cultures, nasal and skin swabs—identification of pathogen

Causes

- Dermatitis
  - Atopic
  - Allergic
  - Venous (stasis, gravitational)
  - Seborrhoeic
- Other skin disease
  - Bullous pemphigoid
  - Cutaneous T cell lymphoma
  - Dermatophytosis
  - Ichthyoses
  - Lichen planus
  - Pityriasis rubra pilaris
  - Pemphigus foliaceus
  - Psoriasis
- Systemic disease
  - Dermatomyositis
  - Lupus erythematosus
  - Sarcoidosis
  - Graft vs. host disease
- Malignancy
  - Lymphoma and leukaemias
- Drugs
  - Allopurinol
  - Amiodarone
  - Antibiotics
  - Antimalarials
  - Anti-TB
  - Aspirin
  - Captopril
  - Carbamazepine
  - Cimetidine
  - Diltiazem
  - Phenytoin
  - Gold
  - Lithium
  - Sulphonylureas
  - Thiazides
  - Over-the-counter herbal medication

Further reading

- Balasubramaniam P, Berth-Jones J. Erythroderma: 90% skin failure. *Hosp Med* 2004; **65(2)**:100–2.
- Neonatal erythroderma: differential diagnosis and management of the red baby. *Arch Dis Child* 1998; **79(2)**:186–91.

Surgery

☠ **Abdominal aortic aneurysm**

Definition

An aneurysm is defined as a permanent localised dilatation of an artery to a width greater than 1.5 times its normal diameter. Aneurysms of the aorta can be either thoracic, thoracoabdominal or abdominal (AAA). AAAs are the most frequent site of aneurysm in the body and may be associated with iliac, femoral or popliteal aneurysms. As such, this section will focus on abdominal aneurysms.

Presentation

Of abdominal aneurysms, 75% are incidental findings, either as a pulsatile epigastric mass or in radiological investigations. The patient with a known or presumed AAA presenting with associated symptoms is a surgical emergency. Leaking or ruptured AAAs demand prompt appropriate management as the consequences for incorrect or untimely intervention are catastrophic.

The symptom profile may be vague and reflect an expanding or rupturing vessel affecting overall perfusion, localised pressure, embolic phenomena and the relationship between the great vessels and the viscera.

The following symptom profile should alert the clinician to the possibility of an AAA:

- Sudden onset abdominal, back or loin pain
- Hypotension
- Pulsatile abdominal mass (may not be apparent in profound hypotension)
- Fresh gastrointestinal bleeding
- Features of distal embolic phenomena
- Evidence of chronic arterial insufficiency
- An apparent renal colic in the elderly

Immediate management

- ABC
- Multiple points of secure, large bore IV access
- Address hypotension—request blood crossmatch and administer fluids to achieve moderate hypotension (≥90 mmHg systolic)
- Obtain 2 units O negative blood (usually kept in A&E or theatres)
- Inform senior colleagues—immediate review is essential
- Discuss with radiology—if not for immediate surgery, CT scan is invaluable
- Analgesia—this will contribute to decreasing force of cardiac contraction and reduce rate of rise of aortic pressure

⚠ The immediate management advocated from here is 'worst case scenario', assuming an unstable patient with leaking rupture who is for operative intervention. Do not allow these steps to take priority over getting to theatre, which is the only definitive solution to the problem.

- Prepare for theatre. Ask the nursing staff to initiate the administrative steps and work through as many of the remaining investigations as time allows
- ECG—ischaemia may be caused either by hypovolaemia or, rarely, by dissection tracking as far proximally as the coronary sinus
- Chest and abdominal X-rays
- Bloods
  - Send crossmatch for 10 units
  - FBC for baseline Hb/haematocrit
  - U&Es—is renal function compromised? (If not, this will give some comparison for the postoperative period)
  - LFTs and coagulation screen will warn of potential complicating factors
- Urinary catheterization for fluid balance (also take catheter urine specimen)
- ABG—if time permits, consider siting arterial line now

Further management

Treatment options
- **Incidental finding in a stable patient.** Referral to a vascular surgeon for consideration of treatment. The decision will be influenced by size of the aneurysm on USS/CT and structures involved, patient factors, co-morbidity and ultimately discussion of risks and benefits with the individual. Repair is either by laparotomy and graft or endovascular stenting
- **Symptomatic but stable patients.** The lead clinician may decide there is benefit in further investigation to assist operative planning. A CT scan will delineate the extent of the aneurysm and structures involved, particularly the renal arteries. Again, repair may be open or endovascular depending upon CT evidence
- **Symptomatic unstable patients.** This group of patients should be transferred to theatre as rapidly as possible. Desirable but unnecessary tests should not delay the move to surgical treatment. In most cases an open graft repair will be performed; however, in some centres endovascular stenting may be performed
- **High risk individuals.** In some cases an operative procedure may not be appropriate. Poor prognostic indicators include age >76 years, Creatinine (Cr) >190 µmol/L, Hb <9.0 g/dL, loss of consciousness and ECG evidence of ischaemia (3 or more = 100% mortality). Therefore, palliation may be more appropriate

Postoperative care
- Following theatre, patients will return to ITU
- Recognised postoperative complications include MI, DVT, PE, chest infection, stroke, ARDS, renal failure, colonic ischaemia, abdominal compartment syndrome and pancreatitis
- Be mindful of infection (the graft will have been put in under emergency circumstances), although this tends to be a problem after discharge

- Early joint care planning between intensivists and vascular surgeons for secondary prevention and rehabilitation is necessary

Further reading
- *OH Clinical Surgery*, 3rd edn. Oxford: Oxford University Press, p. 560.
- Ballard DJ. *Cochrane Database Syst Rev* 2000; **2**:CD001835.
- Izzilo R *et al.* Imaging of abdominal aortic aneurysm; when, how and why? *J Radiol* 2004; **85**(6 pt 2):870–82.
- Hincliffe RJ *et al.* The endovascular management of ruptured abdominal aortic aneurysm. *Eur J Vasc Endovasc Surg* 2003; **3**:191.
- Prance SE *et al.* Ruptured abdominal aortic aneurysm: selecting patients for surgery. *Eur J Vasc Endovasc Surg* 1999; **17(2)**:129–32.

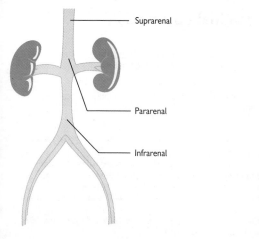

Fig. 11.1 Sites of Abdominal Aortic Aneurysm

☼ Abdominal obstruction

Definition

Impedance of the passage of small or large bowel contents, with or without actual mechanical blockage of the tract.

Presentation

- Abdominal discomfort or pain, often colicky in nature (especially with functional obstruction)
- Bloating
- Nausea
- Absolute constipation (no stool or wind) tends to be a late symptom
- Diarrhoea may be an early symptom
- Effortless vomiting is associated with more proximal obstructions
- Pyrexia and tachycardia are late symptoms often associated with strangulation, particularly if peritoneal signs are present
- Distended, tympanic abdomen (distension will be more pronounced the more distal the obstruction)
- Alteration of bowel sounds (hyperactive initially and hypoactive later)
- There may be an obvious hernia

Immediate management

- ABC. There are several particularly salient points to consider at initial assessment
  - Airway compromise is a risk in several patient groups, given the likelihood of recurrent vomiting. Early nasogastric intubation will obviously not secure the airway, but addresses one of the main risk factors
  - The respiratory rate is a subtle sign, changing early in haemodynamic compromise, as well as warning of ventilation–perfusion mismatches in aspiration or compensation for metabolic imbalances. Thorough auscultation is required to ensure aspiration has not already occurred. ABGs will offer a wealth of information and should be taken as soon as practicable
  - As well as securing IV access and taking bloods, pay close attention to rate and quality of pulse—could there be an associated sepsis?
- Note level of consciousness and temperature. As above, have a high index of suspicion of sepsis in the obstructed patient with warm peripheries and a tachycardia
- Analgesia and antiemetics. ⚠ The 'default' antiemetic often requested by nursing staff is metoclopramide. Its prokinetic action will exacerbate the problem caused by obstruction, and should be avoided
- Check BM
- Initiate strict fluid balance—remember the 'drip and suck' maxim of IV fluids and aspiration of NG tube, in addition to urinary catheterization. Nil by mouth from now
- Is there an operable obstruction? Check hernial orifices and perform PR

Further management

- Senior review—the urgency of your request to be governed by the patient's clinical condition
- Remain vigilant of fluid status
- Request erect CXR, and erect and supine plain abdominal radiographs
- Review the drug chart for medications associated with obstruction (especially opioids)

Investigations

- Erect and supine plain abdominal X-rays—look for fluid levels, sentinel loops and bowel dilatation, all of which may give an idea of the level of obstruction
- Erect CXR—look in particular for subdiaphragmatic free air and evidence of aspiration
- Gastrografin® enema in large bowel obstruction may offer further information about nature of obstruction
- Full blood count
  - Does the WCC and platelet count suggest sepsis?
  - Is there evidence of haemorrhage
- Baseline biochemistry—large fluid shifts may be associated with intra-abdominal obstruction (third space losses) which may compromise renal function, particularly in the presence of sepsis. Metabolic disturbance is itself a cause of ileus, in particular potassium, calcium and urea imbalance
- CRP is a marker of acute inflammatory change and provides a baseline measure for further progress tracking
- G&S should be sent if the patient may be a candidate for surgery
- Urinalysis is useful, particularly in the elderly where UTI is a common source of sepsis. Retroperitoneal disease is a possibility if microscopic haematuria is found
- Consider ABGs if concerned about sepsis or impact on acid–base balance. It will also show an elevated lactate in the presence of ischaemic bowel and should be used as a baseline to assess the degree of metabolic derangement (see p. 422–426)

Causes

Abdominal obstruction can be divided into small bowel obstruction, the most common site, or colonic large bowel obstruction. The obstruction itself may be complete or partial with further subdivision into simple or strangulated obstruction. It accounts for approximately 20% of emergency admissions and is, therefore, commonly encountered on surgical take. Conventionally the causes of abdominal obstruction are divided into two main categories.

Functional obstruction

This is impedance of the normal passage of bowel contents, in the absence of a mechanical obstruction. Paralytic ileus is usually associated with a reflex inhibition of motor activity of the large and small intestine following recent abdominal surgery, spinal injury or retroperitoneal haematoma. It is also seen in metabolic disturbance (especially uraemia, hypocalcaemia and hypokalaemia) and sepsis, associated with drugs (especially opioids, anticholinergics or antidepressants) or as a result of bowel infarction. Symptoms of abdominal discomfort and small bowel dilatation on X-ray are often less pronounced than in other forms of obstruction. Pseudo-obstruction is bowel obstruction for which no cause may be found, seen most commonly in the elderly and immobile. There is a gradual onset of obstruction and distension.

Mechanical obstruction

This is impedance of the normal passage of bowel contents in the presence of a physical obstruction. Primarily seen in the small intestine, the most common cause is adhesions (55% and increasing in frequency owing to the increase in the number of laparotomies performed), malignancies (20%), herniae (10%), inflammatory bowel disease (10%), volvulus (3%) and rare causes making up the remaining 2%. In the large intestine, strictures, diverticular disease and again, malignancy, particularly associated with left-sided lesions, are the main causes.

Further reading

- *OHCM*, 7th edn. Oxford: Oxford University Press, p. 598.
- Bauer AJ, Boeckxstaens GE. Mechanisms of postoperative ileus. *Neurogastroenterol Motil* 2004; **16**(Suppl 2):61–6.
- Bauer AJ, Schwarz NT, Moore BA, Turler A, Kalff JC. Ileus in critical illness: mechanisms and management. *Curr Opin Crit Care* 2002; **8(2)**:152–7.
- Behm B, Stollman N. Postoperative ileus: aetiologies and interventions. *Clin Gastroenterol Hepatol* 2003; **1(2)**:71–80.
- Delaney CP. Clinical perspective on postoperative ileus and the effect of opiates. *Neurogastroenterol Motil.* 2004; **16**(Suppl 2):61–6.
- Ellis H, Calne RY, Watson CJE. *Lecture Notes on General Surgery*, 10th edn. London: Blackwell Science, 2002.
- Holte K, Kehlet H. Postoperative ileus: progress towards effective management. *Drugs* 2002; **62(18)**:2603–15.
- Russell RCG, Williams NS, Bulstrode CJK (eds) *Bailey & Love's Short Practice of Surgery*, 24th edn. London: Arnold, 2004.
- Sajja SB, Schein M. Early postoperative small bowel obstruction. *Br J Surg* 2004; **91(6)**:683–91.

⚙️ **Acute pancreatitis**

Definition

An acute inflammatory process of the pancreas, with variable involvement of other tissues or remote organs.

Presentation

As with all cases of acute abdomen, there is a series of classical signs and symptoms associated with pancreatitis, although atypical presentations do occur. A systemic effect is often seen, thought to be due to inflammatory mediators, which can seriously complicate the situation. The clinician must be vigilant for signs of this multisystem involvement, as well as being cautious to exclude other important differential diagnoses, such as MI, pneumonia and aortic aneurysm.

Features include:

- Tachycardia, tachypnea and hypotension
- Pyrexia
- Abdominal distension, tenderness, guarding, rigidity and absent bowel sounds
- Jaundice
- Lung effusions and ascites
- Grey–Turner's (bluish discoloration of the flanks) and Cullen's (periumbilical bluish discoloration) signs

Immediate management

- ABCs
  - As with obstruction, be mindful of the airway risk with a vomiting, drowsy patient. Is an NG tube sensible here?
  - Good assessment of breathing and oxygenation is required—pancreatitis can cause profound hypoxia. Take ABGs as soon as is practicable—this will also give metabolic indicators
  - Good IV access now is essential. The fluid requirements in pancreatitis are often large, and lines get harder to site as the patient becomes more fluid-depleted
- ❶ If any of the ABC assessment raises concern, hypoxia is correcting poorly on maximal FiO_2 or IV access is impossible, call seniors or critical care outreach now.
- Send FBC, U&Es, LFTs, amylase, bone profile, CRP, coagulation screen and blood cultures
- Check BM—does this show evidence of β cell damage?
- Analgesia and antiemetic
- Fluid balance starts here. Urinary catheterization and supportive fluids, guided by physiological parameters

Further management

- Request old notes—is this a recurring condition?
- Review previous imaging studies if available. Request CXR/AXR for acute abdomen, as well as urgent USS abdomen/pelvis. This has limited ability to visualize the pancreas per se, but offers good screening for local complications
- Review blood tests
  - FBC—anaemia in haemorrhagic pancreatitis, WCC for risk stratification
  - U&Es—derangements secondary to fluid balance (third space losses)
  - Ca^{2+}—hypocalcaemia (secondary to low albumin). If tetany develops, give calcium gluconate IV
  - LFT—is this pancreatitis of biliary origin?
  - Glucose—manage hyperglycaemia with insulin if required
  - Amylase—usually raised >800 units in acute pancreatitis
  - Lipids—particularly triglycerides as a cause of pancreatitis
  - CRP—provides general indication of inflammation and allows monitoring of trends in inflammation
  - Coagulation screen—is there any evidence of liver synthetic dysfunction?
  - Procalcitonin—aids risk stratification
- Consider antibiotics, especially if pyrexial. First line is usually cefuroxime, 750 mg IV with metronidazole 500 mg IV TDS
- Fluid balance check. Is central venous access/arterial access indicated? Serial ABGs are almost certainly an indication for an arterial line
- Ensure a urine sample has been sent off

Causes

I   Idiopathic

G   Gallstones
E   Ethanol, i.e. alcohol excess
T   Trauma (compression of pancreas against vertebrae)

S   Steroids
M   Mumps or other viral infection (Coxsackie, CMV, hepatitis)
A   Autoimmune (NB. polyarteritis nodosa)
S   Scorpion venom. Anyone rash enough to blurt this out on a ward round may be able to redeem themselves by explaining that this is mediated by its effect on Na^+ and Ca^{2+} channels as well as protein kinase C
H   Hypertriglyceridaemia/hypercalcaemia
E   ERCP
D   Drugs (azathioprine, oestrogens, tetracycline, metronidazole, salicylates, erythromycin, H_2 blockers).

In addition to this well known mnemonic the following should also be considered:

- Peptic ulcer disease
- Abdominal or cardiopulmonary bypass surgery (may cause ischaemia of the pancreas)
- Upper gastrointestinal mass lesions (causing outflow obstruction)
- Intestinal parasites (e.g. *Ascaris*, which causes outflow obstruction)
- Ischaemic factors (shock, vasculitis, thromboembolic disease)

Risk stratification

Stratification of risk is important in pancreatitis for directing the level at which care should be delivered. Several scoring systems exist, of which the modified Imrie Glasgow score gives eight independent prognostic factors and is perhaps the easiest to remember.

P	PaO_2 <8 kPa
A	Age >55 years
N	Neutrophils: WCC >15 $\times$ 10^9/L
C	Ca^{2+} <2 μmol/L
R	Renal: urea >16 μmol/L
E	Enzymes: LDH >600; AST >200 units/L
A	Albumin <32 g/L
S	Sugar: glucose >10 μmol/L (unless diabetic).

A score of 3 or more indicates consideration for transfer to HDU/ITU.

Continuing management

Initial management is usually supportive with serial examination, daily bloods and ABGs forming the mainstay of assessment. The clinician should be alert to any deterioration which may herald the onset of haemorrhagic pancreatitis, ARDS or multi-organ failure. Fluid balance should be carefully managed, with a low threshold to transfer to HDU if management in the ward setting is causing concern. A feeding plan should be established early—if recovery is likely to be protracted then consider TPN.

Complications

- Pancreatic sepsis—infection associated with, but not necessarily in, the pancreas. Best managed with percutaneous CT-guided drainage under antibiotic cover
- Pseudocyst—fluid collection with a wall of granulation tissue. Again, best drained percutaneously but if asymptomatic can often be left
- Haemorrhage or haematemesis is a serious finding. Major blood vessels may have been disrupted and prognosis is poor. Stress ulcer may be the cause, requiring urgent gastroscopy and angiography
- Duodenal obstruction is common. If prolonged, TPN may be required
- Colonic necrosis occurs after surgery and may lead to fistulation
- Jaundice, especially in the presence of pyrexia, requires urgent investigation. In the first 48 h after presentation it may represent a stone blocking the ampulla of Vater, necessitating urgent USS and percutaneous drainage or stenting of the duct

Indications for surgery

- Pancreatic phlegmon (non-suppurative inflammatory mass), pseudocyst or abscess may require drainage
- Unstable patients with haemorrhagic pancreatitis may require surgery for haemostasis, although this is uncommon
- Sphincterotomy or cholecystectomy in biliary pancreatitis may be indicated to correct the underlying cause
- Necrosectomies require specialist input

Follow-up

This is variable, depending upon the cause of pancreatitis, but may include cholecystectomy, alcohol awareness, or referral to specialist centres for malignancy. Patients should be made aware of the need to seek immediate medical help if similar symptoms develop.

Further reading

- *OHCM*, 7th edn. Oxford: Oxford University Press, p. 584.
- *OH Clinical Surgery*, 3rd edn. Oxford: Oxford University Press, p. 294.
- Rau B et al. Laboratory markers of severe pancreatitis. *Dig Dis* 2004; **22(3)**:247–57.
- Williams M, Simms HH. Prognostic usefulness of scoring systems in critically ill patients with severe acute pancreatitis. *Crit Care Med* 1999; **27(5)**:901–7.
- Bennett GL, Hann LE. Pancreatic ultrasonography. *Surg Clin North Am* 2001; **81(2)**:259–81.
- Sakorafas GH, Anagnostopoulos G. Surgical management of chronic pancreatitis: current concepts and future perspectives. *Int Surg* 2003; **88(4)**:211–18.

☼ **Appendicitis**

Definition

Inflammation of the vermiform appendix; a vestigial, worm-shaped blind-ended tube originating from the apex of the caecum. It is attached by a fold of peritoneum, the mesoappendix, and is approximately 8 cm in length (although this may vary considerably). It can lie in a number of different positions, leading to variation in the associated symptom profile.

Presentation

Appendicitis is a notoriously subjective diagnosis. Even in the hands of experienced clinicians, 15–20% of the appendices removed are normal. This is due to the highly variable presentation, symptom profile and clinical findings. Diagnosis is particularly difficult in young children (<5 years), the elderly (>60 years), and women of childbearing age where gynaecological causes of pain may confound the clinician. The risk of developing appendicitis is greatest in the young and becomes less common with age, although appendicitis must be considered as a differential in all age groups.

It is important to note that this is the classically described presentation; the astute clinician should be ever alert to more subtle or atypical signs.

- Abdominal pain—initially central with migration to right iliac fossa (McBurney's point, one-third along a line drawn from the right anterior superior iliac spine (ASIS) to the umbilicus)
- 24–36 h history of symptoms
- Anorexia—does the patient feel hungry?
- Nausea
- Vomiting
- Less commonly, altered bowel habit (usually diarrhoea)
- Mild pyrexia
- Tachycardia
- Flushed appearance
- Fetor
- Signs of peritonism over the right iliac fossa
  - Percussion tenderness
  - Rovsing's sign (deep palpation of the left iliac fossa causes pain in the right iliac fossa) may be elicited, but sensitivity and specificity tend to be poor
- Right-sided tenderness on rectal/vaginal examination
- Important to note that some or all symptoms or signs may be absent and none are specific to appendicitis

Immediate management

- ABC
  - Pay particular attention to subtle indicators of systemic illness, such as slight tachypnea
- Bloods as listed later
- Request hourly repeat of observations
- Full history, which must encompass menstruation, period pain and risks of pregnancy in all women of childbearing age
- Full examination—ask patient to put finger on where pain started and where it is now
- Serial examination is often the key; the same clinician should reassess the abdomen after a period of a few hours if the patient's initial condition allows
- Check BM
- Initiate fluid balance regimen (see p. 6–8) and ensure a urine specimen is taken for ward testing and sent for laboratory analysis. Urinary catheterization is not indicated unless the patient is liable to be poorly compliant with fluid balance. Urine pregnancy tests should be performed in women of reproductive age (with consent)
- Make nil by mouth, communicating this to patients, relatives and staff
- Administer analgesia, including opiates if necessary, with an antiemetic as required
- Consider antibiotics if infection seems probable (cefuroxime, 750 mg and metronidazole, 500 mg IV TDS) after taking blood cultures

Further management and investigations

- Review blood tests. FBC and CRP are good indicators of inflammation and infection; LFTs, U&Es, amylase, calcium, blood cultures and glucose tend to be carried out as a 'routine' for acute abdominal pain, possibly helping to exclude other pathology. Serum βHCG should be checked to validate the urinary pregnancy test, as it is not affected by timing of specimen (early pregnancy is detectable only in first voiding of the morning)
- There is little persuasive argument for radiological imaging of all suspected appendicitis. Any peritonitic patients must, though, have standard erect CXR/AXR
- If the patient is well and the senior team are happy to wait, ultrasound imaging can add to the diagnostic process
- There is no indication for ABG sampling in uncomplicated appendicitis; it is, however, a first-line test if the patient appears compromised (see p. 422–424)
- Urinalysis aids identification of genitourinary infection as a cause of pain, and in cases of retrocaecal or pelvic lie of the appendix may show blood and leucocytes
- The bladder must be empty prior to surgery—this may require catheterization
- Senior review—is this patient going to theatre?

- Prepare for theatre. Ask the nursing staff to initiate preparation of the administrative steps for transfer to the operating theatre
- Owing to the variability of the local anatomy, it is essential that the surgeon who will be performing the operation examines the patient prior to induction of anaesthesia
- Diagnostic laparoscopy is particularly useful in young girls, but increasingly accepted as a universal management standard. The availability of equipment and a surgeon skilled in its use is likely to be the limiting factor
- Antibiotics should not be needed beyond a single postoperative dose unless a perforated appendix or gross peritoneal contamination is found at operation. In this situation, 1 day of IV followed by 5 days of oral antibiotics is prudent

Complications

- Perforation of the appendix results in bowel content being lost into the peritoneum, the result of which will be a critically ill patient with peritonitis. This situation demands high dose antibiotics and rapid transfer to theatre
- Appendicular abscesses form when an inflamed or perforated appendix becomes walled off. This often results in a mass in the right iliac fossa. Often the plan will be conservative with no need for surgical intervention

Appendicectomy in pregnancy

- Appendicitis during pregnancy does occur
- Other causes of abdominal pain must be excluded
- USS provides valuable information
- The risks from appendicitis to mother and baby are greater than the risk of appendicectomy; therefore, pregnancy should not influence decision to operate

Further reading

- *OHCM*, 7th edn. Oxford: Oxford University Press, p. 582.
- *OH Clinical Surgery*, 3rd edn. Oxford: Oxford University Press, p. 262.
- Andersson RE. Meta-analysis of the clinical and laboratory diagnosis of appendicitis. *Br J Surg*. 2004; **91(1)**:28–37.
- Russell RCG, Williams NS, Bulstrode CJK (eds) *Bailey & Love's Short Practice of Surgery*, 24th edn. London: Arnold, 2004.
- Ellis H, Calne RY, Watson CJE. *Lecture Notes on General Surgery*, 10th edn. London: Blackwell Science, 2002.

⊙ **Acute cholecystitis**

Definition

Inflammation of the gallbladder, occurring most commonly due to obstruction of the cystic duct by gallstones (calculous cholecystitis). Less commonly there may be acalculous cholecystitis, seen particularly in critically ill patients in the ITU context.

Presentation

- Epigastric pain
  - Localizing with time to the RUQ due to peritoneal irritation
  - Colicky pain less common than constant
  - Referred to the back and/or shoulder tip
  - Often exacerbated by food (particularly fatty food)
  - Exacerbation may occur with palpation over the liver edge on deep inspiration (Murphy's sign)
- Nausea
- Anorexia
- Vomiting
- Tachycardia
- Fever (may be masked in the elderly and diabetics)
- Jaundice—if the hepatic ducts become obstructed either due to external compression or a stone
- Signs and symptoms of pancreatitis (see p. 372–375) if a stone causes obstruction to the pancreatic outflow

Immediate management

- ABC
  - Be alert to signs of systemic illness—the biliary system is a common source of sepsis (p. 304–306 for SIRS and sepsis)
- Inititate fluid balance regimen now
- Consider analgesia and antiemetic
- Make the patient nil by mouth and ensure this is communicated to the patient and other staff members
- Full history and examination
  - Known gallstones confirmed by USS at previous admission? There is a patient population who present frequently with gallstone disease but have yet to have their gallbladder removed
  - History of previous biliary colic, fat intolerance, close association with meal times
  - Is the patient jaundiced, Murphy's-positive or peritonitic?
- Hourly observations
- Urine specimen for ward testing and laboratory analysis
- Pregnancy test if woman of reproductive age—urinary specimen on ward and serum βHCG at lab

Further management

- Request old notes—is this a recurring condition?
- Imaging
  - Review previous imaging studies (particularly USS which may show the presence of gallstones)
  - Erect CXR for air under diaphragm
  - AXR looking particularly for other pathology which may be masquerading as cholecystitis or pneumobilia, suggesting gallstone ileus
  - Urgent ultrasound scan will demonstrate the presence of gallstones, thickening of the gallbladder wall and duct dilatation, all important in further management
  - Consider MRCP/ERCP in ductal dilatation
- Review blood tests
  - FBC for evidence of infection and sepsis
  - LFTs—any hepatic dysfunction?
  - Electrolytes to reflect hydration status
  - Amylase to exclude pancreatitis
  - Calcium
  - CRP—in isolation can only give vague estimate of severity of inflammation, but good progress marker for further management
  - Cholesterol—risk factor
  - Glucose
- ECG—is this an atypical presentation of an MI?
- Consider antibiotics, especially if pyrexial. Cefuroxime 750 mg with metronidazole 500 mg IV TDS
- Review fluid balance now. Is urinary catheterization indicated?
- Review results of ward urinalysis

Causes

Cholecystitis develops due to inflammation of the gallbladder most commonly due to biliary obstruction at the cystic duct or common bile duct by a gallstone. However, it is important to consider other causes of constriction or obstruction of these structures, particularly those of a neoplastic or inflammatory/infective nature.

Approximately one in ten of the population have gallstones although only 20% of these individuals will present with symptoms. The majority of gallstones are composed of a mixture of cholesterol, bilirubin and calcium, although pure cholesterol and pure pigment stones may be found. Essentially, stone formation occurs as a result of an imbalance of bilirubin, cholesterol and lecithin. This results in bile salts coming out of their micelles, allowing salt crystals to precipitate. Only 10% of stones may be seen on X-ray.

Classically described as affecting those who are 'fair, fat, female, fertile, forty and flatulent'. This caricature reflects the facts that gallstone disease is more common in women and the obese, increases in incidence around the menopause and is influenced by hormonal changes. Other risk factors include *Salmonella typhi* infection, Crohn's disease, ileal resection and haemolytic anaemias, which either affect the enterohepatic circulation of bile salts or increase their production.

Complications

- Pancreatitis is one of the most serious complications of calculous gallstone disease (p. 304–306). In simple cholecystitis it is unlikely that LFTs and amylase will be dramatically raised; if they are, it is prudent to assume a stone has left the gallbladder or cystic duct and may be causing outflow obstruction. This may necessitate ERCP to remove the stone—is there ductal dilatation?
- Gallstone ileus occurs when a gallstone erodes through the wall of the gallbladder into the small bowel; its presence subsequently causes an ileus. AXR may show the gallstone within the bowel, which is often dilated and gas in the biliary tree (pneumobilia)
- Ascending cholangitis is infection within the biliary tree, usually due to stasis. It presents as Charcot's triad of pain, fever and jaundice, and is a serious condition which may lead to septicaemia with its accompanying risks. Early recognition and aggressive treatment with antibiotics or a drainage procedure are key to minimizing its impact (see p. 256–257)
- Empyema of the gallbladder is a suppurative infection of the gallbladder, in which the gallbladder fills with infected fluid, eventually leading to pus formation in a contained structure. In infective cases drainage of the gallbladder is essential; this may be done radiologically via a percutaneous approach, laparoscopically or by open procedure

Biliary colic vs. acute cholecystitis

Fundamentally, biliary colic lies to the left of acute cholecystitis on the spectrum of gallstone disease. It does not have the same systemic effects as acute cholecystitis, and is transient pain caused by stone impaction in the cystic duct or Hartmann's pouch. In practical terms, without cholecystectomy the patient is likely to move gradually to the right along this spectrum, as further crops of stones develop and provoke reaction from the gallbladder.

Further reading

- *OHCM*, 7th edn. Oxford: Oxford University Press, p. 590.
- *OH Clinical Surgery*, 3rd edn. Oxford: Oxford University Press, p. 278.
- Russell RCG, Williams NS, Bulstrode CJK (eds). *Bailey & Love's Short Practice of Surgery*, 24th edn. London: Arnold, 2004.
- Ellis H, Calne RY, Watson CJE. *Lecture Notes on General Surgery*, 10th edn. London: Blackwell Science, 2002.
- Indar AA, Beckingham J. Acute cholecystitis *BMJ* 2002; **325**:639–43.
- Moscati RM. Cholelithiasis, cholecystitis, and pancreatitis. *Emerg Med Clin North Am* 1996; **14(4)**:719–37.

⚠ **Acute limb ischaemia**

Definition

Limb ischaemia is defined by its onset:

- Acute ischaemia—onset within 14 days
- Acute on chronic—worsening symptoms in the past 14 days
- Chronic—stable ischaemia for more than 14 days

and severity:

- Incomplete when limb is not threatened
- Complete when limb is threatened
- Irreversible when limb is no longer viable

Presentation

Classically taught as the 6 Ps

- Pain
- Pallor
- Pulselessness
- Perishing cold
- Paraesthesia
- Paralysis

The first four of these symptoms are highly variable; the diagnostic key lies in paralysis and paraesthesia. Further to this, pain on squeezing the forearm or calf suggests muscle infarction and imminent irreversible injury. It is important to attempt to differentiate between embolic and thrombotic causes.

Thrombotic

- More common
- Insidious onset over hours to days, being incomplete in nature owing to collateral blood supply
- Occur as a complication of pre-existing peripheral vascular disease
- History of claudication
- Calcified arteries with bruits
- Contralateral leg pulses likely to be absent

Embolic

- Rapid onset in minutes with complete loss of blood flow and therefore no time for collaterals to develop
- Embolic source most commonly due to an arrhythmia
- History of claudication is less likely
- Contralateral pulses are more often present
- Arteries tend to be soft and tender without bruits

Is there a history of IV drug injection (i.e. one which may have in fact been given intra-arterially) or trauma?

Immediate management

- ABC, being wary of other embolic complications. Take an ABG sample if at all unsure or concerned by physiological parameters
- Full vascular assessment
  - Must include peripheral pulses by palpation and Doppler
  - ABPI will give numerical guide to severity (see box)
- Hourly observations
- FBC, U&Es, LFTs, CRP, coagulation screen, G&S and BM
- Analgesia and antiemetic
- Make patient nil by mouth and initiate fluid balance regimen (see p. 6–8)
- ECG—marked cardiac co-morbidity exists in this patient population

❶ If critical ischaemia is suspected, contact the on-call vascular surgery team immediately. Operative intervention is of the highest NCEPOD urgency classification, being limb-saving, and referral must not be delayed.

Further management

- Review blood tests
  - FBC—baseline Hb is essential prior to embolectomy
  - U&Es—establish baseline renal function and look for evidence of rhabdomyolysis
  - Coagulation screen—patients with known arteriopathies will often be anticoagulated
- ABG may be a useful tool at this point to monitor metabolic effects of ongoing ischaemia
- CXR is indicated by likely cardiac co-morbidity

Further management from here will be under the care of the vascular surgical team and may include:

- Giving an IV bolus of heparin to limit propagation and preserve collaterals, unless there are contraindications such as aortic dissection, polytrauma or serious head injury
- Angiography in incomplete ischaemia to allow a decision on medical vs. operative management
- In cases of complete ischaemia, angiography will only delay embolectomy and lead to a poorer outcome
- Thrombolysis—the introduction of a catheter into the distal extent of the thrombus and the administration of streptokinase or TPA. It is only effective in incomplete occlusions, takes several hours to work, and is associated with complications such as haematoma, bleeding and stroke
- Surgical embolectomy and decompression by fasciotomy

Beyond intervention

- Post-embolectomy, the patient should continue on heparin to mitigate against the formation of further emboli (some surgeons may ask for a 6 h delay to reduce the risk of haematoma formation)
- Warfarin should be commenced after 48 h on heparin unless contraindicated (warfarin initially has a procoagulant effect), and heparin stopped once INR is in the therapeutic range
- A source of embolus should be sought, e.g. by echocardiogram
- Following acute embolus there is a 10–20% mortality rate, usually owing to heart failure, recurrent emboli or stroke. Morbidity and mortality is likely to be higher, however, the longer that is spent agonizing over treatment options
- Reperfusion injury owing to the reintroduction of blood into an area of ischaemia can be more damaging than the ischaemia itself. Endothelium is injured and becomes more permeable, which may cause swelling and eventually compartment syndrome. Systemically, hyperkalaemia, acidosis, cardiac arrhythmias and acute tubular necrosis due to myoglobinuria may result. ARDS is another recognized risk

Further reading

- *Oxford Handbook of Clinical Surgery*, 3rd edn. Oxford: Oxford University Press, p. 548.
- *OHCM*, 7th edn. Oxford: Oxford University Press, p. 596.
- Bendermacher BL *et al.* Medical management of peripheral arterial disease. *J Thromb Haemost* 2005; **3(8)**:1628–37.
- Callum K, Bradbury A. ABC of arterial and venous disease: acute limb ischaemia. *BMJ* 2000; **320**:764–7.
- Dormandy J *et al.* Acute limb ischaemia. *Semin Vasc Surg* 1999; **12(2)**:148–53.
- Katzen BT. Clinical diagnosis and prognosis of acute limb ischaemia. *Rev Cardiovasc Med* 2002; **3**(Suppl 2):S2–6.

Ankle: brachial pressure index (ABPI)

The closing systolic pressure at the ankle divided by that of the brachial artery gives the ABPI.

These measurements are Doppler-assisted and give a measurement of limb ischaemia.

- 1.2–0.9   Normal
- 0.9–0.5   Claudicants
- <0.5   Critical ischaemia

It is wise to have this figure on hand, or a good reason why it has not been performed before calling a vascular surgeon.

Clinical biochemistry

☼ Hyponatraemia

Definition

Numerically defined by serum Na^+ <136 mmol/l, hyponatraemia is essentially a disorder of excess body water relative to body sodium. It is important to note that it is not the plasma Na^+ concentration itself but the rate of fall that is of greater clinical significance.

Presentation

Patients usually remain asymptomatic until serum Na^+ <130 mmol/l. In patients with chronic hyponatraemia, compensatory mechanisms may allow a patient to remain asymptomatic even below this level.

- Plasma Na^+ <130 mmol/l—nausea, malaise
- Plasma Na^+ <120 mmol/l—headache, lethargy, restlessness, disorientation
- Plasma Na^+ significantly <120 mmol/l—seizures, coma, respiratory arrest, brainstem herniation or death

Immediate management

- ABC, as per p. 2–5
  - Secure IV access and send bloods as detailed
- Measure urine sodium and osmolality (in plain universal container, not boric acid; must be before IV fluids)
- Check blood glucose to rule out hyperglycaemia as a cause
  - The osmotic effect of glucose causes dilution of ECF—correction of primary cause will reverse hyponatraemia
  - Look for acidosis or sepsis related to this
  - Fluid resuscitation may be necessary for correction
- Is rapid correction absolutely necessary?
  - Differentiate acute or chronic course by looking at patient's history, previous samples and their clinical condition
  - Rapid correction is only indicated when serum Na^+ is falling rapidly, with associated neurological deterioration, i.e. coma or seizures. This must be discussed with senior colleagues
  - ⚠ Osmotic demyelination (central pontine myelinolysis) may occur, causing irreversible neurological damage and death
  - Patient will immediately need to be transferred to HDU or ICU and advice sought on correction
- If rapid correction is not necessary, ensure that factitious hyponatraemia is excluded. This is commonly from:
  - Hyperlipidaemia—ask lab if previous sample appeared lipaemic
  - Was the sample taken from site proximal to an IV infusion?

Further management

Usually correcting the cause will rectify hyponatraemia. Again, determine if this is acute or chronic course.

All acutely hyponatraemic patients

Assess hydration status. Look at observations (pulse, BP), skin turgor, mucous membranes, eyes (if sunken), JVP, oedema (pedal and sacral), examine chest and note fluid balance charts. Consider catheterization for accurate fluid balance and CVP monitoring. This, in conjunction with urine sodium and plasma urea, should help to elicit a cause.

- Look for any medications introduced recently, particularly diuretics, and consider withholding
- Monitor sodium concentrations regularly during Na^+ correction (every hour if necessary)
- Observe—ensure repeat bloods are taken and reviewed at least every 2 days subsequent to correction
- Ongoing control of fluid balance

Acutely hypovolaemic

Correct volume depletion with IV normal saline. Aim for a rise of not more than 8 mmol/l per day in asymptomatic patients. In symptomatic patients, aim for an hourly rise of 1–2 mmol until patient is asymptomatic, then slow down the correction. Only use hypertonic fluid or loop diuretics with specialist advice.

Treat possible causes as they become apparent. Look for hypotension and postural fall in BP suggestive of adrenal insufficiency. If in doubt arrange a short Synacthen test—this is mandatory before restricting fluid for presumed SIADH, as circulatory collapse may be precipitated if incorrect. If unsure, **do not** administer dexamethasone before seeking senior guidance.

Acutely hypervolaemic

Look for heart failure, cirrhosis with ascites, nephrotic syndrome. Treat any underlying condition, watch fluid balance and consider restriction.

Acutely euvolaemic

Fluid restrict (<1 l/day). SIADH is a diagnosis of exclusion; therefore, when other causes have been eliminated, look for inappropriately concentrated urine (>100 mosm/kg) in the presence of low serum osmolality (<270 mosm/kg).

Renal, adrenal and thyroid function must be normal, and diuretics or IV fluids preclude diagnosis owing to their effect on urinary sodium. SIADH requires fluid deprivation (maximum intake 500 ml/24 h); demeclocycline (600–1200 mg/day) can be considered when fluid restriction alone is insufficient.

All chronically hyponatraemic patients

Investigate as in acute cases; cautious fluid restriction can be implemented once other causes have been excluded.

Investigations

- FBC, U&Es, glucose, lipids, osmolality and TFTs
- Short synacthen test—look at peak cortisol level and rise from baseline
- Urine sodium and osmolality

Causes

Hypovolaemia

- Extrarenal (urine sodium <30 mmol/l)
  - Dermal losses e.g. burns, sweating
  - GI losses, e.g. diarrhoea, vomiting
  - Pancreatitis
- Renal loss (urine sodium >30 mmol)
  - Diuretics
  - Salt wasting nephropathy
  - Cerebral salt wasting
  - Mineralocorticoid deficiency (Addison's syndrome)

Hypervolaemia

- CCF
- Cirrhosis with ascites
- Nephrotic syndrome
- Chronic renal failure

Euvolaemia

- Postoperative
- SIADH
- Hypothyroidism
- Hypopituitarism (glucocorticoid deficiency)
- Water intoxication (primary polydipsia, excessive hypotonic IVT, post-TURP)

Further reading

- *OHCM*, 7th edn. Oxford: Oxford University Press, p. 666.

☼ Hypernatraemia

Definition
Defined by plasma Na^+ >145 mmol/l, hypernatraemia reflects a net water loss or hypertonic gain (excess sodium relative to water).

Presentation
- Restlessness, confusion or irritability
- Anorexia
- Muscle weakness
- Nausea
- Vomiting
- Thirst (may be masked in patients with altered mental status, hypothalamic lesions, children and elderly)

Plasma Na^+ >158 mmol/l can lead to altered mental status, lethargy, irritability and stupor. The acute brain shrinkage at this stage can induce vascular rupture, with cerebral bleeding and subarachnoid haemorrhage.

Immediate management
- ABC, as per p. 2–5
- Secure IV access and send bloods as detailed below
- Measure urine sodium and osmolality (in plain universal container, not boric acid). Must be before fluid treatment is initiated
- A shocked patient should be transferred to an HDU where possible
  - These patients will require normal saline to correct ECF depletion before 5% dextrose to correct sodium balance
- Differentiate acute or chronic course by looking at patient's history, previous samples and their clinical condition
- Where the course is acute
  - Give 5% dextrose and seek advice on further correction

⚠ Rapid correction (falling by 1 mmol/l per hour) must be performed only with specialist input.

Further management
- When the course is chronic (i.e. greater than 48 h)
  - Encourage oral water, but half-normal saline (0.45% saline) can be given in those where this is not appropriate
  - ⚠ Overly rapid correction may precipitate cerebral oedema
- Assess hydration status
  - Is the patient hypovolaemic, hypervolaemic or euvolaemic?
  - Observations (HR, BP, UO, fluid balance charts)
  - Skin turgor
  - Mucous membranes
  - Sunken eyes
  - JVP
  - Confusion, lethargy, ↓GCS
  - Peripheral/sacral oedema
  - Auscultate chest—bibasal crepitations

- Consider catheterization for accurate monitoring of UO
- Consider central line insertion and CVP monitoring if unwell
  - This, in conjunction with urine sodium and plasma urea, should help to identify a cause
- Treat cause as it becomes apparent
- Look for any medications introduced recently and consider withholding
- Ensure repeat plasma sodium levels are reviewed at least every 2 days subsequently
- Ongoing control of fluid balance

Investigations
- FBC, U&Es, glucose, lipids, osmolality
- Urine sodium and osmolality, before fluid therapy
- Overnight water deprivation test (if suspicious of diabetes insipidus, e.g. recent history of head trauma)

Causes
Associated with hypovolaemia
- Dermal losses, e.g. burns, sweating
- GI losses, e.g. diarrhoea, vomiting, fistulas
- Diuretics
- Post-obstruction
- Acute and chronic renal disease
- Hyperosmolar non-ketotic state

Associated with hypervolaemia
- Iatrogenic
  - Hypertonic saline
  - Tube feeds
  - Antibiotics containing sodium (e.g. benzylpencillin)
  - Hypertonic dialysis
- Hyperaldosteronism
- Cushing's disease

Associated with euvolaemia
- Diabetes insipidus
  - Central (consider desmopressin)
  - Nephrogenic
  - Gestational
- Hypodipsia
- Fever
- Hyperventilation
- Mechanical ventilation

Further reading
- *OHCM*, 7th edn. Oxford: Oxford University Press, p. 666.

☠ Hyperkalaemia

Presentation

Like hypokalaemia, this may be an incidental finding on routine biochemistry. It should, however, be considered if the patient has any of the following:

- Muscle weakness leading to flaccid paralysis
- Paraesthesia
- Metabolic acidosis on ABG
- ECG changes—loss of P-waves, wide QRS complexes, peaked T waves.

❶ Arrhythmias may be more marked than this, eventually taking the shape of a sine wave. These are often peri-arrest ☎ 2222.

Immediate management

- ABC, as per p. 2–5
- ECG, looking for peaked T-waves. Take advice on any arrhythmia management. Consider monitoring and transfer to coronary care unit (CCU)
- Secure IV access and send off bloods
- If initial K^+ >6.5 mmol/l give calcium gluconate (10 ml of 10% solution over 10 min). ⚠ This is a short term cardioprotective measure and may need repeating
- ABG—take advice on correcting any acidosis (preferably from the renal team)
- Ensure renal function is thoroughly investigated—it is a common primary cause and may need haemodialysis to correct
- Give 5–10 units soluble insulin with 50 ml of 50% glucose IV
- Consider salbutamol nebulizers 2.5–5 mg
- Set up IV 50% glucose infusion with insulin according to 1–2-hourly capillary blood glucose measurements

Further management

- Consider using calcium resonium (polystyrene sulphonate resin 15 g 6–8-hourly or 30 g in methylcellulose solution PR). Calcium resonium provides longer term potassium depletion but is both highly unpleasant and constipating
- Investigations
- Correct other electrolyte imbalances—coexisting hypocalcaemia, hyponatraemia and hypermagnesaemia can all exacerbate cardiovascular effects
- Treat possible causes as they become apparent
- Observe: ensure repeat bloods are taken and reviewed at least every 2 days subsequently
- Ongoing control of fluid balance: use a fluid balance chart and consider urinary catheterization

Investigations
- FBC, U&Es, glucose
- ABGs—when considering metabolic acidosis. Potassium concentration can also be confirmed, although this is less accurate than lab result
- ECG—loss of P-waves, wide QRS complexes, peaked T-waves, arrhythmias (particularly VF and cardiac arrest)

Causes
Raised plasma potassium levels do not necessarily imply excess of total potassium and may occur in deficit of total body potassium, e.g. DKA.

1. Artefact (common)
- Haemolysis, especially if WCC or platelets high in FBC from same venepuncture. Repeat can be sent in lithium heparin tube to eliminate doubt
- Poor venepuncture technique
- Delay (at lab or on way to lab) in sample being separated
- Repeat sample if in doubt

2. Increased intake
- Parenteral (inappropriate potassium in IV fluid replacement is common)
- Oral (rare)
- Transfusion of old blood

3. Decreased loss—renal
- Renal failure—ARF or CRF with oliguria
- Mineralocorticoid deficiency, e.g. Addison's disease
- ACE inhibitors
- Potassium-sparing diuretics; spironolactone, amiloride, triamterene

4. Extracellular shift
- Rapid tissue breakdown; burns, crush injuries, rhabdomyolysis, cytotoxic therapy
- Massive blood transfusion
- Acidosis
- Digoxin toxicity

Further reading
- *OHCM*, 7th edn. Oxford: Oxford University Press, p. 668.

⊙ Hypokalaemia

Presentation

Even when severe, hypokalaemia may be asymptomatic and so is likely to be an incidental finding. It should be considered if the patient has any of the following:

- Depression/confusion
- Muscle weakness
- Ileus, constipation
- Polyuria (from decreased concentrating ability of distal tubule in hypokalaemia)
- ECG changes—arrhythmias, prolonged PR, u-wave, ST depression, flattening/inversion of T-waves
- Metabolic alkalosis

Immediate management

- ABC as per p. 2–5
- ECG, looking for low, small T-waves. Seek senior or cardiology advice if arrhythmia is apparent; if severe, consider monitoring and transfer to CCU
- Secure IV access and send bloods
- If the initial K^+ is less than 2.5 mmol/l (or less than 3.0 and on digoxin), begin treatment immediately. Give 20 mmol KCl/h at no greater than 40 mmol/l. If a central line is available, 20 mmol/h in 50–100 ml 5% dextrose can be infused but monitor rate
- ABG—take advice on correcting any alkalosis (preferably from the renal team)
- If initial K^+ is between 2.5 and 3 mmol/l, oral replacement should be sufficient unless patient has history of recent MI or is on rhythm control. Cautious (10–15 mmol/h) IV therapy is also an option. Rate of replacement should reflect rate of reduction

⚠ The maximum rate of correction is 0.5 mmol/kg/h. Never give bolus KCl. Do not give K^+ if patient is oliguric—speak to senior colleague or renal physician.

Further management

- If K^+ >3.0 mmol/l, oral supplements are advised if patient is not NBM or vomiting; give 80–120 mmol in divided doses. This can be in the form of Sando-K tablets (12 mmol K, up to 2 tablets QDS), Slow K (8 mmol K and effervescent 12 mmol K)
- Liquid preparations are also available, such as Kay-Cee-L syrup (1 mmol/ml: up to 30 ml KCl added to 500 ml bottle of NG feed)
- Non-effervescent tablets cause gastro-oesophageal irritation
- If oral supplementation is not available, normal IV replacement is 70–130 mmol per 24 h. This can be given as up to 40 mmol of KCl added to each litre of intravenous crystalloid or in TPN
- Monitor K^+ 4-hourly until stable
- Investigations

- Observe—ensure repeat bloods are taken and reviewed at least every 2 days subsequently. Be sure to request that GP monitoring continues in the short term if patient is discharged
⚠ Do not discharge with potassium supplements!
- Treat possible causes as they become apparent
- Ongoing control of fluid balance; use chart, consider urinary catheterization
- Potassium depletion enhances digoxin toxicity—seek advice from cardiologists on any at-risk patients

Investigations
- FBC, U&Es, glucose, magnesium
- ABGs—when considering metabolic alkalosis. Potassium concentration can also be confirmed, although this is less accurate than lab result. Acidosis suggests renal tubular acidosis as cause
- ECGs—arrhythmias, prolonged PR, u-wave, ST depression, flattening/inversion of T-waves
- Urine—potassium concentration (>25 mmol/l suggests renal loss)

Causes
1. Artefact
- Blood taken from the drip arm (common). Repeat sample if in any doubt

2. Inadequate intake
- Parenteral (inappropriate potassium in IV fluid replacement is common)
- Oral (rare but consider eating disorders or alcoholism)

3. Renal
- Diuretics (common, particularly in hypertensive and elderly patients)
- Mineralocorticoid excess, e.g. Cushing's, Conn's syndrome and tumours
- Renal tubular acidosis
- Other medications—ticarcillin, amphotericin B, carbenecillin
- Hypomagnesaemia

4. GI tract
- Vomiting (causes metabolic acidosis)
- Diarrhoea (including lasative/purgative abuse)
- Villous adenoma (of rectum, secretes fluid)
- Intestinal fistulae

5. Intracellular shift
- Insulin and glucose administration
- Alkalosis
- Familial periodic paralysis (very rare, usually males)
- Salbutamol use (in large amounts)

6. Skin
- Diaphoeresis—excessive sweating

Further reading
- *OHCM*, 7th edn. Oxford: Oxford University Press, p. 668.

☼ **Hypocalcaemia**

Definition

Hypocalcaemia is diagnosed when total plasma calcium is <2.2 mmol/l, but of greater clinical significance in hypocalcaemia is the concentration of free, ionized calcium. Around 55% of body calcium is bound to protein (mainly to albumin) and is biologically inert, the rest being ionized and biologically active. This means overt hypocalcaemia may result from an absolute calcium deficiency or a change in distribution.

Presentation

- Tetany
- Muscle cramps
- Stridor (laryngeal)
- Chvostek's sign—tapping of facial nerve anterior to ear producing facial spasm
- Trousseau's sign—tapping or pressure on median nerve in wrist induces carpal spasm
- Prolonged QT interval primarily owing to prolonged ST segment (often found incidentally)

Immediate management

- ABC, as per p. 2–5
- Secure IV access and send bloods as detailed later
- If rapid correction is required when patient is clinically unstable, e.g. tetany, seizures, arrhythmias:
  - Consider an IV injection of 10 ml (2.25 mmol) of calcium gluconate followed by a continuous infusion of about 40 ml (9 mmol)
  - Calcium chloride may also be used but is less well tolerated
  - Take advice from cardiology in patients known to have digitalis toxicity as they are at risk of arrest with rapid correction. Carefully monitor plasma calcium
- Treat hypomagnesaemia if associated
- Oral preparations can be used where correction need not be so rapid, in dosages of 750–1000 mg of elemental calcium per day.
- ⚠ Be careful not to mix calcium solutions with those containing bicarbonate so as not to cause calcium carbonate precipitation

Further management

- Look to correct any hypoproteinaemia and increase dietary calcium. A dietician may be able to advise
- Consider a therapeutic trial of vitamin D metabolites as serum levels may take some time to come back
- Thiazide diuretics cause hypocalciuria and are a useful adjunct in the management of hypoparathyoidism
- Treat cause as it becomes apparent
- Once calcium has been corrected, take thyrocalcitonin levels

- Observe—ensure repeat bloods are taken and reviewed at least every 2 days subsequently
- Ongoing control of fluid balance

Investigations
- Bloods
  - FBC—signs of infection or sepsis, transfusion
  - U&Es
  - LFTs and amylase—does the patient have pancreatitis?
  - Calcium
  - Phosphate
  - CRP
  - Magnesium
  - TFTs
  - Vitamin D metabolites—raised or suppressed?
  - Parathyroid harmone—raised by end organ insensitivity and in vitamin D deficiency, suppressed by Mg^{2+}, etc
- Urine calcium:creatinine ratio for excretion

Causes
- Hypoparathyroidism
  - Surgical (after thyroidectomy—the most common cause of hypoparathyroidism)
  - Genetic (usually presents before adulthood)
  - Idiopathic
  - Magnesium imbalance (chronic deficiency or acute hypomagnesaemia suppress PTH secretion)
  - Acquired destruction of parathyroid (radiation, haemachromatosis, haemosiderosis, metastasis)
- Vitamin D and its metabolites: deficiency or resistance
  - Vitamin D deficiency, nutritional, malabsorption (commonly post-gastrectomy) or lack of sun exposure (particularly in the dark-skinned)
  - 25-Hydroxyvitamin D deficiency—hepatobiliary disease, anticonvulsants (phenytoin, phenobarbital), nephrotic syndrome, glutethimide, malabsorption
  - 1,25-Dihydroxyvitamin D deficiency—renal failure, hyperphosphataemia, PTH deficiency, Vitamin D-dependent rickets (type 1), pseudohypoparathyroidism
  - Resistance to Vitamin D
- Unresponsiveness to PTH
  - Pseudohypoparathyroidism (end organ resistance to PTH)
- Increased calcium deposition (in bone and soft tissue)
  - Osteoblastic metastasis
  - Hypophosphataemia—treatment of lymphoma
  - Acute pancreatitis
  - 'Hungry bone syndrome'—following parathyroidectomy, thyroidectomy and early phase of treatment of rickets
- Miscellaneous
  - Chelation of calcium: massive blood transfusion (>10 units), exchange transfusion, ethylene glycol poisoning, heparin (in vitro)

- Inhibition of bone resorption with drugs—colchicine poisoning, mithramycin, oestrogen, propylthiouracil
- Sepsis
- Cardiopulmonary arrest
- Tumour lysis
- Rhabdomyolysis
- Hypoalbuminaemia (normal ionized calcium)

Further reading
- *OHCM*, 7th edn. Oxford: Oxford University Press, p. 670.

⊙ Hypercalcaemia

Definition

Total plasma calcium concentration >2.6 mmol/l.

Presentation

Hypercalcaemia has many systemic effects aside from moans, groans and stones:

- Weakness, lethargy, fatigue
- Dehydration
- Polyuria or renal impairment (owing to the onset of renal manifestations—nephrocalcinosis, nephrogenic diabetes insipidus, nephrolithiasis or distal renal tubular acidosis)
- Anorexia, abdominal pain, nausea and vomiting
- Constipation
- Altered mental state—depression, impaired cognition, psychosis, personality change/disorders and eventually coma
- Incidental shortened QT interval primarily caused by shortened ST segment
- Clinical pictures of pancreatitis, peptic ulcers, renal stones
- Bone disease
- Eye complications—band keratopathy, conjunctivitis, red eye syndrome
- ❶ Hypercalcaemic crisis/shock (Ca >3.5 mmol/l) associated with:
  - Volume depletion
  - Neurological signs
  - Arrhythmias

Immediate management

- ABC, as per p. 2–5. ⚠ NB. Fluid resuscitation differs in this situation; follow guidelines below
- Secure IV access and send bloods as detailed
- A shocked patient should be transferred to an HDU where possible
- Serum calcium >3.5 mmol/l should be treated immediately, even in the absence of symptoms
- In patients with impaired renal function, haemodialysis may be required; discuss with renal team if available
- Fluid resuscitation
  - 3000 ml normal saline in first 24 h, 2000 ml/24 h thereafter
  - Watch for signs of overload; treat with furosemide if present
  - Continue until urine output better than 2000 ml/day
- Consider administration of bisphosphonates to inhibit bone resorption
  - Only when fully rehydrated
  - Beware risk of hypocalcaemia
  - Monitor renal function
  - Check baselines such as PTH first
- Give IV phosphates if phosphate <0.3 mmol/l, at 10 mmol/12 h

Further management

- Treat cause as it becomes apparent. Consider a therapeutic trial of steroids (usually for vitamin D intoxication, breast cancer or haematological malignancy). This should be given as prednisolone 40–60 mg OD, or hydrocortisone 40 mg TDS
- Observe and ensure repeat bloods are taken and reviewed daily
- Ensure low calcium diet is maintained—a dietician may be able to advise
- Ongoing control of fluid balance, see p. 6–8

Investigations

- Blood
    - FBC—any sign of haematological malignancy?
    - U&Es—be confident of sodium control before prescribing fluid
    - LFTs—is albumin raised?
    - Calcium—confirm result
    - Phosphate—does the patient need intercurrent phosphate replacement?
    - CRP
    - Magnesium
    - TFTs—thyrotoxic?
    - Vitamin D metabolites—intoxication?
    - PTH—raised in primary hyperparathyroidism. Suppressed in other causes of hypercalcaemia
- Urine
    - Calcium excretion
    - Calcium: creatinine clearance ratio—renal causes?

Causes

- Hyperparathyroidism (most common cause amongst general population; in this case hypercalcaemia has chronic course)
  - Primary—from parathyroid adenoma (common), hyperplasia, carcinoma or familial (autosomal dominant)
  - Post-transplant
  - Tertiary (e.g. in cronic renal failure)
- Malignancy-associated (most common in hospital inpatient population), both from lytic bone metastasis and mediated by humoral agents (PTH-related peptide, transforming growth factor, circulating prostaglandins and $1,25(OH)_2D_3$). Usually severe hypercalcaemia with associated hypophospataemia
- Granulomatous diseases (e.g. sarcoidosis and tuberculosis)
- Exogenous—Vitamins A and D, lithium, thiazides, phosphate-binding antacids, betelnuts, oestrogens and calcium. 'Milk-alkali syndrome' is from excessive milk and antacid ingestion, and is associated with hypercalcaemia
- Endocrine—thyrotoxicosis
- Addison's disease
- Immobility
- Sampling error (pseudohypercalcaemia)—prolonged application of the tourniquet causes transient hyperproteinaemia with hypercalcaemia

Further reading

- *OHCM*, 7th edn. Oxford: Oxford University Press, p. 672.

☼ **Paracetamol overdose**

Definition

Ingestion of any more than 4 g of paracetamol in 24 h is by definition an overdose; serious toxicity is unlikely in doses below 150 mg/kg in 24 h, however.

Hepatocellular necrosis is the major toxic effect of paracetamol poisoning, rarely seen in doses below 250 mg/kg or around 12 g.

Presentation

- Gastrointestinal symptoms and signs of toxicity are common, particularly in the first 24 h:
  - Anorexia
  - Nausea
  - Vomiting
  - Pallor
  - Diaphoresis
  - Malaise
  - Right upper quadrant pain (usually 24–72 h)
- Suspect paracetamol in any overdose, particularly polypharmaceutical or if taken with alcohol
- It is important to remember that patients may be asymptomatic until onset of fulminant liver failure (ALT >1000 u/l) around 72 h after ingestion

Identifying high risk patients

Patients are at risk of severe liver damage if more than 150 mg of paracetamol/kg body weight or 12 g has been ingested (whichever is the smaller). It is unlikely that severe liver damage will occur at lower paracetamol levels unless the patient:

- Has a history of regular alcohol excess
- Is on enzyme-inducing drugs (commonly carbamazepine, phenytoin, phenobarbitone, primidone, rifampicin and St John's Wort
- Has a condition causing glutathione depletion (malnutrition, eating disorders, cystic fibrosis, HIV infection)

In these patients, treatment should be considered at lower doses (75 mg/kg).

Immediate management

❶ ABC. Be aware of risk of polypharmaceutical overdoses ± concomitant alcohol excess: ↓GCS and ↑risk of vomiting. Do not allow concern over biochemistry to detract from basic resuscitation principles. Discuss with senior or anaesthetist if airway protection is likely to be a problem.

1. Patients presenting within 8 h of ingestion

- Give 50 mg activated charcoal if paracetamol greater than 150 mg/kg body weight is thought to have been ingested *and* it is <1 h since the overdose
- There is little evidence for the efficacy of gastric lavage
- Take blood for plasma concentration as soon as possible after 4 h since overdose (within 4 h is not significant as continued absorption and distribution of the drug will occur)
- Many hospital policies now advocate salicylate levels in tandem with all paracetamol levels. Discuss with senior if any other substances are to be sought at this stage, particularly if polypharmacy is suspected
- Assess risk of severe liver damage (high or low risk)
- Do not treat if the plasma paracetamol concentration is below the relevant line on the treatment graph and the history is consistent with <150 mg/kg body weight paracetamol having been ingested
- Start treatment with N-acetylcysteine (NAC; see below) if plasma paracetamol concentration related to the time from ingestion is above the relevant line on the treatment graph

2. Patients presenting 8–15 h after ingestion

The efficacy of NAC declines progressively from 8 h after the overdose. If at risk of severe liver damage (>150 mg/kg or 12 g ingested), start NAC immediately without waiting for plasma paracetamol concentration.

3. Staggered overdose

- Beyond 15 h post-ingestion, risk estimates are less reliable and clinical judgement becomes more important in management. Patients who present at this point tend to be more severely poisoned and at greater risk of developing serious liver damage
- FBC, U&Es, LFTs, INR, venous blood acid–base balance
- Treat patient as serious risk and consider for treatment with NAC. Plasma paracetamol concentration is meaningless in relation to the treatment graph in these cases

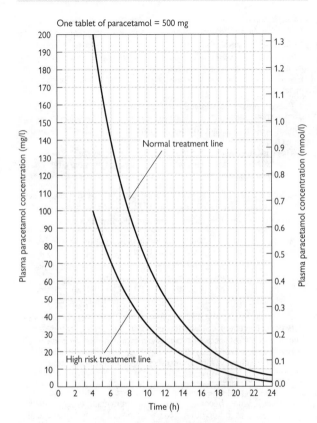

Fig. 12.1 Treatment curve for paracetamol overdose. From *OHCM*, 7th edn. p. 829

N-acetylcysteine

IV administration is recommended, particularly if the patient is vomiting or urgent treatment is necessary.

⚠ The maximum dose permissible is for patients of 110 kg—all patients heavier than this should receive this dose regardless.

NAC infusion doses (based on patients >12 years of age)

Dose	NAC (mg/kg)	5% Dextrose (ml)	Infusion duration
1	150	200	15min
2	50	500	4 h
3	100	1000	16 h

NAC may elevate INR (to around 1.3 or less) but this is incidental and does not require further treatment. NAC treatment should persist if both ALT and INR are elevated.

⚠ Previous anaphylactoid reaction to NAC is not an absolute contra-indication. Pre-treat with antihistamine (chlorphenamine, 10 mg IV) and ensure first dose is given no faster than advised rate.

Further management

- Any evidence of continuing liver dysfunction (LFT or clotting derangement) requires immediate attention—discuss with team senior or liver team. Assessment for transplant may be required
- Patients can be discharged subsequent to NAC treatment or 24 h after the last paracetamol was ingested, provided they are asymptomatic and the INR, plasma creatinine, plasma bicarbonate and ALT are normal
- If plasma creatinine is raised at presentation, admit for monitoring of renal function. Isolated renal failure is rare
- Patients should be advised to return to hospital if vomiting or abdominal pain develop or recur
- The reasons for overdose should be explored thoroughly and psychiatrists involved where overdose was deliberate. Dosette boxes may be useful if overdose is accidental

Further reading

- *OHCM*, 7th edn. Oxford: Oxford University Press, p. 828.
- For further advice on NAC or the management of overdose, contact National Poisons Information Service (NPIS):
  Tel: 0870 600 6266 (UK), Dublin 01 837 9964 or 01 809 2566.
- TOXBASE at http://www.spib.axl.co.uk

☼ Salicylate overdose

Declining in incidence owing to popularity of other analgesics, salicylate (most commonly found in aspirin) poisoning has its metabolic effect by uncoupling oxidative phosphorylation, thereby disrupting the Krebs cycle.

Presentation
- Minor overdose
  - Vertigo
  - Tinnitus
  - Nausea
  - Vomiting
  - Diarrhoea
- ❶ Major overdose (substantial ingestion with potential to require ITU admission)
  - Neurological abnormalities—seizures, reduced conscious level or coma
  - Acid–base disturbance—respiratory alkalosis (early), potential later metabolic acidosis
  - Pulmonary complications such as non-cardiogenic pulmonary oedema
  - Coagulation defects
  - Fever
  - Hypotension
  - Hypoglycaemia and low CSF glucose
  - Hypokalaemia
  - Sodium disturbance (can be ↑ or ↓)

Immediate management

- ABC, as per p. 2–5. Bear in mind the additional airway implications of reduced consciousness and vomitus; perform basic airway manoeuvres and seek anaesthetic assistance early
- Establish a time and quantity of overdose if possible. If acute and the dose is greater than 125 mg/kg, gastric lavage with activated charcoal may be of benefit. Chronic overdose is more likely in the elderly, owing to miscalculation or misadministration of tablets
- Send urgent bloods as detailed, helping to guide treatment
- ABG to assess acid–base status
- Empirical administration of 5% dextrose may help correct CSF glucose
- The Done nomogram is no longer recommended as a treatment guideline as it fails to account for variability in speeds of uptake and mechanisms of overdose

Further management

- Urinary alkalinization increases renal clearance of the drug, decreasing half life by as much as 16 h. HDU care is desirable; regular ABGs need to be performed (2-hourly) for both pH and potassium surveillance (hypokalaemia reduces the efficacy of alkalinization). Target pH for arterial blood during alkalinization is 7.3–7.5, with a urinary pH of 7.5–8
- The definitive treatment for acute, large overdose is haemodialysis. If the patient's clinical condition is of concern, the renal team should be involved early. Although plasma levels are generally reliable, condition must be the ultimate arbiter of treatment, and dialysis takes time to organize. A level of 700 mg/l warrants rapid dialysis even if the patient is well
- Although urinary alkalinization enhances clearance, forced diuresis shows no benefit in clearance and should be avoided
  - Alkalinization is likely to be of benefit in overdoses between 450 and 700 mg/l
  - 1 l of 1.26% sodium bicarbonate should be infused over 3 h
- Mild overdose can be treated with rehydration orally or IV, with administration of activated charcoal until plasma salicylate has peaked
- Careful screening for sequelae is important; intracranial bleeds, GI bleeds and pancreatitis may all result from salicylate toxicity, and require early diagnosis and intervention

Investigations

- FBC, U&Es, LFTs, amylase and coagulation profile to assess end organ damage and clotting dysfunction
- Paracetamol level—is this polypharmaceutical?
- Sequential ABGs (2-hourly)
- Sequential glucose (2-hourly)
- Repeat U&Es 4-hourly
- Sequential plasma salicylate levels (until clearance)
- Sequential urinary pH (2-hourly)
- ECG—may show changes consistent with hypokalaemia (see p. 396–398)
- CXR if suspicious of pulmonary oedema

Further reading

- *OHCM*, 7th edn. Oxford: Oxford University Press, p. 828.
- *OH Emergency Medicine,* 3rd edn. Oxford: Oxford University Press, p. 187.

☼ **Tricyclic antidepressant overdose**

Tricyclic antidepressants (TCAs), such as amitryptiline, are commonly prescribed in primary care for both mood disorders and refractory neuropathic pain. They are, unfortunately, a common drug for overdose—good management is essential due to their metabolic impact and cardiotoxicity.

Presentation
- ECG features (often most pronounced sign)
  - Prolonged PR, QRS and QT intervals
  - Non-specific ST and T-wave changes
  - AV block
- Commonly
  - Sinus tachycardia
  - Dry skin, mouth and tongue
  - Dilated pupils
  - Drowsiness
- Rarely
  - Ataxia
  - Nystagmus
  - Divergent squint
  - Coma
  - Respiratory depression
  - Increased tone and hyper-reflexia
- Very rarely, deep coma leading to areflexia
- Other features
  - Metabolic or mixed acidosis (metabolic effect of drug complicated by respiratory depression)
  - Hypotension
  - Hypothermia and rhabdomyolysis in unconscious patients

❶ ECG changes, unconsciousness or significant metabolic derangement should be dealt with as a peri-arrest situation. Anaesthetic, medical emergency or arrest team presence is desirable.

Immediate management

- The principles of ABC management (see p. 2–5) are vital here. The airway in this patient population is inherently unsafe owing to the common combination of vomiting and drowsiness. Call for help early and remember that simple manoeuvres save lives; turning a patient on their side or basic jaw thrust application will help provide adequate patency until anaesthetic assistance arrives
- ABG—is there an acidosis?
- Plasma alkalinization will reduce the amount of free drug
  - Indications are: systolic BP <90mmHg, QRS duration >160 ms, pH <7.1, recurrent seizures or arrhythmia
  - Bolus doses 1–3 ml/kg 8.4% sodium bicarbonate IV every 3–5 min, aiming for plasma pH 7.5–7.55, titrated against clinical response

- Maintain pH using either boluses or infusion 1.26% sodium bicarbonate
- Patients remaining hypotensive despite alkalinzation must be discussed with chemical toxicologist and intensive care team— inotrope support and hypertonic saline may be required
- Some of these patients will have taken either another medication or alcohol. Detailed history from either patient or relatives is required, as well as plasma paracetamol and salicylate levels 4 hours after overdose
- Close observation of GCS and airway is required, with early involvement of critical care team. Semi-urgent intubation is frequently required with an overnight ITU admission whilst the drug is cleared
- There is a risk of seizures from TCA toxicity. These are normally self-limiting and rarely require benzodiazepines, but may in the worst cases require propofol sedation or general anaesthetic to guard against the hyperthermia and rhabdomyolysis of status epilepticus

Further management
- A 6-hour observation period is mandatory in TCA overdose, the location of which will be dictated by clinical condition
- Further ABGs will be required if acidosis is present at first. If the accepting ward is happy, consider placing an arterial line to avoid repetitive radial sampling
- Cardiac monitoring must be ongoing throughout the 6 h. Bear in mind that bedside monitors offer only one trace (usually lead II). If further analysis is required, ECGs should be taken as appropriate
- Follow-up in mental health terms is also important. Once medical obstacles are overcome, patients are frequently discharged with insufficient attention being paid to the intentional nature of the presentation. Discuss with on-call psychiatrist in sufficient time to allow assessment to be made whilst an inpatient, and try to involve family where possible
- Haemodialysis is rarely effective in TCA toxicity, as the volume of distribution is extremely large

Investigations
- Serial temperatures
- ECG—to be repeated if any evidence of QRS changes
- ABG—to be repeated if acidosis requiring treatment
- U&Es—hyperkalaemia or renal failure suggestive of rhabdomyolysis (if it is possible that the patient has had seizures)
- CXR if aspiration risk
- Paracetamol and salicylate levels
- Alcohol level if conscious or mental state precludes honest history from patient

Further reading
- *OH Emergency Medicine,* 3rd edn. Oxford: Oxford University Press, p. 192.
- *OHCM,* 7th edn. Oxford: Oxford University Press, p. 822.

① **Methanol poisoning**

Methanol, an alcohol found in windscreen washer fluid, cleaning solvents, 'moonshine' and antifreeze exerts its toxic effect by being metabolized to formic acid and formaldehyde by alcohol and aldehyde dehydrogenases in the liver. These metabolites are particularly toxic to the CNS, and as little as a mouthful of methanol can cause irreversible toxicity.

Presentation

- Poorly reactive or fixed and dilated pupils. Atrophied optic discs may be seen, but complaints of altered visual field are frequent without visible pathology on fundoscopy
- Lethargy, seizures, confusion and coma. Parkinsonism may be established if the overdose was less recent
- Abdominal pain
- Abnormal respiratory pattern (sometimes Kussmaul pattern may be notable)
- Cardiovascular stability is normally maintained until abrupt respiratory arrest

Immediate management

- ABC, as per p. 2–5. NB. Increased risk to the airway from conscious level and potential vomiting
- Bloods as detailed
- Capillary blood glucose—hypoglycaemia is common
- ABG—severe metabolic acidosis in overdose context with significant anion gap should be treated as methanol toxicity until actively disproved
- Urinalysis—may be abnormal odour due to formaldehyde
- The key to protection against methanol is ethanol administration, which has affinity in the order of 100 times that of methanol for alcohol and aldehyde dehydrogenases

  ⚠ All treatment for methanol poisoning should be discussed with national poisons information service (NPIS) before commencing

  - Oral administration should be avoided because of the airway risk and gastric irritation
  - Load with 10 ml/kg 10% ethanol in 5% dextrose
  - Maintenance infusion is 0.15 ml/kg/h in non-drinkers, 0.3 ml/kg/h in regular drinkers, with plasma target of 17–22 mmol/l ethanol
- Fomepizole is available on a named-patient basis in liaison with NPIS
  - Also a competitive inhibitor of alcohol dehydrogenase
  - Load with 15 ml/kg IV, 12-hourly boluses of 10 ml/kg
  - Continue therapy until concentration <200 mg/l
  - If still infusing at 48 h after first dose, boluses increased to 15 ml/kg to counteract development of fomepizole induction
- Ensure nursing staff perform regular neurological observations, and that patient is kept under extremely close supervision

Further management

- Reproducible neurological deficits will require further investigation, best discussed with a neurologist. MRI has been shown to demonstrate several changes associated with this poisoning
- ITU admission for close observation and haemodialysis is likely to be required
- Monitor ABG frequently (ideally via an arterial line)
- Monitor methanol level until cleared
- Sequential neurological examination is indicated if there is a fluctuating symptom course

Investigations

- Bloods
  - FBC—may be anaemic
  - U&Es—absence of anion gap excludes methanol toxicity. Needs repeating regularly to monitor renal function
  - LFTs—liver damage?
  - Methanol (only check if anion gap present)—<20 mg/dl unlikely to be harmful, 20–50 mg/dl requires treatment and >150 mg/dl is likely to be fatal if untreated. Serum formic acid levels may actually be a more reliable guide than methanol levels in terms of actual toxicity
  - Ethanol levels 2-hourly to monitor treatment levels
  - Amylase can be raised without pancreatitis in this presentation
  - Coagulation screen
  - Regular creatine kinase for rhabdomyolysis
- CXR if suspicious of aspiration
- Neurological follow-up as advised

Further reading

- *OH Emergency Medicine*, 3rd edn. Oxford: Oxford University Press, p. 200.
- *OHCM*, 7th edn. Oxford: Oxford University Press, p. 822.

ⓘ Benzodiazepine overdose

With a mortality rate in the region of 0.003%, benzodiazepine overdose is rarely fatal due to toxicity. Care must be taken, however, to ensure that basic supportive measures are taken throughout the period of altered consciousness it will cause.

Presentation
- Dizziness
- Confusion
- Visual disturbance
- Paradoxically, anxiety or agitation
- Ataxia
- Nystagmus
- Amnesia
- Slurred speech
- Respiratory depression
- Hypotension
- Clouded cognition

Immediate management

- Basic ABC care is, as always, first line (p. 2–5)
- ABG if respiratory depression has been noted in primary survey
- Bloods as detailed
- CXR if concerned about aspiration
- Start antibiotics if CXR consistent with this. Is ITU assessment required for ARDS sequelae of aspiration?
- ECG—polypharmaceutical overdoses are not uncommon, so the cardiotoxic effects of TCAs must be screened for
- Serum glucose, with treatment of any derangement
- Single-dose activated charcoal may be of use if within 4 h of ingestion. Should co-ingestion of potentially lethal substance be suspected, lavage may be attempted if within 1 h of ingestion
- Close observations, including neurological assessment, until consciousness improves. Emphasis must be placed on nursing in such a way that airway protection is paramount

⚠ Flumazenil is a benzodiazepine reversal agent, rarely indicated in this scenario. Its action is very short-lived, producing a transient, rapid rise in conscious level. The concern with this is that in a polypharmaceutical overdose, the benzodiazepine component may be suppressing seizures induced by another drug, such as TCAs. Reversing the benzodiazepine effect may, therefore, precipitate seizure. There is little purpose to reversal other than confirming diagnosis of benzodiazepine overdose—an indefensible position should further harm be caused.

Further management
- Continued observation until consciousness is regained and maintained
- Persisting GCS of 8 or below warrants ITU admission to allow time for the overdose to be overcome
- Further bloods at 4 h post-overdose for paracetamol and salicylate
- Continued treatment of any respiratory sequelae, liaising with chest physicians where necessary
- Psychiatric follow-up should be considered mandatory prior to discharge

Investigations
- FBC, LFTs and U&Es—screen for effects of any other components of overdose, in addition to effects of chronic alcohol use (commonly associated)
- CXR if aspiration likely
- Serum glucose

Further reading
- *OHCM*, 7th edn. Oxford: Oxford University Press, p. 826.
- *OH Emergency Medicine*, 3rd edn. Oxford: Oxford University Press, p. 194.

☼ **Opiate overdose**

Traditionally, teaching has been that opiate tolerance is an individual characteristic, governed partly by the amount of pain the patient is experiencing. In addition to iatrogenic overdose, however, there is a substantial patient population who present having overdosed on heroin. Although the mechanisms are very different, common principles of management apply.

Presentation
- Depressed consciousness
- Respiratory depression
- Pinpoint pupils
- May have mild hypotension (owing to peripheral vasodilatation)
- More rarely, CNS features of unpleasant hallucinations, agitations and seizures may be seen
- There may be an obvious route of administration—either patient-controlled analgesia in inpatients or evidence of IV injection sites in recreational users

Immediate management
- ABC as per p. 2–5
- If there is a controllable source of administration, such as a PCA device, stop it, or remove transdermic patients
- Oral ingestion may be at least partially counteracted up to a fairly late stage with activated charcoal, owing to the lowered GI motility it causes
- The effect of the overdose can be reversed with naloxone (400 µg IV initially). Consider the requirement for reversal carefully; profound CNS and/or respiratory effects obviously warrant it, but a peaceful patient with stable physiological parameters and a patent, self-managed airway may gain little benefit from this abrupt reversal
- ABG—is there acidosis suggestive of prolonged hypoventilation?
- Unless this is known iatrogenic overdose in an inpatient, further steps need to be taken. Is this overdose polypharmaceutical? Standard 4 h bloods for paracetamol and salicylate, in addition to drug-specific tests for anything else the patient may be prescribed. If there is a high opiate dose, causing confusion at home, for example, there is a real risk of significant disarray in drug administration
- Any suggestion of aspiration should be confirmed by CXR, after which appropriate antibiotics (consult local guidelines) should be administered. If significant effect of aspiration seen on CXR, liaise with ITU outreach or respiratory physicians early on

Further management
- Close observation during recovery of consciousness
- A period of hypoxia during the episode raises the likelihood of non-cardiogenic pulmonary oedema, so this patient group should be observed for at least 24 h

⚠ If reversal has been made, further administration is required, as naloxone has a typical half life in the region of half an hour. Infusions can be prescribed, or IM depots (400 μg) administered.

- Careful attention to any sequelae, especially aspiration
- Known IV drug abusers are at extremely high risk of endocarditis— check for murmurs
- Check renal function for rhabdomyolysis
- Reversal may precipitate opiate withdrawal in frequent users, usually seen as:
  - Myalgia
  - Vomiting
  - Yawning
  - Chills
  - Diarrhoea
- Substance abuse specialists should ideally meet the patient during this time, with the goal of avoiding opioid augmentation or relapse
- Secondary prevention in recreational use may be considered by some to be idealistic, but it should always be discussed with the patient, offering referral to drugs and addiction services
- Equally, psychiatric follow-up in deliberate self-poisoning is mandatory

Further reading
- *OHCM*, 7th edn. Oxford: Oxford University Press, p. 826.
- *OH Emergency Medicine*, 3rd edn. Oxford: Oxford University Press, p. 186.

Arterial blood gases

Arterial blood gas (ABG) analysis allows for an assessment of respiratory function and acid–base status, and is invaluable in guiding therapy on the ward, in theatre and in critical care areas. Modern analysers commonly provide assays estimating numerous additional values (e.g. Hb, glucose, lactate, Na^+, K^+, Cl^-, Ca^{2+}). These can provide vital initial guidance, pending the availability of formal biochemistry and haematology results. If repeated sampling is required, an indwelling arterial cannula should be sited; these must only be used in patients who are being nursed in a critical care area.

⚠ The estimated additional values provided by the analyser are significantly less reliable than those provided by formal lab results, and so should only ever be an adjunct.

Interpretation

It is important always to look at blood gases in the context of the patient's clinical condition. The classic example of this is in acute severe asthma, where an apparently normal $PaCO_2$ is an indicator of life-threatening illness.

The following is a guide to basic initial ABG interpretation.

1. What is the acid–base status?

- Acidaemia (pH <7.35)
  - With $\uparrow PaCO_2$ (>6.0 kPa)   Respiratory acidosis
  - With $\downarrow$BE (more negative than −2) Metabolic acidosis
  - With $\uparrow PaCO_2$ + more negative BE Mixed acidosis
- Alkalaemia (pH >7.45)
  - With $\downarrow PaCO_2$ (<4.7 kPa) Respiratory alkalosis
  - With $\uparrow$BE (>2)   Metabolic alkalosis
  - With $\downarrow PaCO_2$ + $\uparrow$BE Mixed alkalosis

The body attempts to compensate for the primary pH abnormality by altering ventilation (i.e. $PaCO_2$) in metabolic conditions, and by altering renal H^+ excretion/HCO_3^- retention (i.e. BE) in respiratory conditions. Overcompensation for any acid–base change will not occur, therefore look for the pH abnormality. For example, if there is an acidosis but the $PaCO_2$ is low, then there is a primary metabolic acidosis with respiratory compensation.

2. How well is the patient oxygenating?

PaO_2 should always be interpreted in the light of the FiO_2. A 'normal' PaO_2 with a high FiO_2 indicates difficulty in transporting oxygen from the alveolus to the blood (a high A/a gradient).

- Increased gradient occurs when there is inefficient gas exchange, e.g. because of parenchymal lung disease or V/Q mismatch (e.g. pulmonary embolism, intracardiac shunts)
- This helps distinguish between hypoventilation and other pathologies
- Normal gradient increases with age and with increasing FiO_2

Causes

Respiratory acidosis

Usually caused by acute ($\leftrightarrow$BE) or chronic ($\uparrow$BE) hypoventilation

- Structural and mechanical pulmonary disease
  - COPD
  - Life-threatening asthma
  - Large airway obstruction
- Neuromuscular or mechanical problems
  - Gross obesity, sleep apnoea syndromes
  - Guillain–Barré syndrome
  - Myasthenia gravis, motor neurone disease, muscular dystrophies
  - Traumatic flail chest
  - Ankylosing spondylitis, severe kyphoscoliosis
- Muscle relaxant drugs
- Respiratory centre disorders
  - Organic disease affecting respiratory centres
  - Respiratory depressant drugs (e.g. opioids)
  - Respiratory arrest

Metabolic acidosis

The anion gap estimates the contribution of unmeasured ions (e.g. lactate) and can be useful in determining the cause of a metabolic acidosis.

$$\text{Anion gap} = (Na^+ + K^+) - (Cl^- + HCO_3^-)$$

- Normal anion gap (10–18 mmol/l)—loss of bicarbonate or ingestion of acid
  - Gastrointestinal HCO_3^- loss (diarrhoea, pancreatic fistula)
  - Renal tubular acidosis
  - Ingestion of acidifying agents (hydrochloric acid, ammonium chloride, arginine hydrochloride, TPN with excess basic amino acids)
  - Rapid IV hydration (dilutional acidosis)
  - Drugs
  - Addison's disease
- Raised anion gap (>18 mmol/l)—increased production of acids.
  KUSsMAuL is a useful mnemonic (Kussmaul's respiration is a clinical sign of metabolic acidosis)
  - **K**etoacidosis (DKA, starvation, alcohol)
  - **U**raemia
  - **S**alicylate poisoning
  - **M**ethanol poisoning
  - **(A)**ethylene glycol poisoning
  - **L**actic acidosis ($\uparrow$metabolism $\pm$ $\downarrow$tissue oxygen delivery— e.g. sepsis, shock, ischaemia, hypoxia)

Respiratory alkalosis

- Spontaneous/psychogenic hyperventilation
- Pain or fever causing hyperventilation
- Reflex hyperventilation (e.g. PE)
- Respiratory centre stimulation

- Via chemoreceptors—$\downarrow FiO_2$ (e.g. high altitude), alveolo-capillary diffusion block (e.g. fibrosing alveolitis), right → left shunt, carbon monoxide poisoning
- Via drugs or metabolites—salicylate poisoning, acute liver failure, chronic liver disease
- Brain haemorrhage, stroke or meningitis

Metabolic alkalosis

- Ingestion/infusion of excess HCO_3^-
  - Iatrogenic—over treatment of acidosis
  - Milk–alkali syndrome
- Inappropriate acid loss
  - Pyloric stenosis, self-induced persistent vomiting
  - K^+ depletion (other than renal tubular acidosis or laxative abuse)
  - Cl^- depletion
  - Hyperaldosteronism (primary or secondary)
- Contraction alkalosis
  - Rapid diuresis
  - Other causes of mild extracellular fluid depletion
- Fulminant liver failure

Reference ranges

- pH   7.35–7.45
- pCO_2 4.7–6.0 kPa
- pO_2 10.6–13.3 kPa
- HCO_3^- 20–24 mmol/l
- Base excess   −2–2 mmol/l
- Anion gap   10–18 mmol/l
- Lactate   0.5–2.0 mmol/l

Further reading

- *OHCM*, 7th edn.Oxford: Oxford University Press, p. 148.
- *Oxford Textbook of Medicine*, vol, 2, Section 11.11. Oxford: Oxford University Press, p. 139.

ⓘ **Beta blocker toxicity**

One of the most commonly prescribed cardiac medications, the β blocker class of drugs, is a less common intentional overdose, but can be accidentally taken in confused elderly patients in whom polypharmacy is a risk.

Presentation
- Cardiac
  - Hypotension
  - Bradycardia
  - AV block
- Non-cardiac
  - Lethargy
  - Coma
  - Seizures
- More rarely
  - Bronchospasm
  - Hypoglycaemia
  - Hyperkalaemia

Immediate management

❶ Inducing vomiting is absolutely contraindicated, owing to potential precipitation of cardiovascular collapse.

- ABC, as per p. 2–5. Cardiac monitoring is mandatory, even when patient is stable
- Any history is valuable, especially time of ingestion and which β blocker has been ingested. Later management is divergent, dependent on this
- Activated charcoal may be of benefit in the first hour after ingestion, but there is no evidence to support serial administration
- CXR if there is evidence of pulmonary oedema or heart failure
- ECG—variable AV block, atrioventricular junctional rhythm, widening QRS or torsade de pointes
- Glucagon, 2–10 mg IV over 1 min followed by infusion of 50 µg/kg/hour has a positive inotropic and chronotropic effect, mediated by calcium influx into the myocardium. It may also be diagnostic if confirmation of β blocker as the overdose is required
- ABG if evidence of respiratory compromise (respiratory acidosis) or seizures (metabolic acidosis)
- Basic investigations should be for assessment of end organ damage from hypotension, e.g. U&Es for kidney damage (see later list)
- Plasma concentrations of β blocker have been shown to have little predictive value; degree and duration of hypotension are of greater prognostic significance

Further management
- Atenolol (and sotalol) exhibit low lipid solubility and protein binding, so elimination can be expedited by haemodialysis; this treatment is of no value in metoprolol or propranolol overdoses. Dialysis should be reserved until failure of pharmacological measures
- External pacing should be considered if pharmacological measures fail or peri-arrest rhythms such as torsade de pointes are present on ECG
- As mentioned previously, maintenance of adequate cardiac output is the key to survival of this overdose. Atropine, adrenaline and dopamine may all be used to support this, in consultation with critical care teams
- Significant overdose requires invasive monitoring; central venous and peripheral arterial access should be gained at the earliest opportunity, giving beat-on-beat indication of haemodynamic status

Investigations
- U&Es for renal damage secondary to hypoxia
- Paracetamol and salicylate levels for exclusion of mixed overdose
- ABG for acidosis (respiratory or metabolic)
- CXR for pulmonary oedema
- Serial ECGs
- Capillary blood glucose

Further reading
- *OHCM*, 7th edn. Oxford: Oxford University Press, p. 826.
- *OH Emergency Medicine,* 3rd edn. Oxford: Oxford University Press, p. 196.

☢ Digitalis toxicity

As a second-line drug for symptom control of atrial fibrillation, the cardiac glycoside digoxin is another drug widely used by an ageing patient population more prone to errors in dosage and administration. In combination with a fairly narrow therapeutic window (dependent on overall electrolyte balance), overdose is therefore easily inadvertently achieved. Digoxin's mechanism of action is inhibition of the Na^+/K^+ ATPase, leading to raised intracellular calcium and sodium, and decreased intracellular potassium. The net effect of this is increased myocyte automaticity and decreased conduction.

Presentation
- Lethargy and fatigue
- Syncope, dyspnoea, chest discomfort or palpitations
- Somnolence, confusion or (more rarely) seizures
- Characteristic yellow-tinged vision, blurring or halos
- Nausea, vomiting (infrequently) abdominal pain

Immediate management

- The immediate management of this condition is almost purely by principles of ABC (see p. 2–5)
- ABG for oxygenation and any metabolic imbalance (the toxicity may be caused by primary electrolyte imbalance)
- Initial ECG and cardiac monitoring
- Dysrhythmias should be treated by universal ALS algorithm. Heart block of all degrees is a common finding, as is bigeminy and trigeminy. VT is prognostically poor

❶ Rhythm changes to heart blocks causing cardiovascular compromise or VT are peri-arrest and should be treated as such. ☎ 2222 or cardiologist on call for assistance in management.

- Full secondary assessment and history. Look for signs of hypothyroidism (reduced threshold for toxicity) or evidence of acute renal impairment (urinalysis, temperature, etc). Is there any possibility of non-pharmaceutical administration (digitalis is a plant derivative from foxgloves; toxicity from ingestion has been known for centuries)
- Initial biochemical investigations as detailed

Further management

- Cardiovascular compromise or ischaemia is an indication for Digibind, an antibody to digoxin. Discuss with cardiologist on call before prescribing. Other indications include persistently altered sensorium, severe symptomatic hyperkalaemia, and steady state digoxin levels >10 ng/l. Doses may be calculated as follows:
  - *When quantity ingested is known*
    Number of vials = total amount ingested (mg) × 0.8/0.5
  - *When quantity ingested is not known*
    Initial administration of 10 vials, with repeat dose of 10 vials if no or inadequate response seen
- Magnesium is a good temporising measure in VT/VF if Digibind is not immediately available—4 g IV bolus followed by 1–2 g/h infusion
- Patients exhibiting dysrhythmia with no cardiovascular compromise may be treated by discontinuation of digoxin and observation until ECG, clinical condition and plasma digoxin are all normal
- Cardioversion must not be attempted—the background increased excitability involves serious risk of precipitating VF arrest
- Investigate and treat any associated electrolyte imbalance. Note that the normal treatment of hyperkalaemia with calcium agents is to be avoided owing to their cardioactive nature. Glucose and insulin will be safer in this instance
- Treat any other underlying causes, such as urological sepsis, dehydration, etc.
- Any intentional overdose of digoxin must be followed up by psychiatric services

Investigations

- Plasma digoxin concentration; the therapeutic dose should be below 2 ng/l and levels >10 ng/l must be reversed with Digibind. It should also be noted that the digoxin assay is immunologically based, and so is specific for the drug itself. Plant digitalis will not register on the assay; do not discontinue treatment of a patient with a good history and clinical features of poisoning on the basis of this blood result
- U&Es—is this primarily caused by electrolyte disturbance? If available, old U&Es results will give an indication of premorbid renal function— is this an acute event or one impending through months of renal impairment? Early involvement of a nephrologist is desirable if renal primary causes are identified, as treatment will need to be modified in light of this presentation
- ECG—the classically taught 'reverse tick' of deep S-waves scooping up through the ST segment is neither consistently present nor pathognomonic in diagnosing toxicity. Although no arrhythmia is diagnostic, those more commonly associated are varying degrees of block, paroxysmal atrial tachycardia with 2:1 block, polymorphic VT and sinus bradycardia

- ABG—a good immediate assessment of oxygenation and metabolic status. The electrolyte estimation is accurate enough to permit early treatment of hyperkalaemia, etc. pending return of U&E results from the labs
- Troponins or cardiac enzymes as per local protocol if ECG or history are suggestive of a period of cardiac ischaemia

Further reading
- *OHCM*, 7th edn. Oxford: Oxford University Press, p. 826.
- *OH Emergency Medicine*, 3rd edn. Oxford: Oxford University Press, p. 197.

Index